Family in America

Family in America

Advisory Editors: David J. Rothman

Professor of History,
Columbia University

Sheila M. Rothman

Child Care
In Rural America

ARNO PRESS & THE NEW YORK TIMES

New York   1972

Reprint Edition 1972 by Arno Press Inc.

Reprinted from copies in
The University of Illinois Library and
The State Historical Society of Wisconsin Library

LC# 70-169360
ISBN 0-405-03884-4

Family in America
ISBN for complete set: 0-405-03840-2
See last pages of this volume for titles.

Manufactured in the United States of America

CONTENTS

U. S. DEPARTMENT OF LABOR
CHILDREN'S BUREAU
JULIA C. LATHROP, Chief

MATERNITY AND INFANT CARE

IN A RURAL COUNTY IN KANSAS

By

ELIZABETH MOORE

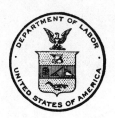

RURAL CHILD WELFARE SERIES No. 1

Bureau Publication No. 26

WASHINGTON
GOVERNMENT PRINTING OFFICE
1917

CONTENTS.

LETTER OF TRANSMITTAL.

U. S. DEPARTMENT OF LABOR,
CHILDREN'S BUREAU,
Washington, June 25, 1917.

SIR: Herewith I transmit a report entitled " Maternity and Infant Care in a Rural County in Kansas." This report is the first in a series undertaken for the purpose of learning what safeguards are available for the physical welfare of mothers and young babies in typical rural communities. The study was made under the supervision of Dr. Grace L. Meigs, the head of the division of hygiene of the Children's Bureau. This series of field studies is a direct sequence of the statistical report upon Maternal Mortality in the United States, made by Dr. Meigs last year. In that work the grave urgency of this subject is clearly shown. The outline for the inquiry was prepared chiefly by Miss Viola Paradise, research assistant, and the field work was done by Miss Elizabeth Moore and Miss Frances G. Valentine; the text was written by Miss Moore.

Special mention should be made of the assistance of the State board of health, at whose request the study was undertaken; Dr. S. J. Crumbine, secretary of the board, secured the cooperation of physicians, social workers, and officials, and through the press made clear the purpose of the study. Mr. W. J. V. Deacon, the State registrar, prepared all the preliminary data needed as to vital statistics. Dr. Lydia A. Devilbiss, director of the Kansas division of child hygiene, was of much assistance. The study is based upon interviews with individual mothers, and the general approval with which it was received is shown by the fact that not a single interview was refused the bureau's agents.

In the detailed statements given such changes have been made as prevent identification without impairing the accuracy of the illustration.

The bureau is indebted to Dr. J. Whitridge Williams, Johns Hopkins University, for advice with regard to technical matters connected with maternity care and especially for help in drawing up the standards suggested.

Respectfully submitted.

JULIA C. LATHROP, *Chief.*

HON. WILLIAM B. WILSON,
   Secretary of Labor.

MATERNITY AND INFANT CARE IN A RURAL COUNTY IN KANSAS.

INTRODUCTION.

OBJECT OF THE SURVEY.

In 1916 the Children's Bureau began its projected studies of maternal and child welfare in country districts. Three of these investigations were undertaken during the year in selected areas in North Carolina, Wisconsin, and Kansas. In the latter two States the studies were planned and carried out upon the same basis and with the same purpose, and both are confined to a much more limited range of topics than the study in North Carolina.

In Kansas, as in Wisconsin, the investigation is an extension of one phase of the study of the causes of infant mortality which the bureau has been carrying on in cities for the past four years. The one aspect of this wide subject which has been especially emphasized in these rural surveys is the conditions affecting the health of the mother during pregnancy and at the time of childbirth. The points covered are the general living conditions of the family, the work done by the mother, the care she received during pregnancy and at confinement, and the cost of such care. The care and health of the babies during their first year of life also are considered.

This question of the care of the childbearing mother was selected for special attention out of the many problems connected with infant mortality because of its great importance in connection with the loss of infant life through premature birth, injuries at birth, congenital weakness, and associated causes, leading to stillbirths and to deaths in the first weeks of life. Statistics show that this group of causes is responsible for about two-fifths of all infant deaths.[1] To this number should be added the loss from stillbirths[2] and the unmeasured but very great waste of potential life through miscarriages, making altogether a heavy charge against the prenatal and natal causes of death. Obviously any saving at this period can be effected only through the mother, by bringing her and her baby through the period of pregnancy in better health and by giving them

---

[1] Deaths under 1 year of age in 1915 in the registration area, all causes, 148,561; malformations, premature birth, congenital debility, and injuries at birth, 61,082 or 41.1 per cent of the total. Mortality Statistics, p. 645, Bureau of the Census, 1915.

[2] In the seven cities in which infant mortality studies have been made by the Children's Bureau the stillbirth rate was found to be 3.5 per cent of the total legitimate births.

7

both better care at the time of birth. In addition to these general considerations, many letters coming to the bureau from country women, as well as many of those written to the Secretary of Agriculture about the needs of farm women, have made it evident that the problem of securing adequate medical and nursing care at confinement is an extremely serious one for country mothers; that for many of them such care is practically inaccessible, either because of actual isolation or because of the expense resulting from distance from physicians and nurses. Consequently it appeared that the bureau would be neglecting its obligations if it delayed further the study of the conditions surrounding maternity in rural districts.

The information on which the Kansas survey is based was secured through interviews with mothers in the selected territory who had had children born within the two years preceding October 1, 1916. The object held in view in the use of this information has been to present a picture of maternity and infant care in the district studied; and no attempt has been made to show the relationship of particular conditions to the infant mortality rate, as has been done in the bureau's city investigations.

FIELD OF THE SURVEY.

The investigation was located in Kansas, partly because that State was considered typical of a large area of plains country west of the Missouri River which had previously been untouched in the bureau's work; and partly on account of the urgent invitation of the Kansas State Board of Health, which believed that a study by the Children's Bureau would stimulate the rural communities of the State to increase their efforts on behalf of mothers and babies. A certain county recommended by the secretary of the State board of health as typical of the western farming country was chosen for investigation. The study was confined to the farming area of this county— the open country—all of which was covered in the inquiry; the one city and all the villages were excluded.

METHOD.

So far as possible a record was made concerning every birth— whether live birth or stillbirth—during the period of two years from October 1, 1914, to September 30, 1916, occuring in families resident in the country districts of the selected county at the time of the birth. As a first step toward securing these records the names of the parents of all babies whose births or deaths were registered were obtained from the State and local registrars' offices. A canvass was made to find additional unregistered births. In all, 353 schedules were secured, representing 331 families; among these were 4 pairs of twins, so that the records cover the history of 349 confinements.

None of the mothers visited refused to give the desired information, and almost always their cooperation was most cordial. A large proportion of the parents had heard about the investigation through newspaper articles or from friends or neighbors and were ready to welcome the agents when they came. In all but 10 cases the main part of the information was given by the mother herself, with supplementary information from the father in many instances. The remaining 10 records were furnished by others—6 by the grandmother, 2 by an aunt, 1 by the baby's married sister, and 1 by the attending midwife, who was also a relative.

Mothers who had had miscarriages but no live-born or stillborn children within the period of the investigation were not interviewed, and no records were secured for such miscarriages except in two instances where the miscarriage resulted in the death of the mother. These two are not included in the figures for the county. Furthermore, no attempt was made to secure records about illegitimate births. A birth certificate was found for only one illegitimate child in the country districts in the two years covered by the survey, and the agents heard of no others in the course of their canvass.

Schedules were not secured for 78 of the registered births in the country districts, for the following reasons: In 60 cases the family had moved out of the county; in 10, the family was not at home at the time of the agent's visit and it was impossible to revisit; in 8, the family could not be located. Among these births there was 1 stillbirth, and 5 of the children are known to have died.

Instead of reproducing here the schedule used the following typical story is given to indicate the kind of information secured in an interview. The names are of course fictitious, and substitutions from other records have been made in order to prevent identification of the family.

Mrs. Green has a baby, Robert, 15 months old, who was born in September. He weighed 9 pounds at birth and has always been well except for two attacks of diarrhea in the summer, when he was 9 months old, and a bad cold now. He is still nursing, but his mother began to give him bread and milk, crackers, and cereals when he was 6 months old.

There are four children living, all in good health. Mrs. Green, who is now 35, was married when she was 22. The next year she had a stillborn baby, a girl. Two years later her oldest boy, now 10 years old, was born; the following year she had a three months' miscarriage. These first three confinements occurred on a farm in eastern Kansas; for the first two Mrs. Green had a midwife, and after the miscarriage her mother took care of her. The last three children— a boy 8 years old, a girl of 4 years, and the baby—were all born on this farm, and Mrs. Green had a doctor each time.

The day after the stillbirth she called a doctor, because the baby was "mortified" and she feared blood poisoning; he performed a curettage, but did nothing for the severe laceration which had occurred. This laceration has given so much trouble since the last baby was born that her present physician advises an operation. The second pregnancy almost resulted in a miscarriage at three months and the third one did so. Although no serious complications followed, she was weak for a year afterwards. The last three confinements have been normal.

Mrs. Green has suffered from nausea, varicose veins, and swollen hands and feet during every pregnancy, and especially during the last two. During the pregnancy for which the record was secured she had no prenatal care whatever.

When the baby was born Mrs. Green was attended by the doctor from the nearest village, 7 miles away. She was in labor about 18 hours, during which time the doctor made two visits; he also made one postnatal visit. This fee was $18.

Mrs. Green stayed in bed 10 days. One of her neighbors came in every day, washed the baby, and " fixed up. the bed "; otherwise her husband took care of mother and baby, and did the necessary housework for two weeks. He also did the washing (with the washing machine) during the winter, both the year before and the year after the baby was born; he is too busy to do much during the summer or fall, but he always carries the wash water from the windmill about 40 feet away, even in the busiest times.

Except for such help as her husband and the boys can give, Mrs. Green does all the housework and the family sewing; she does nothing outside the house except to care for the chickens. She is evidently a good housekeeper, as indicated both by her house and by the children's neatness.

Harvest occurred two and a half months before the baby was born, and Mrs. Green had six extra men to board for two weeks; but she had a hired girl for that time. The thrashing crew came three weeks before the baby was born, just when the oldest boy was having the measles; but Mr. Green arranged so that none of the men boarded at the house. In the summer after the baby's birth she could get no help at harvest. It was then that the baby got diarrhea because she was unable to watch what he ate. That fall Mrs. Green cooked for the four grain haulers for three days. Aside from this she has not had to board any hired men.

Mrs. Green has always lived in the country. As a girl she helped with the housework from the time she was 10 years old, but " never did a washing till she was 13 "; she also helped with the outdoor chores and " drove teams " in the fields from the time she was 8 years old. After she was 14 or 15 she frequently " worked out " among the neighbors for short periods, and the last two years before she was married she did housework in the city. She has never had any serious sickness, except pneumonia at the age of 12; but while she was working in the city she never felt well.

The Greens have lived on this farm 9 years; during this time Mr. Green has paid for one quarter section (160 acres) of good wheat land and has recently purchased a second quarter, which is still heavily mortgaged. He has built a good barn and granary and a comfortable five-room house. Mr. and Mrs. Green were both born in Kansas of native American parents.

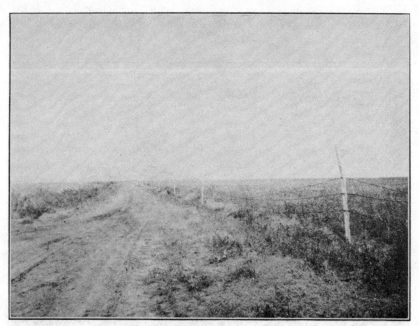

A COUNTRY ROAD ACROSS THE PLAINS.

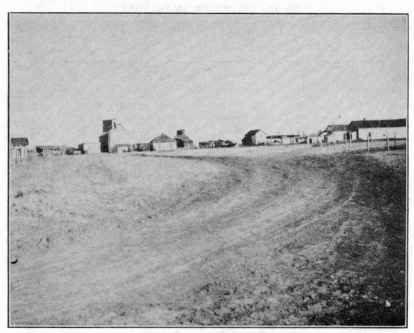

A SMALL VILLAGE IN THE WHEAT COUNTRY.

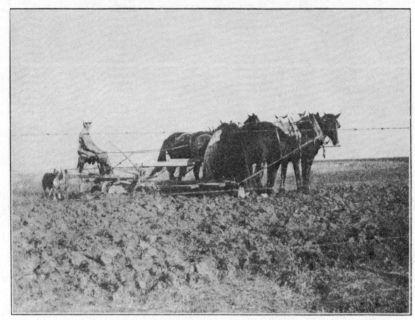

DISKING THE GROUND FOR THE WHEAT.

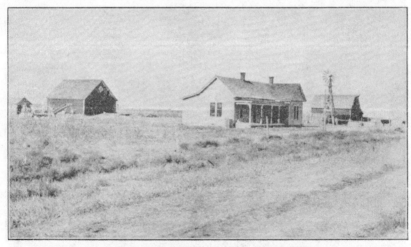

A TYPICAL WESTERN KANSAS FARM HOME.

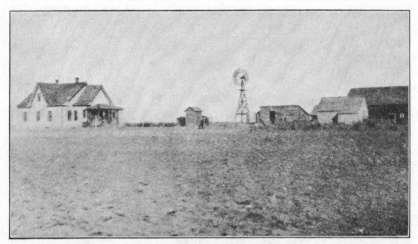

THE HOME OF A PROSPEROUS LANDOWNER.

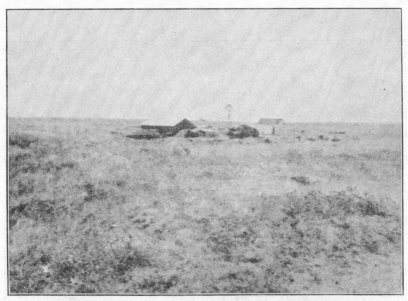

A RENTER'S HOME, WHERE THE FAMILY LIVES IN THE GRANARY.

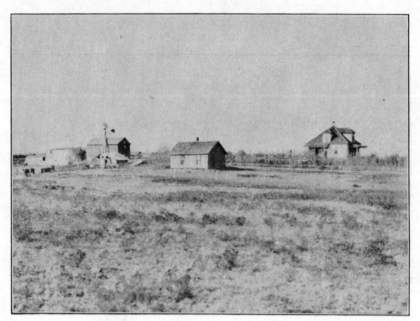

OLD AND NEW HOUSES ON A PROSPERING FARM.

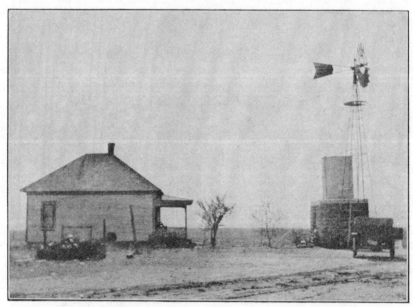

A MODEST HOME WITH RUNNING WATER FROM THE WINDMILL TANK.

THE COUNTY.

Before the findings of the survey are discussed a brief description is given of the chief economic and social factors—such as the physical characteristics of the county, character of the population, means of communication, type of farm life, and conditions affecting health—bearing on maternity and infant care in the area studied.

LOCATION AND TOPOGRAPHY.

The county studied is situated near the southern boundary of Kansas, about one-third of the way across the State eastward from the Colorado line. In other words, it belongs in the western half of the State, which has a semiarid climate and a comparatively sparse population. It is one of the larger counties in the State, being 30 by 36 miles in extent. With the exception of the valley of the Arkansas River, which crosses it from west to east, and the valleys of a few minor creeks, the whole county is a high, treeless, rolling plain—part of the Great Plains, which extend across half of Colorado and Kansas as well as adjacent States north and south, sloping gradually eastward from the Rocky Mountains. Very little of this plain is absolutely flat, but the variations are slight except in the neighborhood of the streams, where the ground often drops or "breaks" abruptly. The landscape in most places gives an effect of limitless expanse in which the scattered homesteads, with their struggling hedges, are often hardly noticeable. As one approaches the villages the tops of the grain elevators are visible on the horizon long before there is other sign of habitation.

The general level of the plain drops from between 2,600 and 2,700 feet elevation at the western border of the county to 2,400 feet near the eastern border; about half of the river bottom is below the 2,400-foot level.

SOIL AND CLIMATE.

The soil of this high plain, comprising fully two-thirds of the county, is what is called by the Bureal of Soils [1] Richfield silt loam—a soil "well adapted to the growing of wheat," though "the average yield of wheat when calculated for a series of years is somewhat low, probably not exceeding 10 bushels, and for the average farmer this is barely within the limit of profitable production." The soil is undeniably fertile; it needs no fertilizer and in some places has produced wheat steadily for 30 years with no apparent exhaustion.

---

[1] Reconnoissance Soil Survey of Western Kansas, p. 58. U. S. Bureau of Soils, Washington, 1912.

The reason why fertile soil, well adapted to wheat, gives such low average yields is largely a matter of rainfall. In this part of Kansas the average annual rainfall is only between 20 and 23 inches,[1] and crop yields are uncertain because of droughts. A good year, one of more than average rainfall, gives fine crops, while an unusually dry year may bring total failure. The selected county is just on the edge of what appears to be the profitable farming belt, at least under present methods of farming; and there is a distinct difference in rainfall and in the resulting prosperity between the eastern and western ends of the county. Moreover, within the same year local showers will sometimes make a considerable difference in crops in neighborhoods not far apart.

The Arkansas River valley, which separates the northern from the southern half of the county, presents very different conditions from the upland plains. The river itself carries little water in the channel; but it has a large subsurface flow which irrigates the adjacent strips of alluvial soil and makes them very valuable, especially for raising alfalfa. This strip of rich land is narrow, not more than a mile or two wide at most. North of this bottom is an irregular strip of rough stony land rising steeply to the bluffs a couple of miles back from the river. South of the river bottom runs a similar strip of sand hills and sandy soil, largely worthless except for pasture.

HISTORY OF SETTLEMENT.

Most of the land in the county, except in the northwestern corner, was taken up in quarter-section tracts by homesteaders about 30 years ago, at the time of the western Kansas boom beginning in 1885. Few of these early settlers are left, however, as nearly all were driven out during the dry years following the boom. It is a common saying that almost every quarter was taken up and relinquished six or seven times before it was finally " proved up." Much land went into the hands of cattle ranchers and speculators after the boom, and only in recent years has been put under cultivation again.

East of the county seat the exodus was not so general as farther west; and in the eastern end of the county there is a large German settlement which dates from the eighties. These families migrated from Ohio to Kansas as a group 30 years ago and have remained largely separate from their neighbors ever since. They intermarry to a considerable extent within " the settlement," and have their own churches. Although in the early days they went through very hard times, they held on to their land; and to-day this neighborhood has the best-developed farms in the county as well as the largest proportion of home owners.

---

[1] Reconnoissance Soil Survey of Western Kansas, p. 58. U. S. Bureau of Soils, Washington, 1912.

Another and even more distinct community is formed by two small Amish colonies in the southern part of the county. These people are German in origin, a sect of the Mennonite Church; they have a distinctive costume and strict rules as to simplicity of living and hold very little intercourse with outsiders. Within their own group they are closely bound together by relationship as well as by church ties. The Amish families in this county came chiefly from Indiana, most of them less than 10 years ago. They are thrifty, and, in spite of having been poor in the beginning, they have made creditable progress toward farm ownership. A visitor is impressed by the unusual neatness and cleanliness of most of the homes, which go far to compensate for their absolute lack of adornment. German is still the language of family life among these people, though they have been in America for generations. The women are hard workers, following the German custom of helping with the farm work in addition to the housework and care of the children.

PRESENT POPULATION.

Nationality.

As a whole this is a predominantly native American community. Out of the 662 parents in the families visited 505, or 76.3 per cent, were native white of native parentage, while only 19, or 2.9 per cent, were foreign born, 16 of whom were German. Only 4 of the parents could not speak English; these were Russian Germans, 2 of the second generation.

Literacy and intelligence.

The population of the county is also predominantly literate. The 1910 census shows only eight-tenths of 1 per cent of the native white population 10 years of age and over illiterate. Among the farming population there are practically no illiterates; in fact, only one was found among the parents in the families visited. The general level of intelligence—of interest in public affairs, in questions of health, and in the education of the children—also is high. A large proportion of the mothers had read some kind of literature on infant care and were keenly interested in taking their babies to the various "Baby Days" held in the county. The country schools are of the one-room type, but the buildings are well built and well kept; innovations like playground apparatus are not uncommon, and a general interest in school efficiency is manifest. There is a high school in each of the incorporated villages as well as in the county seat, and these high schools are well attended by country children.

Community centers.

The county seat, a city of about 4,100 inhabitants, is the community center for the whole northwestern section of the county. Besides this one city there are three incorporated and three unincorporated villages. These are all small villages according to urban standards, ranging from 76 to 778 inhabitants. But the two largest are important local business and social centers and boast of "city" water supplies. All of these villages, in fact, except the smallest one, are important to their surrounding communities, providing churches, stores, physicians, and mail and shipping facilities.

Density.

According to the Kansas State census for 1915 this county had 13,152 inhabitants—an increase of 15 per cent since 1910.[1] The six villages, together with the county seat and the State soldiers' home, had a combined population of approximately 6,900,[2] which leaves 6,250 people in the open country—that is, the area covered by the survey—or a rural density of 5.8 persons per square mile. The density of the rural population in the three townships on the eastern border of the county is 7.6 per square mile, while in the four townships on the western border it is only 4 per square mile, illustrating the increasing sparsity of settlement as one goes westward. In the extreme northwestern township, which is the most arid and least thickly settled of all, there were only 2.2 persons per square mile.

MEANS OF COMMUNICATION.

Railroads.

Two transcontinental railroads and two branch lines cross the county, with stations at intervals of not more than 10 miles and one or more grain elevators at every station. Consequently the county is well provided with means of travel; and the shipping facilities would be sufficient if it were not for shortages of railroad cars, which often prevent the farmers from marketing their grain when they wish.

Roads.

The roads in this district, as throughout western Kansas, are usually in excellent condition, thanks rather to the climate and the nature of the soil than to any work put upon them. No attempt is made to surface the country roads in any way (except for a few miles of sandy road along the river which have been covered with cinders), and a heavy rain makes them almost impassable. Such rains, however, are infrequent, and the dirt packs hard and smooth again in a surprisingly short time. Certain of the main roads are designated "county roads" and are kept well graded and dragged; the rest receive practically no attention except that necessary culverts are

---

[1] The population more than doubled in the preceding decade, 1900–1910. (U. S. Bureau of the Census.) According to the State census the increase between 1915 and 1916 was 4 per cent.

[2] Incorporated places from State census. Unincorporated places from postmasters' estimates. Soldiers' home from commandant's statement.

built and kept up. But in this fortunate country a mere wagon track across the plains soon makes a good road. A large proportion of the country families, especially among the land owners, have automobiles to enable them to take advantage of their good roads.

Telephones.

Telephone facilities extend throughout the county; more than two-thirds of all the families visited had telephones in their homes, only four were farther than a mile and a half away from a telephone, and none had to go more than 3 miles to reach one. This is particularly advantageous in a community where the distances are so great and the homes so widely scattered.

CHARACTER OF FARM LIFE.
Size of farms.

It has been shown already how sparse the population is—hardly one family to the square mile in the western part of the county and less than two in the eastern end. The census of 1910 shows that of the farms in the county three-fourths contained at least 260 acres and nearly one-third were as large as 500 acres. Of the farms visited two-thirds were farms of 320 acres or more; and the consensus of opinion is that 320 acres—a half section—of reasonably good land is the least upon which a farmer can expect to make a comfortable living. All this means that next-door neighbors are often a mile or more apart, and "town" may be anywhere up to 20 miles away. Although houses may be easily distinguished from a distance of 2 or 3 miles, yet from many places out on the plains there is hardly a dwelling in sight in any direction.

Chief crop.

Winter wheat is far and away the main crop of this part of the country. According to the report of the Kansas State Board of Agriculture for 1914 four-fifths of the acreage of planted crops in the county was in wheat; and 85 per cent of the total crop values were due to the wheat crop. Oats and spring crops—corn, kafir corn, etc.—are raised on most farms, mainly for feed; but none of these grains, nor all of them together, approach anywhere near the importance of the wheat. In fact, wheat stands in almost as predominant a relationship to the material well-being of the farmers of this territory as cotton does in the cotton States. In discussing how he is getting along, almost any farmer or his wife will tell of his wheat crop—its acreage, yield, and price—with hardly a thought of anything else.

The life of the typical farm revolves around the wheat crop. Work is active in the fall when the wheat ground is being plowed or disked and the wheat is being sown; after that there is not much to do, unless an unusual amount of stock is kept on the farm or spring crops are raised, until the following June when the wheat again demands attention. At this time comes the great work crisis of the year—the wheat harvest, employing from 3 to 15 men for two or three weeks—men whom the farmer must usually snatch from the incoming trains and whom the housewife must manage to board. Wheat thrashing usually follows some time in the summer, but lasts only a few days. If spring crops are raised to any great extent, the busy season extends through a much longer period, from spring through corn husking or kafir thrashing, which often comes late in the winter; but there is no such time of concentrated stress as the wheat harvest.

Economic situation.

At the time of the survey wheat crops had been satisfactory for the past few years, and wheat was bringing in the neighborhood of $1.75 a bushel, which was then regarded as a phenomenally high price. Consequently a general atmosphere of good times prevailed in spite of the total failure of the corn crop in the current year. Aside from the car shortage there seem to be no marketing difficulties, as farmers' associations own cooperative grain elevators at nearly every railroad station. Average wheat crops for the current year ran about 13 to 15 bushels, though some farms produced as much as 20 bushels or more to the acre.

Tenantry.

A serious feature of social conditions in this county is the large proportion of farms in the hands of tenants. At the time of the 1910 census this proportion was 34 per cent of the total; among the families visited in the survey it was 38 per cent, not including those who rented land from their parents. In the decade between the 1900 and 1910 censuses the number of tenant farms increased from 73 to 374, while the number in the hands of owners increased from 484 to 722; that is to say, the majority of the newcomers were tenants and the proportion of tenants rose nearly threefold. At present tenantry is distinctly more prevalent in the western or more recently settled half of the county than in the eastern half. This fact seems to indicate—as do many individual histories—a wholesome tendency for the new settlers who start out as tenants to become landowners. Whether this tendency will continue in the face of the rise in land values remains for the future to show. It must be borne in mind in this connection that many of the older settlers homesteaded their land, but that now there is practically no free land left. At present, the customary rental charge of one-third of the grain crop allows an enterprising and capable farmer to " get ahead " and buy land in the course of time. But many of the renters move about from place to place, forming a transient, unattached, thriftless element in the community, their very names unknown to many of the neighbors. For example, one family moved four times in 13 months, another three times in 7 months. The houses on most rented farms are decidedly inferior to those occupied by landowners; many of them are poorly built and in wretched condition. And it frequently happens that, in addition to the handicap of inadequate farm buildings, renters have insufficient capital to farm profitably, and their whole standard of living is much below the general level.

Many landowners rent land in addition to that which they own, in order to extend the scale of their farming; but they are by no means in the same economic status as the tenants and are not so counted; for they are not transients, and they usually own the homes in which they live. For similar reasons those farmers who operate land belonging to their parents—an appreciable number among the younger folk—do not belong in the tenant class, whether or not they pay rent, for they have a permanent interest in the community and usually have the advantage of farm buildings and dwellings such as an owner ordinarily puts up for himself but not for tenants.

HEALTH.

No investigation of general sanitary conditions was included in this survey. It is worth noting, however, that the general climatic conditions—the elevation and the dry atmosphere—are favorable to good health. So also is the character of the water supply. Practically all the water used throughout the county is taken from drilled wells more than 100 feet deep, which draw from uncontaminated ground-water strata.[1] Open wells, such as are found in many country districts, are very rare. Hence, though the water is hard it is reasonably safe from pollution.

Vital statistics.

The death rate for this county has been for several years somewhat above that for the State. But it should be noted that Kansas as a whole has a remarkably low death rate, about 2 per thousand below that for the rural part of the registration States. Moreover, the rates for the county are stated by the secretary of the State board of health to be increased by the deaths of patients brought from outside the county to the hospitals in the county seat.

---

[1] Statement of the secretary of the State board of health.

3698°—17——3

TABLE I.—*Death rate per 1,000 population.*[a]

	1912	1913	1914	1915	1916
Selected county	11.8	12.4	13.5	19.9	13.5
State of Kansas	10.2	10.6	10.5	10.7	11.7
Rural part of registration States [b]	12.4	12.7	12.3	12.3	

[a] Derived from Second Biennial Peport of the Central Division of Vital Statistics, Kansas State Board of Health, 1914–15; from data furnished by the State board of health; and from Mortality Statistics, Bureau of the Census, 1913, 1914, and 1915.
[b] Includes all places of less than 10,000 population in 1910 in the death-registration area.

According to the State birth-registration figures this county has a birth rate which is not only one of the highest in the State but also is considerably in excess of that for the State as a whole, or for the birth-registration area of the United States which was 24.9 per 1,000 in 1915.[1] As shown in Table II, the rate for the county studied was 29 per 1,000 or higher every year for the past five years. Of the six other Kansas counties which had birth rates higher than 29 more than once in the four years 1912–1915, all but one are immediately adjacent to the one studied, so that evidently a high birth rate is characteristic of this part of the State. In each of the past three years the county seat appears to have a higher birth rate than the rest of the county; possibly this is due, at least in part, to more complete birth registration in the city.

TABLE II.—*Birth rate per 1,000 population.*[a]

	1912	1913	1914	1915	1916
Selected county	35.4	29.0	33.2	29.9	31.0
County seat			37.9	35.8	35.2
Rest of county			31.0	27.2	28.9
State of Kansas	22.5	21.0	21.2	22.2	24.0

[a] Derived from Second Biennial Peport of the Central Division of Vital Statistics, Kansas State Board of Health, 1914–15, and from data furnished by the State board of health. Rates for the rural part of the registration area are not available.

In this community a high infant mortality [2] rate does not accompany a high birth rate. In contrast to its general death rate, the county of the survey had in 1914 a lower infant mortality rate than the average for the State, and also in both 1914 and 1915 a rate lower than those found in other States. The rate for the birth-registration area of the United States in 1915 was 100 per 1,000 births; only one State—Minnesota—had a rate lower than 85, while in 6 of the 10 birth-registration States the rate was higher than 100.[3]

[1] Birth Statistics for the Registration Area of the United States, p. 10, U. S. Bureau of the Census, 1915.
[2] Infant mortality rate, as the term is used in vital statistics, means the ratio between the number of deaths under 1 year of age and the number of live births in the same period.
[3] Birth Statistics for the Registration Area of the United States, p. 10, U. S. Bureau of the Census, 1915.

TABLE III.—*Infant mortality rate per 1,000 live births.*[1]

	1914	1915	1916
Selected county	62	71	92
County seat	75	88	113
Rest of county	55	61	79
State of Kansas	77	70	69

[1] Derived from Second Biennial Report of the Central Division of Vital Statistics, Kansas State Board of Health, 1914–15; from data furnished by the State board of health; and from birth and death certificates for the county.

The figures in Table III show that the rate for the county seat was over one-third higher each year than that for the rest of the county; but here again the real facts are obscured to some extent by deaths of children brought from the country to the city hospitals.

It should be noted that the rates for the county and also for both subdivisions were higher in 1915 than in 1914, and much higher in 1916 than in either of the preceding years; also that in this last year this county had a higher infant mortality rate than the State.

Causes of infant deaths.

In the two years 1914 and 1915, 22 of the 53 infant deaths occurring in the county were due to malformations and diseases peculiar to early infancy; outside of the city 13 of the 29 deaths were due to this group of causes, or about the same proportion. In 1916, 14 out of 39 deaths in the county and 7 out of 21 outside of the city belonged in the same group. Taking the three years together, or any one year, malformations and "early infancy" are responsible for a larger number of deaths than any other group of causes; but they are not responsible for the sharp rise in the mortality rate in 1916.

Both in the county as a whole and outside of the city the number of deaths from gastric and intestinal diseases in 1916 alone exceeded the number in the two preceding years. That is to say, in 1914 and 1915 there were 10 deaths from these causes in the county, but in 1916, 12 deaths; and similarly outside of the city, 4 deaths in the two years but 6 in 1916. In July, August, and September of that year there occurred in and around the county seat an outbreak of infantile diarrhea, which loomed large in the minds of parents, doctors, and nurses. In fact, 11 children under 2 years old died from diarrhea in these months; but only 4 of these were under a year old, which number will not account for the high infant mortality rate for the year. On the contrary, the records show that deaths from diarrheal diseases were excessive throughout the year and throughout the county.

Contagious diseases.

During 1916 there were reported to the county health officer 229 cases of measles, 28 of scarlet fever, 24 of chicken pox, 10 of diph- theria, 7 of whooping cough, 1 of infantile paralysis, and 87 of small- pox. Measles seems to be unusually well reported; but the same can hardly be said of whooping cough, for the mothers visited told of fully as much whooping cough as measles in their families. An epidemic of measles which occurred earlier in the year in the city and in the southwestern quarter of the county was responsible for most of the cases of that disease reported.

The cases of smallpox were due to two outbreaks in the spring, in the city and in one of the villages. The latter was widespread, but no deaths resulted.

Compared with the fatalistic attitude common in many localities, the parents in this community seem as a rule to be careful in avoid- ing exposure of their children even to the milder contagious diseases. At the time of the survey little trouble was experienced from any of the ordinary children's contagious diseases, except for a diphtheria scare in the city from which only five or six cases developed.

Public-health activities.

In Kansas the county is the local unit for rural public-health ad- ministration. The county board of health consists of the county commissioners and a county health officer appointed by them. There are no township health officials, consequently the county officer has an extensive field to cover.

At the time of the survey this county was fortunate in having an active, interested health officer—a local physician who had obtained special training for his duties by attending the course for county health officers given by the State board of health. Unfortunately the low salary paid—$250 a year—threatened to deprive the county of his services for the following year.

The health officer's duties embrace the inspection of stores, restau- rants, slaughterhouses, etc., the sanitary inspection of schools, and the control of contagious diseases. During his term the officer of this county had twice inspected the stores, restaurants, and slaughter- houses throughout his territory and had visited " about half a dozen " of the 67 schoolhouses of the county. His activities were largely concentrated on the prevention of the spread of contagious diseases. He visited promptly every locality where there was an outbreak and had done much traveling for this purpose. In addition, he took an active part in the " Baby Days " held in the county. Obviously, he had performed far more service than the community was justified in expecting for the salary paid.

The social-service league of the county seat employed a visiting nurse—who was a graduate of the State board of health's training course for public-health nurses—during six months of 1916 and expected to continue this work in 1917. The city and the county each contributed $15 a month toward the nurse's salary; the remainder was raised by private subscription. Her work was confined almost entirely to the city.

The most significant undertaking of the year, from the standpoint of children's health, was the series of "Baby Days" inaugurated by the visiting nurse and carried out by local physicians and dentists in the county seat and three of the villages. Young children were given physical examinations according to a plan recommended by the State board of health, in which the American Medical Association score card was used; but no prizes were given. These examinations aroused a great deal of interest throughout the county; more children were brought to each examination than could be admitted. At the largest meeting 60 children were examined by 4 physicians and 2 dentists.

The spontaneous response to this opportunity, as well as the enthusiasm of the doctors in face of the arduous work involved, indicates a very promising field for public-health work. It seems probable that the project of inducing the county commissioners to employ a public-health nurse for work throughout the county, which is being discussed in the city, would be received with favor by the country constituency.

FINDINGS OF THE SURVEY.

FATHER'S OCCUPATION.

All but 3 of the heads of the 331 families visited were engaged in farming; 317 were farmers, 2 farm managers, 8 farm laborers, and 1 had as his chief means of livelihood the operation of a thrasher. Five of the farmers also worked as farm laborers part of the time; 6 operated thrashers; and 9 had some other supplementary occupation. Of the 3 fathers not engaged in farming, 1 was a storekeeper, 1 a railroad station agent, and 1 a rural mail carrier.

The small number of families found who depended upon farm laborers' wages is a reflection of the extremely seasonal character of farm work in this district. Wages are high during a few months in the busy season, but during the winter a laborer of any kind finds almost nothing to do; hence the bulk of the hired labor is done by a migratory class.

PLACE OF CONFINEMENT.

As has been stated, all the mothers with whom this study is concerned were resident in the country districts of the selected county at the time of confinement. Some of them, however—17 in all—went for their confinement care outside of the area covered in the survey; 3 of these went to relatives outside of the county, 10 went to hospitals in the county seat, and 4 stayed with relatives in the county seat or in one of the villages in the county. Five others went away from their own homes in order to be with relatives but stayed within the country districts of the county.

MATERNITY CARE.

Attendant at birth.

Almost all (95 per cent) of the 332 births in the rural districts were attended by a physician; but in 42 cases the doctor did not arrive until after the birth of the child; and in 10 of these not until an hour or more afterwards. Twelve births were attended by a midwife, 3 by a neighbor, and 3 by the father only; 1 was attended by both a physician and a midwife.

Midwives.

Kansas makes no provision for licensing midwives; the only law in which the existence of such persons is recognized is the birth-registration act. There are no professional midwives in this territory, for no one could possibly make a living from the few obstetrical cases to which midwives are called. The 12 births mentioned above were attended by 7 different women, who are classed as midwives because they have had experience in this work, take charge of confinement cases on their own responsibility, and are considered by the neighborhood competent so to do. Three of these women had 2 cases each in the 2 years, and 1 had 3 cases; the others had only 1 each in that period. Of the 3 who were interviewed the first had attended 11 cases in 10 years, the second 6 cases in 10 years, the third 15 cases in 7 years. The last—a young native-born woman who had taken a course in midwifery—would gladly have had more practice; the others did the work primarily as a neighborly accommodation, making no regular charge but often receiving presents for their services.

In the 12 families served by midwives, however, they have been an important factor and are evidently preferred to physicians. Out of 76 confinements in the history of these families 53, or more than two-thirds, had been attended by midwives and only 18 by physicians; of the 49 children born to these 12 families in this county 29, more than half, were delivered by midwives and only 13 by physicians.

Obstetrical service by physicians.

The county is well supplied with physicians. Twenty-five doctors attended the births included in this study; 10 of them attended 10 or more cases each, or 273 cases in all. Eighteen of these doctors are located in the county and the others in near-by towns in adjacent counties. The county seat has 8 practicing physicians; each of the villages of 100 population or more has at least 1, while the two largest each have 2.

Probably no home in the county is more than 20 miles from a doctor. All but four of the families visited had a doctor within 15 miles when the baby was born; more than 80 per cent had a doctor within 10 miles and 32 per cent within 5 miles. Even 20 miles is not a prohibitive distance in this country of smooth level roads where, under normal circumstances, the doctor's automobile can cover that distance within an hour of receiving a call. More than one mother remarked, in discussing the subject, that since the coming of the telephone and the automobile distance made no particular difference in getting the doctor. Nearly half (19) of the physicians, it is true, who were late in reaching their obstetrical patients came 10 miles or more; but two-thirds (13) of these were less than an hour late— several only a few minutes. Some chance, such as a flood in the river, a winter storm, the doctor's being " out on a case," a delayed summons, or a brief labor is more likely to be the cause of the doctor's failure to arrive on time than is distance.

That distance is not a serious obstacle to securing medical care in this territory is further indicated by the fact that for 46 confinements some other than the nearest physician was called, from a distance averaging 7 miles greater than that to the nearest doctor. In 17 instances the attendant physician came from 15 miles or more away, though, as has been seen, only 4 families needed to send so far for a doctor.

The fact that a physician can serve a large area makes a choice of doctors possible to most families in the county—a privilege not always available even in much more densely settled districts than western Kansas. This seems to be a factor in the general satisfaction with the medical situation.

The available evidence tends to indicate a comparatively high standard of obstetrical service at the time of confinement. None of the mothers complained of neglect during the period covered by the survey. Instrumental deliveries were rare, only 16 cases out of 349; and the stillbirth rate is low. With one exception all the lacerations which seem to have been severe were repaired.

On the other hand, postnatal supervision of obstetrical patients is much less common than might be expected from the general high level of medical practice. In 136 out of 314 confinements attended by physicians in the open country no return visit was made; in 128 cases one visit; and in only 48 cases more than one visit. In part this failure to make return visits depends on distance from the patient, for the proportion of cases receiving no postnatal visits increases markedly as the distance increases. (See Table IV.) In part, also, it is a matter of the habit of individual physicians; some doctors make return visits to almost all their obstetrical cases, while others revisit almost none.

TABLE IV.—*Number of postnatal visits, by distance from physician.*

Distance from attending physician.	Mothers attended by physicians in country districts, receiving specified number of postnatal visits.					
	Total.	No visits.		One visit.	More than one visit.	Not reported.
		Number.	Per cent.			
Total	314	136	43	128	48	2
Less than 3 miles	31	2	6	15	14	....
3 to 4 miles	61	14	23	37	10	....
5 to 9 miles	134	57	43	56	20	1
10 to 14 miles	71	48	68	18	4	1
15 miles or more	17	15	88	2	....	....

The most common fee for attendance' at childbirth is from $15 to $20, which was the charge in half of the 266 cases for which this information was secured; in over three-fourths of the cases the physician's charge was from $15 to $25. The fee is seldom less than $15 or as high as $30. Except in complicated cases the number of visits made by the physician does not seem to influence his charge, nor does the distance he travels unless it exceeds 15 miles. (This is true only of obstetrical fees, for the rate for an ordinary visit is usually based on a mileage charge.)

Hospitals.

The county has three hospitals—two of 16 and 25 beds in the county seat, and one of 10 beds in one of the villages. All are physicians' private hospitals. These hospitals reported caring for 60 obstetrical cases in 1916,[1] the great majority in one hospital.

Ten country mothers went to the hospitals for confinement during the two years of the survey. Neither mother nor baby died in any of these cases. Four of these women went to the hospital as the most convenient arrangement. Two were in poor health, one with symptoms of toxemia and the other much weakened by a miscarriage and repeated lacerations. The other four had more serious complications, including one case of convulsions, one Cæsarean operation, one premature birth following a fall, and one case where the doctor expected to use instruments; each of these women was taken to the hospital from a distance of 10 to 16 miles, after labor began. On the whole, therefore, the hospital still seems to be generally regarded as a last resort; the custom of making use of hospital facilities is hardly as well developed as might be expected in view of the community's intelligence upon health matters and the availability of hospitals.

The ordinary hospital charge is $20 a week with physician's fee ($15 for normal labor) in addition, or $25 a week including the doctor's services. This makes the usual expense of a confinement at a hospital amount to between $50 and $60. In this district, therefore, hospital care costs but little more than does care at home if the family pays for nursing instead of relying on unpaid help. For example, one mother paid $50, including doctor's fee, for two weeks at the hospital when her first baby was born; when the second baby came, she stayed at home, paying $18 for one visit from the doctor and $26 for a practical nurse who also did the housework for three weeks. Of course, where there are other children some provision must be made for the housework whether or not the mother goes to a hospital.

---

[1] The reports cover 12 months for one hospital, 11 months for another, and 5 months for the third, which opened in July, 1916.

Nursing care and household help at confinement.

Trained nurses are not impossible to secure for those who can afford them, since both of the city hospitals give nurses' training courses. Eighteen mothers who did not go to a hospital had a trained nurse, in most instances at the standard rate of $25 a week, or a total expense in different cases of from $25 to $60. As might be expected, the incurring of such an expense is confined to the more prosperous families; 16 out of these 18 families belonged to the land-owning class; and in all of them the father was farming at least a half section (320 acres) of land.

Several of the doctors, when attending confinements, frequently take a trained nurse or a hospital pupil nurse along with them to act as an assistant at the delivery; such a nurse washes the baby and makes the mother comfortable before leaving, but does not stay with the patient. One doctor who had a large practice did this regularly, making no extra charge for the nurse; other physicians usually charged $3 or $5. When, as often happens, the household provides only inexperienced assistance—a daughter or husband or a more or less incompetent hired girl—the services of a nurse even for this short time are of the greatest value both to the doctor and to the mother.

In addition to the mothers who had a trained nurse, 53 others had at least partially trained care by a midwife or a practical nurse (usually called in this neighborhood an "experienced woman"). Such attendants, however, are scarce and often difficult if not impossible to secure. In the great majority of cases the mother had to depend upon an untrained hired girl, a member of the family, a relative, or a neighbor. A very common arrangement is for a neighbor to come in daily to wash the baby, while some member of the household gives all the rest of the nursing care.

The amount of nursing done by the fathers is worth noting. In 16 cases the father took all the care of the mother, though usually—but not always—some one else attended to the baby. One father said: "I have waited on my wife both times according to the doctor's directions, thereby saving the price of a nurse"; this same father did the housework for two or three weeks after the first baby came; but the second time the family had a hired girl. In two large families visited the father had delivered most of the children, and in another family the mother insisted upon his officiating at the last two births, because it worried her to have an outsider around. In 19 cases the father did all the housework while the mother was sick.

As has been said, the absence of a competent "experienced" nurse is often due not to considerations of expense so much as to difficulty in getting anyone to help. For instance, in one prosperous family the mother said that, as she could get no one to come in, she took care of the baby herself from the day after it was born, while her oldest girl (15 years old) waited on her and brought her what she wanted. Another mother's account was that her daughter of 15 did all the housework and that she took care of herself and the baby; the daughter brought things to the bed for her to wash and dress the baby with, and under her direction did whatever she could not do herself. In another instance a neighbor came in the day the baby was born and once afterwards to "fix things up"; after the third day the mother got up and attended to the baby and even made the bed herself.

About half of the mothers visited had hired household help at the time of childbirth; nearly one-fifth had help during the latter part of pregnancy. Such help is rather more common on the larger farms (320 acres or more) than on the smaller ones, but usually absence of hired help is not to be attributed to poverty. Sometimes, it is true, the help which relatives can give seems sufficient; but more often the family would have had a hired girl if a good one could have been found. As in all country districts, household help is scarce; but the dearth does not seem to be as absolute as it is in many places, partly perhaps because the farmers are able and willing to pay fairly good prices for such help at times of stress.

So few women except trained nurses were employed to do nursing exclusively that they hardly count in an estimate of the nursing expenses of childbearing. Most of the "experienced women" and nearly all the hired girls who did childbed nursing did the housework also. The usual wage for a woman taking charge of the household at such a time and doing more or less nursing was $1 or $1.50 a day; a girl doing ordinary housework without taking much responsibility was commonly paid $4 or $5 a week.

Considering only those (332) confinements which took place in the country we find that in 142 cases the mother had no expense for either nursing or household help at that time; that is, all such work was done by members of the family, relatives, or neighbors. In the other 190 cases some expense was incurred for these services, either for nursing or housework, or both. In more than half of these cases where the cost was obtained this item in the budget was less than $20; in nearly two-thirds it was less than $25; in only one-eighth was it greater than $50. The amount spent depends mainly upon the length of time for which help is kept; the figures given above cover a maximum period of 12 weeks—6 weeks before and 6 weeks after confinement; but the minimum was sometimes as short as 3 days. As a matter of fact, 19 mothers had help for more than 6 weeks before confinement and 18 for more than 6 weeks afterwards; but the expense for these additional weeks has not been included in considering the costs of childbirth.

Prenatal care.

In one-third (119) of the pregnancies which occurred in the two years of the survey the mother had *some* prenatal care from her physician. How adequate this supervision was, however, is a different question.

In order to be able to classify the care received by mothers during pregnancy the following outline has been drawn up, after consultation with Dr. J. Whitridge Williams, professor of obstetrics, Johns Hopkins University, as representing a fair standard for *adequate* medical prenatal care:

1. A general physical examination, including an examination of heart, lungs, and abdomen.

2. Measurement of the pelvis in a first pregnancy to determine whether there is any deformity which is likely to interfere with birth.

3. Continued supervision by the physician, at least through the last five months of pregnancy.

4. Monthly examinations of the urine, at least during the last five months.[1]

Though this standard is no higher than is necessary to insure the early detection of abnormal symptoms and conditions, it is not a standard which is generally attained in private or public practice, either in cities or in rural districts.

Comparing conditions as reported by the mothers with this standard, we find that six of the patients who are counted as having prenatal care because they sent the urine to the doctor for examination never saw the doctor at all during pregnancy, though in some instances he sent them medicine. Sixty-nine patients who saw the doctor had no general examination. Fifty-nine had no analysis of the urine. In no case was the pelvis measured with the calipers, in spite of the fact that 42 of these patients were carrying their first babies. About two-fifths of the patients saw the doctor only once; in 28 of these cases the one consultation with the doctor, with no general examination, was all the prenatal care given.

In only two cases, neither of them a first pregnancy, could the care received be counted as adequate; in four other cases it would have been adequate, since there was continued supervision and repeated urinalyses, except for the fact that the patients were primiparae and no measurements of the pelvis were made. In 18 cases, none of which was a first pregnancy, there was a physical examination, one or more urinalyses, and some supervision, though not enough to make the care adequate; these are classed as having fair care. All the rest (99) of the women either were primiparae and had no measurements taken, or else they lacked one of the other essentials. For example,

---

[1] See Maternal Mortality, pp. 12–13. U. S. Children's Bureau publication No. 19.

a women in her first pregnancy, in poor health and under the doctor's care all the time, had no general examination and no urinalysis. Another mother, who sent the urine for examination daily during the last two months of her first pregnancy, never saw the doctor until the time of confinement. Another mother, who was bloated, vomited, and had dizzy spells all through her first pregnancy, went to the doctor in the second month. He made no examination nor analysis of the urine, though he told her she had kidney trouble; he merely gave her some medicine " which did no good," so she never went back. At eight months she had eclampsia.

As a rule the mothers who feel themselves to be in poor health during pregnancy are the ones who resort to the doctor. Among the 119 who had prenatal care, only 22 reported that they felt well during pregnancy; 34 had minor ailments such as backache, nausea, cramps, headaches, swollen hands and feet, or varicose veins; and the rest had some more serious trouble. Few women in this community recognize that it is wise to consult a physician during pregnancy whether or not they feel normally well. On the other hand the fatalistic assumption that a pregnant woman may expect to be thoroughly miserable is much less common than in many other places. Most of these women, if they feel sick, make some attempt to get relief from the doctor even if only by sending for medicine. Doctoring with patent medicines is occasionally tried but is not common.

The cost of prenatal care in this community is difficult to determine, because it is frequently either included with the doctor's obstetrical fee or lost track of in the general family bill. In the majority of cases where a report could be obtained the cost was less than $5. Apparently no charge is ordinarily made for urinalysis; most consultations with the doctor take place at his office, for which the fee is never high; and only when some serious complication calls the doctor to the home is any considerable expense involved. That cost is seldom a determining factor in calling upon the doctor is further indicated by the fact that in this district prenatal care is no more common among the well to do than among the poorer families.

Cost of childbearing.

An attempt was made to find out how much it costs to have a a baby in this part of the country. This estimate of costs covers only the services connected with the birth—prenatal care, obstetrical fee, nursing, and extra household help for the confinement period—and does not include equipment of any kind, such as medicine, nursing supplies, or the baby's clothes.

The ordinary range of the different items of cost thus included has been already described. The total cost for these services was obtained for 249 cases [1] (the other mothers being unable to give this information), and was as follows:

Cost of confinement.	Number of confinements.
Total	249
Less than $50	198
Less than $25	114
No cost	4
Less than $5	1
$5 to $9	6
$10 to $14	13
$15 to $19	53
$20 to $24	37
$25 to $29	28
$30 to $39	39
$40 to $49	17
$50 to $59	18
$60 to $69	11
$70 to $79	7
$80 to $89	5
$90 to $99	4
$100 or more	6

From these figures it appears that nearly half (46 per cent) of the babies cost their parents less than $25; that four-fifths (80 per cent) cost less than $50; and that the expenses of the birth of the large majority (63 per cent) came to between $15 and $40.

Of the 22 cases where the costs were markedly higher than the general rule—that is, $70 or more—2 were hospital cases with serious complications; in 4 cases the cost for physician's services outside of the hospital exceeded $25; in 7 cases a trained nurse was employed; and in 9 cases the expenditure for household help and nursing (exclusive of trained nurses) was $50 or more. Apparently, therefore, unusually high expenses of childbirth are much more apt to be due to the cost of nursing and household service than to medical fees.

COMPLICATIONS OF CONFINEMENT.

Among the 349 confinements concerning which records were secured in this study there developed 2 cases of eclampsia. Four of the children were stillborn. Sixteen deliveries were effected with instruments. One Cæsarean section and 2 versions were performed. In the rural parts of the county during the period studied 3 deaths occurred from puerperal septicemia, 2 following miscarriages, and 1 following a full-term birth. So far as could be learned, these were the only deaths in this area from causes connected with childbirth.

During their whole child-bearing history the 330 [2] mothers had had 1,269 pregnancies, of which 63 (5 per cent) resulted in mis-

---

[1] Including confinements in a hospital, but excluding others where the mother went away from the country district of this county.

[2] The history for one mother, secured from the grandmother, was too incomplete to use.

carriages and 23 (1.8 per cent) in stillbirths. Of the 1,216 children carried to at least seven months' term 73 were delivered with instruments; 48 of these were first-born children. That is, 14.5 per cent of the first-born children of these mothers and only 2.8 per cent of the subsequent children were delivered with instruments. There was only one fully developed case of eclampsia besides the two in the survey period, but in one other instance the doctor forced an eight-months' birth "because he feared spasms."

MOTHER'S WORK.

The work which a mother does during pregnancy and within the first months after childbirth is a possible direct cause of injury to her and to her baby. So, also, her ordinary duties and the work which she did in girlhood have an important influence upon her health, and presumably therefore affect her children's vitality.

As would be expected in a farming community, the mothers of this study did practically no work away from home; two laborers' wives hired out for a few weeks to cook for harvest hands or thrashers, but that was all. Consequently the problem of the work the mothers did during the period of the survey resolves itself into a question of housework and work on the home farm. Of these, housework is much the more important in this district.

Cessation of work before childbirth.

It already has been shown that about 1 in 5 of the country mothers had hired help with her housework during the last weeks of pregnancy. Often such help is primarily a precaution to insure having some one on hand when needed, but in some cases the hired girl relieves the mother of most of her work. Generally, however, pregnant mothers keep up their usual round of duties until labor begins, unless they are disabled by serious ill health.

Resumption of work after childbirth.

In this community two weeks is well established as the shortest period that should elapse after confinement before a woman undertakes any great amount of work; and often the heavier housework such as washing and ironing, and the out-of-door chores, are not resumed for two or three months. Ten days in bed is the prevailing standard for recuperation after childbirth, but normally a mother who gets up after 10 days does no work within the fortnight.

Less than 1 in 10 of the mothers visited got up from bed before the tenth day; less than 1 in 40 under a week. Pressure of work does not often seem to be an important factor in inducing the women of this part of the country to get up too soon, for out of 7 who were up in less than a week, 3 did no work for two or three weeks; 3 did some work after one week but had help for two or three weeks; only 1 did any of her regular work within the first week, and she did nothing but the cooking during the first two weeks.

Usual housework and help.

Leaving out of account the period immediately preceding and following confinement, we find that only 16 mothers—1 in 20—had a hired girl as a regular or usual assistant; 73 had a sister, mother, or daughter 14 years or older to help them; and 33 reported that they had more or less help from their husbands. The rest—about two-thirds of the whole number—managed their housework alone or with some help from the boys or younger girls. The amount of work the mother has to do depends also to a great extent upon the size of the family. Moderately large families—of seven or eight people—are numerous, forming almost as large a proportion (28 per cent) of the total as do the small families of three or four (30 per cent). The typical family has several children who are too small to be of any help to the mother but are, on the contrary, a decided addition to her burdens.

The farmhouse.

The typical farmhouse[1] has from three to six rooms, most commonly four, all on one floor. Most of the houses, except on some of the tenant farms, are fairly well built and in good repair; but many are needlessly inconvenient for the housewife. As one renter's wife said when asked about conveniences, "I mostly had *in*conveniences." Occasionally one comes upon a farmer who has just taken hold of his own land, and is temporarily housing his family in a one or two room shack; but such pioneer conditions are rare. Probably the most serious housing problem is the difficulty some renters have in finding any house to live in or, at least, any decent accommodations.

Room crowding is fairly common in these farm homes, and the inevitable confusion must add appreciably to the housewife's labors. Nearly half (45 per cent) of all the homes had more than one occupant per room, counting all the rooms in the house and not including the baby; one-sixth (16 per cent) had two or more occupants per room, which makes a distinctly overcrowded household. As might be anticipated, the homes on the smaller farms (under 320 acres) are more often crowded than on the larger ones.

Water supply.

Almost every farm is provided with a windmill; in spite of the fact that a drilled well with its mill is an expensive piece of equipment, it is fortunately accepted as essential. And as the western plains are

---

[1] All house information is for the house where the parents were living when the baby was born.

notoriously windy, the water seldom has to be pumped by hand; except that, as one farmer explained, "The wind 'most always gives out at harvest, just when you need the water most." In the majority of cases the windmill is located within 50 feet of the house; nearly one-fourth of the houses have their mills within 25 feet. On the other hand, 1 in 8 of the homes without water inside is 100 feet or more away from its water supply. For the most part, however, the carrying of water is not such a task as in districts where it must be brought from a spring or creek.

As the pumping power is already provided, it is comparatively easy to pipe water into the house; in a typical instance, where running water had recently been put in, the installation cost only $100. Nevertheless only 60 families, or less than 1 in 5, had water in the house when the last baby was born. But the idea of installing "waterworks" is evidently spreading, for several families had made this improvement within the year; and more were planning to do so in the near future, especially when building new houses. One mother expressed a common sentiment when she said, "We sure will have water when we are settled on a place to stay."

When people have water in the house they usually have running water from a tank filled by the windmill. This tank is sometimes in the house and sometimes on the windmill frame. But some builders have been so misguided as to arrange the tank *under* the house so that the water must be lifted into the kitchen by a hand pump. A number of families have piped water available in the summer, but the tanks or pipes are not protected from freezing in the winter.

One in four of the landowning fathers had water in his house, but only 1 in 10 of the renters.

Other conveniences.

Sinks for the disposal of waste water are as scarce as inside water, and even more markedly confined to the homes of landowners. Eighteen families had bath tubs—most, but not all, with running water; only 2 had water-closets.

Although conveniences which are taken as a matter of course in the ordinary city home—sinks, running water, set tubs, and lights—are scarce, the housewives are well supplied with other labor-saving devices such as oil stoves, sewing machines, washers, and mechanical churns. Nearly every one has a sewing machine. Four in every 5 women have washing machines, and 1 in every 8 has a washing machine run by an engine.

Boarding hired men.

By far the most serious aspect of the housework problem in this community is the necessity of boarding hired men. About one-third

(114) of the families visited kept a regular hired man for whom the housewife must provide for at least six months through the summer and fall. During their last pregnancy 263 mothers had occasional farm laborers to board. These extra hands appear for the busy seasons, almost always for harvest and thrashing, often also for plowing and sowing in the fall, and sometimes for the spring work.

One mitigating feature of the situation is that it is not the custom in this district for the housewife to do the washing for the hired men, particularly not for men who are employed for only a short time. Even men employed for the season are usually expected to do their own laundry work.

Harvest and thrashing crews.

Of all the "hands" the harvest crew is the greatest burden. Wheat harvest comes in the latter part of June and the early part of July and ordinarily lasts for from two to three weeks, occasionally for a month; and life is strenuous during that time. The smallest number of men who can handle the reaping is 3—called a half crew— which means 2 men besides the head of the family, unless there are grown sons or brothers in the household. A standard crew for work with a header—the almost universally used type of reaping machine—is 6 or 7 men, and this is the number most commonly employed; but the larger farms not infrequently need a double crew of 12 to 15 men. To have such a crew to cook for, even with the help of a hired girl, for about three weeks in the middle of summer is plainly no light task and is especially trying when it comes near the time of confinement. The women recount that during harvest they have to begin work about 4 a. m. and get through about 10 p. m., with possibly a short rest after dinner. The work is acknowledged to be so hard that hired girls regularly get more than their standard wages at this time—sometimes as much as $2 a day.

The housework at thrashing time is not regarded as so arduous, even when a larger number of men (thrashing crews usually number 12 to 15 men) has to be provided for, because thrashing ordinarily lasts only a few days, and "you can get a lot of things cooked up in advance to last that long." Furthermore, many of the thrashing outfits feed their own men—the "machine men"—from a portable kitchen called the "cook shack," an arrangement which relieves the housewife of all responsibility so far as these men are concerned. Then all she has to provide for, in addition to her family, are the few men who haul the grain; and when, as is often the case, the haulers are neighbors who are "changing work," she has to give them only their dinners. Obviously the cook shack is a great boon to the housewife. The reason it is not always employed is that under the standard scale of charges it constitutes a large addition to the farmer's thrashing expense; he can save a good deal of money by getting an outfit without a cook shack and providing for the men himself.

How the situation works out for a representative group of farm mothers is shown in the following illustrations:

On a farm of 160 acres, where the family consisted of the father, mother, and two children of 3 and 5 years, the baby was born in June, at the beginning of the harvest season. For a week before her confinement the mother had to house and board 4 men; and when the actual harvesting began, 10 days after the baby was born, she had 6 men to board for 8 days. Six weeks later came the thrashing, with 5 men for 3 days. This extra burden of work came at a time when the mother most needed her strength, at the end of a trying pregnancy which was complicated by swollen feet, varicose veins, and dizzy spells. While the confinement was normal, the recovery was slow. Although for 2 weeks before and 3 weeks after the baby was born she had a hired girl who did most of the work, and although her sister came to help during thrashing, nevertheless the mother attributes her slow recovery to the fact that she had to work "harder than she would have liked" after the baby was born.

The mother on another 160-acre farm had 4 children, the eldest 8 years old. She was miserable with pain and nausea all through the latter months of her fifth pregnancy, and was weak for more than a month afterwards. Harvest began the day before the baby was born. The two "hands" stayed 15 days; but they got part of their meals at a neighbor's, and the mother did not have to cook for them herself because she had a hired girl who did all the work for 2 weeks before and 5 weeks after the baby came. At thrashing time the mother had only two meals to give.

In another case, on a farm of 640 acres, the mother, who was badly bloated and troubled with headaches and vertigo during the last month of pregnancy, had to board during that month 3 carpenters and 6 men for the barley harvest, in addition to the 1 man employed for the season. Though she had a hired girl for the last 2 or 3 weeks, she helped with the cooking up to the last day and had the care of her three small children. The baby was born the very day the wheat harvest began; that day there were 15 hired men on the place. Harvest lasted 12 days; the next day the hired girl left; and the day after that came the thrashing, with 6 men to provide for. It is not surprising that the mother reported that she recovered her strength slowly.

The baby on a 450-acre farm—the youngest of 5 children under 9—was born in the winter. The mother had had a stillborn child less than a year before, and she vomited badly all through this last pregnancy. Every year she has 6 men for harvest in July for about 3 weeks, and 6 grain haulers in October for about 8 days; her husband keeps 1 hired man all the time and usually 2 all summer. The mother has had no help for the past three seasons.

The family on a 520-acre farm consisted of 9 people; 2 boys were grown, but the oldest girl was only 12, and there were 3 children under 5. The last baby was born in the fall, 3 months after harvest; the mother was troubled during pregnancy with pains and dizziness. Harvest brought 2 hired men for 10 days early in July; later in the month thrashing brought 3 men for 2 days. The mother had no help with the housework except her daughter.

On a farm of 200 acres where the baby was born early in the fall the mother had 3 harvesters to board for 2 weeks in June; at thrashing in August she had 4 men for dinner 2 days only. She had no help either time and she reported that she felt "extra well" throughout the summer. In addition to her work for the men she had two little children, 2 and 3 years old, to care for.

On a 160-acre farm the mother, whose baby was born late in the fall, boarded 6 men for 2 weeks at harvest beginning the last of June; at thrashing in August she boarded 5 men for 2 days. She always has to be careful of her strength during the early months of pregnancy, but fortunately was in excellent health during the busy season. Her daughter of 18 helps her with the housework; she has only one other child besides the baby, but she is caring for two of her sister's children.

On a 380-acre farm the baby was born in the latter part of May, the sixth child in a family whose eldest was only 8 years old. The mother was in excellent health through her pregnancy and recovered from childbirth so well—"felt better than ever before"—that she kept her hired girl only two weeks, after which she did all her regular work, including milking, gardening, and the care of chickens. Harvest came when the baby was 3 weeks old, bringing 5 "hands" for 2 weeks; at thrashing, immediately after harvest, 2 haulers were boarded for 2 days. The mother had no help with the housework during this time, but she did no milking or gardening through the harvest period; as far as possible she had "got her work done up ahead" the first week she was up from bed.

The mother on a farm of 240 acres had three children, the oldest 7, before her last baby was born. This birth occurred in the winter, which made the trying latter months of pregnancy—the mother suffers from swollen feet and varicose veins—easier than if it had come in the summer. In the previous summer she boarded 6 men at harvest for 6 weeks; and almost immediately after that she had the "whole crew" of 12 thrashers to cook for for 3 or 4 days. From the time the baby was 3 weeks old she had 1 hired man to board; 6 harvesters again in the summer, but for only 2 weeks; and 12 thrashers in August. She had help each summer, however.

Another mother, whose baby was born in the fall on a 640-acre farm, had to board 4 harvest hands in July and 12 thrashers for 6 days in August in both the preceding and following summers; she had no outside help with the housework, but her 2 grown daughters do much of the work. She was in good health throughout this time except for varicose veins during pregnancy. Another baby was born the second spring, and the varicose veins were "worse than ever." That year the mother had the usual 4 harvesters for 2 weeks when the baby was 10 weeks old; but the thrashers brought a cook shack, so that she had only 3 or 4 grain haulers to provide for. The father keeps 1 hired man nearly all the time. This mother has 11 children, of whom 5 were less than 10 years old when the last baby was born.

The baby on one 560-acre farm was born in the winter. The mother was troubled with vomiting throughout pregnancy. One hired man was employed steadily that year. The six harvesters stayed until the end of July, but the mother had help then. For the last three months before the baby was born she had a hired girl all the time and did no work except cooking and sewing. The cooking in itself was no light task during this period, as her husband thrashed three different times that fall, the last time only a month before the baby was born; and each time the mother cooked for the whole crew of 12 to 14 men. Ever since this confinement—her first—she has been almost disabled with uterine trouble. The following summer there was 1 hired man before harvest; 6 harvesters for 2 weeks; and only 3 or 4 haulers for 3 days at thrashing, because the thrashers brought a cook shack. The mother could not get a hired girl that year, but her sister helped her through harvest and thrashing.

A mother who lived on a 640-acre farm had four little children before this baby came, of whom the oldest—twins—were only 4. The baby was born in the winter, five months after harvest time, and the mother had good health all through her pregnancy except in the first two months. At harvest that summer she had a hired girl to cook for the 7 men, but no help at thrashing in September, when she had to do the cooking for 15 men for 3 days. One man is employed all the time. The year following the baby's birth the mother cooked for 3 harvesters and later for 3 haulers at thrashing, and then for 2 hired men until November; she could not get a girl at all that year, although the 2-year-old was sick at harvest time and the mother was barely able to struggle through with the work. This family plans to give up farming, partly because the harvest work is too hard for the mother and they have found it almost impossible to get household help.

Four-fifths (272) of all the farm mothers worked for harvest crews, of at least 3 men, either before or after confinement; 43 of them within 1 month of confinement, 81 within 2 months, and 124 within 3 months. That serious harm may result from the strain of such work is illustrated by the experience of two mothers during former pregnancies, in each instance a little over a year before the last baby was born. Each had a miscarriage that summer, one at 2 months and one at 5, which she attributed to overwork at harvest time. Both of these women evidently were hard workers. One of them had a gang of carpenters in addition to the farm hands to provide for the summer of the miscarriage, and besides her own work she did the washing and baking for a bachelor neighbor.

It is markedly true of this country that prosperity comes hard on the farmer's wife, because prosperity here means practically always a larger farm and more wheat, and therefore more men to board for a longer time. One woman expressed the situation succinctly by saying: "We have so many men because we farm so much land." She had a double crew of 15 harvesters to board both the year her baby was born and the year after, and 10 thrashers immediately after harvest; also 2 men through the rest of the summer and fall, and a gang of carpenters for a good part of both summers. Though she had a hired girl during harvest and thrashing, her work was nevertheless much heavier than that of the wife on a quarter-section (160-acre) farm whose only "hands" were a single crew of harvesters for a couple of weeks and a few haulers for two or three days. It also happened that in her case the difficulties of the situation were aggravated by an uncomfortable pregnancy, with much vomiting, and a difficult instrumental delivery—the birth occurring two weeks after thrashing—resulting in injuries which troubled her for a long time afterwards.

Another mother, whose husband farms a section and a half (960 acres), had a crew of 17 men on the place for three months the summer her baby was born and 1 or 2 men all the time. A third, on another 960-acre farm, had 4 men for a week, then 12 men for six weeks (finishing one week before her baby was born), and after that from 1 to 4 men for two months more until the next crop was sown. Each of these women had a hired girl through the summer.

Mothers' work for harvest crews is not only heavier on the larger farms but also falls to the lot of a larger proportion of the mothers. Where the father farmed less than half a section 72 per cent of the mothers had this work to do either before or after confinement; on farms of from one-half to three-quarters of a section the percentage of mothers having such work was 85; and on farms of over three-quarters of a section 87. This relation holds true of all work for farm hands; where the farm was smaller than one-half section 79 per cent of the mothers had to carry this burden during pregnancy; on the medium-sized farms, one-half to three-quarters of a section, 90 per cent; and on the larger farms (over 480 acres) 95.5 per cent of the mothers had hired men to work for.

Renters' wives have many inconveniences to bear, but they fare a little better than owners' wives when it comes to working for the hired men; 84 per cent of the former boarded some hired men during pregnancy and 92.4 per cent of the latter. Farm laborers' wives, of course, usually escape this kind of work, but sometimes they have to board some of the employer's hands.

Summer work is likely to fall heavily upon the wife of the man who owns and runs a thrasher. There were 7 of them among the mothers included in the survey. Among these 2 ran the cook shack for the husband's crew for about 2 months; 2 did the husband's farm chores for 2 or 3 months while he was away with the thrasher; 1 had the crew to feed at the house most of the time for 2 months; and another had the crew at the house over Sundays all through the thrashing season.

Dairy work.

Dairying is a minor factor in agriculture in this part of Kansas; most farmers keep a few cows and many sell some butter or cream, but very few make any large part of their income from this source. Though half of the women visited did some churning, the large majority of these made butter only for their own use. Neither milking nor running the separator is customarily regarded as women's work, and a goodly number of the men even do the churning; in most families the mother does the milking only when the men are away or particularly busy, just as she would help with their other chores at such times. As the heaviest milk production comes in the winter while there is wheat pasture for the cattle, and as the men are least busy at this time, the situation works out very conveniently for the women.

Poultry raising.

The most common outdoor work done by the women is poultry raising. Almost every farm has its flocks of chickens and turkeys. Eight out of every 10 women visited kept chickens; and most of them raised at least 200 a year, while flocks of 400 or more are not uncommon. Most of the mothers do not regard the work of caring for the chickens as onerous, for in this climate chickens seem to thrive with very little care except in the spring, and therefore do not aggravate the summer rush.

Gardening.

Less than half of the mothers reported having done gardening during the period covered by the survey. Many had no garden (it is a discouraging task to try to raise vegetables in this climate), and in other families some one else—husband, children, or grandmother— took care of the garden. The men as a rule are helpful about doing the harder part of the work, such as preparing the ground, and often the cultivating also.

Other farm work.

Other farm chores—feeding the stock, etc.—rarely fall to the lot of the mother of the family; only 13 women reported doing this kind of work. And field work is even more unusual, only 7 mothers having helped in the fields during the last pregnancy or the year following. One woman expressed the general standard when she said: "I had rather do outside work than housework, but I won't do both." In this community few women would think of neglecting their housework in order to help in the fields.

Farm work during girlhood.

The situation is very different when one inquires as to the work which these same mothers did when they were girls. Ninety per cent of them lived in the country for at least two years of their girlhood (after they were 10 years old); and of these, four-fifths did more or less farm work. About one-third of the country girls did chores only—milking, gardening, care of chickens, feeding stock—while nearly half of them, in addition to their chores, did some work in the fields. For the girls raised in western Kansas this field work usually consisted of driving teams or herding cattle; but the list includes women who as girls did many other kinds of work in other places.

INFANT WELFARE.

Infant mortality rate.

The term "infant mortality rate" is used in the Children's Bureau studies to mean the number of children out of each 1,000 born alive within a given period who die before they are 1 year old.

In the group of 349 live-born children included in the survey, 175 were born at least a year before the agent's visit; and of these 7 had died before reaching their first birthday, giving an infant mortality rate of 40 per 1,000, or 1 death for every 25 births. For the other 174 born within the year preceding the visit no definite rate can be computed, because some of those who were still alive when they were visited may have died afterwards before they were a year old. There were 8 known deaths among this group, so that the infant mortality rate was at least 46 per 1,000. According to the death records of the county, no others of these children died up to the close of 1916, when all of them were at least 3 months old and had therefore passed the age when most infant deaths occur. Hence it seems probable that the actual rate for this group would not be a great deal higher than this figure.

An infant mortality rate of 40 per 1,000 is the lowest found in any of the Children's Bureau studies and less than half of the lowest rate found in any of the cities studied; the rate found in the same way for selected country townships in Wisconsin was 54 per 1,000. It must be remembered that the figures upon which this rate is based are so small that one or two deaths more or less—which might easily have happened without any real change in conditions—would make a considerable difference in the rate. Still it is improbable that chance variation would bring the rate much above 50.

The mothers of these babies had had altogether 1,193 live-born children. Excluding the 174 who were born within a year of the date of visit, there remain 1,019 children in these families for whom the infant mortality rate can be computed. Among these children 56 died before they were a year old, which gives an infant mortality rate of 55 per 1,000, or a little over 1 in 20. Evidently, then, the low rate for the survey period is not sporadic; the causes which produce a low rate among the babies in these country families have been in operation throughout the family history.

It is encouraging that in a prosperous, intelligent, farming community the infant mortality rate can be brought so low as this. Nevertheless, the existing rate should not be regarded with complacency, for, as Sir Arthur Newsholme says, "If babies were well born and well cared for, their mortality would be negligible." In other words, there is no inherent reason why *any* babies should die in a community which has all the advantages possessed by this county—country life, healthful climate, high standards of living, a high level of intelligence about matters of health, and means wherewith to provide for its mothers and babies.

Causes of death.

Of the 15 deaths under 1 year of age which occurred in the group of babies for whom schedules were secured, 2 occurred under 1 day, 4 under 2 weeks, and 6 under 1 month. Five of the deaths were due to causes peculiar to early infancy, 5 to diarrhea and enteritis, 3 to respiratory diseases (1 of these was bronchitis following whooping cough), 1 to measles, and 1 to marasmus.

Feeding customs.

Practically all the babies in this study were breast fed at least for a few days. Of the 349 live-born babies 2 died before they were fed at all; only 2 were fed from the bottle from the beginning; and only 7 were weaned before the middle of the first month. On the other hand, 311 or 92 per cent of the 340 babies for whom the record covers the first month of life were exclusively breast fed through the greater part of that month, and another 20 or 6 per cent were partly breast fed. The proportion of exclusively breast-fed babies then drops month by month to 71 per cent at 5 months and to 61 per cent at 6 months. After that the percentage naturally falls off more rapidly, but 23 per cent or nearly one-fourth of the babies were still exclusively breast fed during the ninth month, and a small number (8 per cent) had no other food than breast milk until after they were a year old.

Breast feeding in combination with other food is continued longer even than these figures would indicate. At the end of the ninth month only 19 per cent of the babies were weaned, i. e., wholly taken off the breast, and at the end of 12 months only 30 per cent or less than one-third. In fact, for the majority breast feeding continues well into the second year; at the end of 15 months 45 per cent or nearly one-half were not yet weaned; and at the end of 18 months 24 per cent or about one-fourth. Medical authorities agree that this custom of late weaning is not to be recommended. Though less dangerous than the opposite practice of too early weaning, nevertheless it is not advantageous either for the mother or for the baby. In most cases the baby should be weaned by the end of the first year.

If the feeding history of these country babies in Kansas is compared with that of the city babies of native mothers in Johnstown, Pa., and Manchester, N. H.—the first two cities where this study was made by the Children's Bureau—and in Akron, Ohio, the larger of the cities of the Middle West, we find that exclusive breast feeding is much more common through the first nine months in this Kansas county than in any of these cities (with the exception of the last three months in Akron), and, conversely, that artificial feeding is even more markedly absent. Since breast feeding, especially in the early months, is proved and acknowledged to be an important factor in protecting a baby's chance of life, this fact of the unusual prevalence of breast feeding probably accounts, in part at least, for the low death rate among this group of country babies.

TABLE V.—*Breast and artificial feeding, by month and locality.*

Locality.	Percentage of infants who were exclusively breast fed.				Percentage of infants who were artificially fed.			
	During first month.	During third month.	During sixth month.	During ninth month.	During first month.	During third month.	During sixth month.	During ninth month.
County in Kansas....	92.0	83.2	60.8	23.3	2.1	6.1	12.5	19.3
Johnstown, Pa.[1]......	....	66.9	41.1	11.8	....	20.3	26.1	34.1
Manchester, N. H.[1]...	81.7	60.9	36.3	17.1	15.4	32.5	47.4	55.1
Akron, Ohio [1]........	87.9	73.3	54.5	27.7	8.1	18.5	26.9	32.3

[1] The percentages for Johnstown, Manchester, and Akron are given only for the babies of native-born mothers, because in the Kansas county practically all the mothers were native.

A mother may be obliged for some reason to resort to supplementary feeding or even to wean her baby altogether; but necessity does not excuse the giving of solid food in the early months, as is often done by ill-advised mothers. The mothers of this community are on the whole careful in such matters. Only 10 babies (out of 310 whose feeding records for three months were obtained) were given any solid food before they were 3 months old, including as solid food gravy, or milk thickened with flour, crackers, etc. Only 59 (out of 263) began to eat solid food before they were 6 months old. And 79 children (out of 202) had no solid food until after they were 9 months old.

PERCENTAGES OF ALL BABIES RECEIVING DIFFERENT KINDS OF FEEDING, BY MONTH
OF AGE.

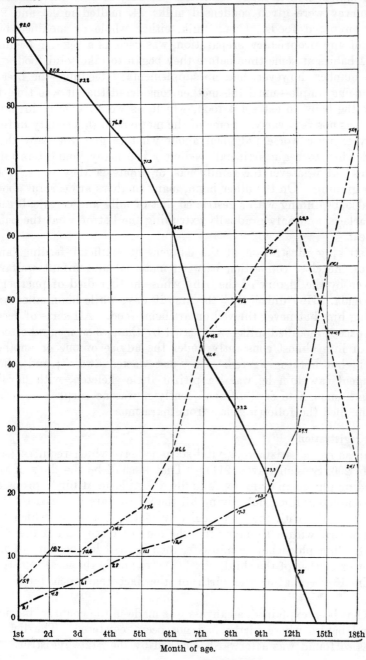

Month of age.

——————————— Breast feeding.
— — — — — — Mixed feeding.
— · — · — · — Artificial feeding.

The use of proprietary foods and condensed milk for babies is less common than in many localities. Twenty-four of the babies of the survey were given condensed milk; 14, malted milk; and 26, other prepared foods. Cows' milk, either whole or modified but without any proprietary preparation, was used as a regular feeding for 51 babies at some time before they began to take solid food. A large number, however, had no supplementary feeding—the breast milk being ample—until the mother considered that it was time to allow the baby to eat solid food, which, as we have seen, in most cases was not very early. Some of the mothers in this county unfortunately exercise worse judgment about what to give the baby than about when to begin artificial feeding. Too many youngsters take "tastes" of whatever the family has, or whatever they want, from the beginning. On the other hand, many mothers are careful about this also, beginning with a restricted diet of milk and cereals, bread, or crackers, and only gradually extending the list of what the baby may eat.

A striking illustration of the dangers of artificial feeding, and also of the close connection between maternal and infant welfare, is given by the history of the baby whose mother died of puerperal septicemia. He " did finely " the first 10 days while his mother was nursing him but never thrived on artificial food. All sorts of feeding—except modified milk—were tried by the two women who took care of him almost constantly under the advice of one or another doctor; but nothing agreed. He "just wasted away"; and when the agent saw him he was "a pitiful little skeleton, with hardly strength enough to cry." Consequently it was no surprise to learn that he died the following day from marasmus.

Birth registration.

Kansas has a satisfactory vital-statistics law which requires (sec. 10, ch. 296, Session Laws 1911) : " That it shall be the duty of the attending physician or midwife to file a certificate of birth, properly and completely filled out, giving all the particulars required by this act, * * * with the local registrar of the district in which the birth occurs, within 10 days after the date of birth, and if there be no attending physician or midwife, then it shall be the duty of the father or mother of the child, * * * to notify the local registrar within 10 days after the birth of the fact that such birth occurred * * *."

As has been explained, a canvass was made in the country districts to find babies whose births had not been registered. The list of names so found was afterwards checked by the State registrar.

In this way 35 [1] unregistered births were discovered. Fourteen of the 350 children born in the county were born in town and all of these 14 were registered; but of the 336 births which occurred out in the country, these 35 or 10.4 per cent were unregistered. If this county may be taken as a fair sample of the completeness of birth registration in Kansas, only a slight improvement would be necessary to bring the State up to the standard required for admission to the birth-registration area, viz, that at least 90 per cent of all births shall be registered.

Twenty-six of the unregistered births were attended by physicians, 5 by midwives, and 4 by other people. As midwifery in this county is on such a nonprofessional basis, it is fair to say that the duty of reporting all these 9 births where there was no physician devolved upon the parents. Six of the 10 physicians who did the bulk of the obstetrical work in this district reported all their births; and 3 of the others were responsible for half of all the failures to register.

No record was secured as to promptness of registration except for the 19 births which occurred in September, 1916. All of these were registered; but 8 of the 19 were registered more than 10 days after the birth took place, and therefore the requirement of the law on this point was not fulfilled.

Township, village, or city clerks act as local registrars in Kansas and are required not only to secure complete registration from their districts but also to keep local records of all births and deaths. According to the provision of the law (sec. 3, cit.), which authorizes the State board of health to establish registration districts, this county is divided into eight districts of varying size. Five consist of only one township, while the largest contains five townships. Apparently the purpose is so to arrange the districts, by grouping the townships around the larger towns, that the registration office shall be as convenient as feasible to the local physicians. But this arrangement must interfere, where the districts are large, with the registrar's ability to keep track of events through his own acquaintance. The problem of registration is further complicated by the fact that in some cases births are not registered in the districts where they occurred but in the physicians' home towns. This practice is unnecessarily confusing to the registrar of the district in which the birth did occur, if he is making an effort to carry out his duties and see that the births in his territory are registered.

---

[1] Including one which was registered several months after the canvass was made, possibly, therefore, as a result of the canvass; but excluding one which had been registered in the local office but the certificate not forwarded to the State registrar.

SUMMARY AND CONCLUSIONS.

The findings of this survey of the rural area of one county have a meaning not only for the county itself but also, because this county is a typical one, for large tracts of western farming country. The circumstances affecting the care of mothers in childbirth here have therefore a wide significance. The fact that every year in the United States thousands of mothers die needlessly from childbirth compels attention to this subject. The favorable conditions described in this report suggest measures to be taken by other communities interested in the prevention of suffering and death of mothers and babies. The less favorable conditions reported will doubtless be recognized as typical of large numbers of rural districts throughout the country.

The farming population of this county is almost entirely of native birth and predominantly of native parentage. The general standard of living and of education and intelligence is high, especially among the two-thirds of the population who own land. For several years the all-important wheat crop has been satisfactory and prices high, so that the community is in a prosperous financial condition. Consequently most families are not debarred by poverty from obtaining such care for mother and baby as seems to them necessary.

The infant mortality rate of the group of babies studied in this district is low—40 per 1,000 births. Though this is only half of the lowest rate found by the Children's Bureau in any of the cities it has studied, nevertheless the community should not rest satisfied with this record but should set as its aim the saving of all its babies. Nearly all the babies seen were strikingly sturdy, active, and apparently well developed. It is significant that these indications of good health occur in a community where only 1 baby in 5 is weaned before he is 9 months old, and where the mothers as a rule are careful of the feeding of their babies and are interested in learning all they can about the best methods of infant care.

The interest shown by the mothers of the county in having their babies examined at the "Baby Days" indicates a field for further endeavor. Such examinations might well be held by physicians at regular intervals at accessible centers throughout the county. A county public-health nurse could assist the physicians at the "Baby Days" or baby-health conferences. She could also establish headquarters at the county seat and at accessible substations throughout the county in smaller towns and rural schools, where she could weigh babies and talk with mothers who wish her advice. How to keep the baby well through the hot summer; what to do before the doctor comes, in an emergency such as croup or convulsions; how to nurse a sick child or a mother and newborn baby at home—these are all questions about which women are anxious to learn all they can. The simple equipment necessary for these meetings and baby-health conferences throughout the county—scales for weighing the babies, exhibit material, and apparatus for giving demonstrations—could easily be moved from one center to another if an automobile were available for the nurse's transportation.

The study shows that approximately 1 in 10 of the babies in this county born in the open country will be unable to get a birth certificate if one is needed later in life. Such a percentage is a fairly low one, but it shows that a still greater appreciation of the importance of birth registration on the part of parents and physicians is necessary. No community should be content until every birth is registered.

Except at harvest the ordinary run of work which the mothers have to do is not overhard. Although such conveniences as running water, sinks, and indoor toilets—which a city woman considers indispensable—are too often lacking, nevertheless mechanical labor-saving devices are fairly common. Few mothers do any field work or any farm chores except poultry raising and gardening. But at wheat-harvest time, and often at thrashing, there comes an almost overwhelming rush of work because of the necessity of boarding the crews. This is always a great burden and may be a serious matter if it happens at a time when the mother's strength should be spared.

Trained nursing care at confinement is seldom obtained. Only a few of the mothers went to a hospital at this time or had a trained nurse together with a helper for the housework at home. Even the so-called "experienced" nurses are rare; most of the mothers visited depended upon relatives, neighbors, or hired girls for their nursing care.

There is an evident need in this community for trained attendants—competent women who have had some training and experience in home care of the sick, and who can do the necessary housework for the mothers and the nursing under the supervision of a trained nurse. In several communities it has already been proved that women can be found willing and anxious to do this work. Training courses have been established, and registries of properly qualified and supervised trained attendants are conducted in several cities and towns. The supervision of the work of these attendants by registered nurses is an essential part of the plan. Visiting nurses are acting in this capacity in several communities. A nurse, or a group of nurses, employed by this county could well include this work of supervision in their program.

The situation as to medical care in connection with childbirth is better than in other country districts studied by the Children's Bureau. Almost all the mothers were attended by a physician at confinement. Roads which are nearly always good made medical care accessible even in this country of widely scattered farms. The necessary cost of medical service is not prohibitive to the majority of families. Hospitals, accessible to all parts of the county by means of the good roads, are available for complicated cases. The mother in the group of families studied who had to be delivered by Cæsarean section might have been lost, and her baby also might have died, if she had lived in a rural district where, either because of distance or because of impassable roads, no good hospital was within reach.

The question of the prenatal care obtained by this group of mothers is important. Only of late and to a limited degree has it been realized that expert supervision is necessary for every woman during pregnancy, if complications of this period and of confinement are to be prevented or cured. Such supervision is essential for the reduction of the maternal mortality rate of any community. That physicians should realize these facts is not enough; women and their husbands must realize them also. Otherwise women will not consult their physicians early and regularly during pregnancy, nor will their husbands be willing to pay for this added service. In this rural county one-third of the mothers secured some prenatal care from physicians. In few cases was this care adequate or even fairly adequate; nevertheless, a beginning has evidently been made toward the realization that medical supervision during pregnancy is necessary. During the last few years it has been proved that trained nursing service is invaluable in supplementing medical supervision during pregnancy. If this is true in the city, where it is comparatively easy to consult a physician, it is still more true in the country where the distance from the physician makes it more difficult to see him regularly. A nurse who has had special training and experience in prenatal work, and who is especially equipped to discern the danger signs of pregnancy, can be of great help to the prospective mother in the country and to her physician. She will advise the mother about daily details of her care of herself so that she can avoid much discomfort and disability; she will urge her to see her physician early for a thorough preliminary examination and later when necessary; she will urge her to send samples of urine regularly to be examined, or, if asked to do so, she will make examinations of the urine and report the results to the physician. Such prenatal work may be one of the most important phases of the duty of a county public-health nurse.

The fact that in more than one-third of the confinements the mother did not receive a visit from the physician after the day of the birth, and the fact that in another third she received only one visit, are evidence that the importance of after-care for the mother is also not realized.

The Children's Bureau in a recent publication [1] has suggested a plan for securing adequate medical and nursing care for mothers and babies in a rural county, which should include:

1. A rural nursing service, centering at the county seat, with nurses especially equipped to discern the danger signs of pregnancy. The establishment of such a service would undoubtedly be the most economical first step in creating the network of agencies which will assure proper care for both normal and abnormal cases. * * *

2. An accessible county center for maternal and infant welfare at which mothers may obtain simple information as to the proper care of themselves during pregnancy as well as of their babies.

3. A county maternity hospital, or beds in a general hospital, for the proper care of abnormal cases and for the care of normal cases when it is convenient for the women to leave their homes for confinement. Such a hospital necessarily would be accessible to all parts of the county.

4. Skilled attendance at confinement obtainable by each woman in the county.

In the county studied progress has evidently been made in securing certain of these suggested essentials for the care of mothers and babies. It will be evident that in this county and others of similar type the next step may well be the establishment of a nursing service for the rural parts of the county. The ways in which a nurse could be of help to the mothers of this district have been pointed out.

A number of public-health nurses in the United States are now employed by county boards of supervisors or boards of education. Their work is no longer an experiment; its value has been definitely proved. In certain counties the work was established at first through private subscriptions; enough money was raised in this way to support a nurse for a period of 6 to 12 months; after the value of the work had been demonstrated the county authorities appropriated money to continue it. This was in recognition of the fact that public-health nursing is not a charity but is a measure for health protection to which all the people of the community have a right. In one county in a Middle Western State a federation of women was formed which included all the organizations of women in the county—women's clubs, ladies' aid societies, and parent-teacher associations, as well as small neighborhood groups of rural women. Largely through the efforts of this federation a tax was levied by referendum vote and a

---

[1] Maternal Mortality from All Conditions Connected with Childbirth in the United States and Certain Other Countries, p. 27. U. S. Children's Bureau publication No. 19. 1917.

large sum of money provided for health work. Two nurses are now employed by this county.

In many counties the nursing service has been established through the employment of a nurse for the rural schools, and this method has proved very successful. In other counties the nurse has begun her work as a tuberculosis nurse; in others as an assistant to the county health officer. Whatever the beginning of the work, the nurse soon finds that the assistance which she can give to mothers in the care of themselves and of their babies is one of its most important developments.

In planning a rural nursing service two things are essential:

1. Every effort should be made to get the right nurse. The nurse employed should have had training in public-health or visiting nursing such as is given now in many training courses, and should also have practical experience. Nurses who have had hospital training only are not fitted to carry out public-health nursing successfully.

2. Ample provision must be made for transportation through the county.

In Kansas, county boards of commissioners have the authority to employ county nurses if they see fit. There is therefore no legal obstacle in the way of this measure for the promotion of the public welfare, and this county could in no way better demonstrate its progressiveness nor more effectively protect the health of its citizens than by providing such nursing service for the whole county.

O

U. S. DEPARTMENT OF LABOR

CHILDREN'S BUREAU

JULIA C. LATHROP, Chief

RURAL CHILDREN

IN SELECTED COUNTIES OF NORTH CAROLINA

BY

FRANCES SAGE BRADLEY, M. D.

AND

MARGARETTA A. WILLIAMSON

RURAL CHILD WELFARE SERIES No. 2

Bureau Publication No. 33

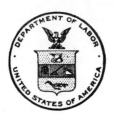

WASHINGTON

GOVERNMENT PRINTING OFFICE

1918

CONTENTS.

3

CONTENTS.

LETTER OF TRANSMITTAL.

U. S. Department of Labor,
Children's Bureau,
Washington, September 25, 1918.

Sir: Herewith I transmit a report entitled "Rural Children in Selected Counties of North Carolina." This study was made at the request of the North Carolina State Board of Health in cooperation with State and local authorities and volunteer organizations. The purpose was to secure information as to the rural child—his well-being, surroundings, needs, and opportunities.

The study was under the direction of Dr. Frances Sage Bradley with the assistance of Miss Margaretta A. Williamson.

Julia C. Lathrop, *Chief.*

Hon. William B. Wilson,
Secretary of Labor.

7

RURAL CHILDREN IN SELECTED COUNTIES OF NORTH CAROLINA.

INTRODUCTION.

This inquiry into the conditions surrounding rural children was undertaken with the purpose of studying at first hand the everyday life of the rural child of the South, at home, at work, at school, and at play—his health, environment, needs, and opportunities. Since three-fifths of the children of the United States are rural children, it is obvious that the problems of the rural child must meet with careful consideration in any program of child conservation.

At the request of the State board of health it was decided to con- ·duct the study in North Carolina, which may fairly be considered a typical Southern State, with its characteristic population, customs, climate, soils, and crops. The inquiry was necessarily confined to definite and limited areas, and an effort was made to choose sections representative of rural conditions in different parts of the State.

North Carolina is clearly divided into an eastern coastal plain of low-lying land, intersected by many streams, partly swamp land but mainly sandy and fertile loose loam soils; a central or piedmont region of higher altitudes and a greater variety of fertile soils;[1] and a western or mountainous region in the heart of the Appalachian system. Cotton raising is the leading industry of the coastal and pied- mont regions; in the mountains little crop farming is done and the chief dependence of the people is live-stock raising and the develop- ment of timber interests.

A lowland county, lying at the junction of the coastal and pied- mont sections, was selected as representative of conditions in the cotton belt, and a mountain county in the extreme western part of the State was chosen as a typical mountain county embodying charac- teristics not only of western North Carolina, but also of other moun- tainous sections of the Southern Appalachian system.

The inquiry was initiated in the lowland county by a children's health conference and a child-welfare exhibit at the county seat, and followed by a series of conferences in each township of the county.

Following the children's health conferences an intensive detailed house-to-house study of the children was made in one rural township of the lowland county (in the cotton belt), and in three smaller rural townships of the mountain county.

---

[1] Thirteenth Census of the United States, 1910, Vol. V, Agriculture, p. 895.

In the townships chosen every home in which there was a child under 16 was visited; the survey included in the lowland county township 127 white families with 340 children, and 129 negro families with 404 children under 16; in the three townships of the mountain county 231 white families with 697 children under 16 were visited. The inquiry, which was made in 1916, covered a period of approximately three months in each county. During this time the bureau agents lived in homes in the townships visited rather than maintaining headquarters at the county seat, in this way gaining a somewhat fuller experience of particular rural conditions and problems than could otherwise have been possible. In the lowland county a Ford car was used for travel; in the mountains, owing to the condition of the roads (with the exception of the main road to the county seat), the agents rode horseback.

Whenever possible the mother was interviewed, otherwise the father, grandmother, or other nearest relative. Information was obtained concerning various phases of child care, together with a comprehensive history of each family in its relation to the well-being of the children of the family. The questions covered the number of children the mother had borne; the number lost, with the causes of their deaths; the mother's prenatal, obstetrical, and postnatal care; distance from physician; nursing care; infant feeding; diet of older children, their physical condition, education, work, and recreation; the mother's household and farm duties; and the housing, sanitation, and economic status of the family.

The inquiry was confined to normal children, no attempt being made to cover dependency, delinquency, illegitimacy, or other problems of abnormal children except a brief survey of State facilities for their care.

Certain phases of child welfare were covered by supplementary studies. Information as to the neighborhood midwives of the four townships was obtained by visiting every midwife who had attended a case within the past five years; a test of birth registration was made and also a brief survey of school facilities in the townships covered.

During the course of the inquiry, various State and other organizations—the State board of health, State board of education, State university, State Normal and Industrial College, States Relations Service of the United States Department of Agriculture, and the staff of an important farm journal—were most helpful in their cooperation, assisting in choosing the counties to be studied, in planning the work, and helping to assemble material for the report.

Local officials and organizations in the counties chosen—the county physician, county superintendent of schools, county medical society, women's clubs, and the press—also showed an active interest in the inquiry and gave every possible assistance.

The success of such an inquiry necessarily depended upon the good will of the community, especially of the families interviewed. Mothers in the sections visited showed the same desire to secure the best possible results in rearing their children and the same cordial interest in the efforts of the Children's Bureau to study the problems of childhood that have been found elsewhere. A friendly, hospitable reception was accorded at every home, both mothers and fathers giving every possible assistance. In fact notes, messages, and remonstrances were sent by mothers whose homes had not yet been reached and who feared they might be overlooked. At one home a note was found pinned to the front door, directing the agents to the field where the mother would be found at work.

The results of the inquiry fall under the five following heads: (1) Children's health conferences, (2) and (3) the survey of conditions surrounding children in the lowland and mountain counties, (4) summary and conclusions, and (5) the State and its relation to child welfare (see Appendix, p. 101).

PART I.

CHILDREN'S HEALTH CONFERENCES.

The children's health conferences, held first at the county seat and later in rural sections, were a series of consultations of physicians with mothers concerning the physical development of their children and were in charge of a physician from the Children's Bureau.

The purpose in view in holding the conferences was (1) to call the attention of mothers to methods of improving the condition of their children, (2) to demonstrate to the communities the value of periodic examination and sustained supervision of young children, and (3) to stimulate local authorities to various forms of follow-up work as suggested by the conference.

CONFERENCE AT THE COUNTY SEAT.

The conference met with a cordial response from local organizations. The mayor, clergy, school officials, and other prominent citizens offered every possible assistance. The civic association, the county medical society, local hospitals, and other organizations gave practical expression of their interest in the work.

Ample publicity was obtained through the courtesy of the State and local press, which gave generously of their space; also through the health bulletins of the State board of health. A letter addressed to all mothers of young children was sent through the cooperation of schools into every home where there was a child. Attractive cards announcing the conference appeared in the windows of schools, churches, stores, railway stations, and elsewhere. Notices announcing the conference and inviting mothers to bring their young children to it were read from every pulpit. To attract the school children, a prize of a five-dollar gold piece was offered by the Children's Bureau for the best composition written by a child under 12 on the conference and its accompanying exhibit.

The conference at the county seat was held at a rest room maintained by the civic association for the use of rural women from the surrounding country when they come to town to do their Saturday's shopping. It extended over 10 days, including two Saturdays, in order to reach as many as possible of the rural women. After the conference for white children, one was held for negroes in an assembly hall of their own, with negro doctors and nurses assisting the Children's Bureau physician.

13

Children under 6 years of age, brought by their parents, were examined by a physician of the Children's Bureau or by local physicians. Each child was weighed, measured, and examined, and the mother given a record of his present condition with written suggestions for his improvement; when necessary the mother was urged to take the child to her own or the best available local physician. The examinations were conducted in view of the audience, that the mothers might observe and profit by the practical demonstration. but with a partition of netting separating the examining room from the audience, to protect the child from the crowd and confusion beyond.

It was made clear that the conference was neither a contest nor a clinic. No prizes were offered, and there was no other incentive than the desire of parents for finer children; nor were sick children admitted, or those recently exposed to communicable diseases. The conference was intended rather for the average child who though apparently well is yet rarely free from defects which may often be corrected if discovered in time.

Accompanying the conference was a child-welfare exhibit of material, part of which had been prepared by the Children's Bureau and part loaned by various organizations or constructed (under the direction of the agents of the bureau) by local women's clubs. A set of panels covered such subjects as prenatal care, infant care, infant mortality, and the visiting nurse. A series of charts on flies, typhoid fever, and malaria was loaned by the State board of health and one on the care and eruption of teeth by a local dentist. Models added greatly to the value of the exhibit. An electrical device showing the infant mortality of the State was loaned by the State board of health; in a village of 100 miniature homes lights went out, one by one, as babies died, showing the infant mortality for the State. Another electrical model warned against the danger of "doping" the baby. A sleeping basket, bathing equipment, and suitable clothing for the baby of a family of limited means were shown; also a homemade playing pen and simple homemade toys. In a glass case was displayed a home with flies and mosquitoes breeding in the neglected back yard and outhouses. A homemade fireless cooker, iceless refrigerator, and flytrap were loaned by the home demonstration agent of the Department of Agriculture.

The care and preparation of modified milk for the baby was demonstrated by a nurse from a local hospital, and a representative of the home economics department of the State Normal Industrial College demonstrated food values and the preparation of food for the growing child.

In a series of informal talks, the physician of the Children's Bureau discussed with the mothers such subjects as prenatal care, obstetrical care, care of the baby and the young child, care of the sick child, school lunches, medical inspection of the schools, and the value of a visiting nurse.

Through the courtesy of the local moving-picture houses a Children's Bureau film, "A Day in a Baby's Life," was shown; also public-health slides loaned by the State board of health and other organizations.

The attendance at the conference was drawn not only from the county seat but from the surrounding country as well, farmers leaving their fields in the midst of the busy plowing and planting season and driving 12 and 15 miles to bring their children for examination. Doctors came with small patients, parents brought children, and teachers came for help with their problems. A number of mothers and babies were brought into the conference each day from a near-by mill village by the manager of the mill. One father at first thought the conference only an excuse for the mothers to go to town and refused to have his child examined, but when he saw the record given his brother's child he insisted that his own son be brought for examination. The mothers admitted that they carried their babies' records around in their pockets and compared notes at leisure moments.

The attendance often taxed the accommodations to the utmost, and the increasing number of children brought for examintion was perhaps the best evidence of its growing hold upon the public. One hundred and forty children were examined at the white conference and 49 at the conference for negroes. The value of the conference, however, can not be measured wholly by the number of children examined. Not only those who brought children for examination, but also many others—children and adults—were in attendance; and the interest they displayed in all that was said and done can but lead to good results.

CONFERENCES IN RURAL COMMUNITIES.

After the conference at the county seat, each of the 12 townships of the county was visited and an afternoon or evening conference held. In 1 township, because of the crowd, it was necessary to repeat the white conference; and in 2 townships a second one for negroes had to be arranged; in all, 27 rural conferences were held, and, in addition, 4 in small mill villages.

As a rule the district school was the chosen meeting place, though occasionally the church was selected when it was more centrally located or would better accommodate the crowd.

As at the county seat, the conference was cordially received in rural communities, preachers, teachers, doctors, and other leading citizens all assisting in every possible way. Several ministers came repeatedly to ask that their districts be included in the circuit. More than one good negro meeting was due to the efforts of the negro midwife. Like the preachers and the teachers she is an autocrat in her community, and mothers naturally shy about bringing children for examination would obey her arbitrary summons. One was heard to insist that the mother "take that child to the doctor and see what makes her have sore eyes." (At a later private interview this midwife was urged to write to the State board of health for a proper solution of silver nitrate with instructions for its use.)

In a preliminary visit to the townships, prominent persons had been consulted in regard to convenient dates and places for conferences. Window cards had been placed in the windows of country schools, churches, and stores, or tacked to conspicuous trees. Notices had been read in schools, churches, and Sunday schools. In one community publicity had been secured by a flourishing woman's club. For the most part, however, the news traveled by word of mouth— the usual medium of communication in rural districts.

The rural conference differed from that held in the county seat only in size and in the ability of the agents to meet the mothers on a more intimate footing in their own immediate neighborhood than in the more formal town conference. The mothers felt freer to ask questions and compare experiences with their neighbors and friends.

Although it was obviously impossible at the rural conference to use the original exhibit previously described, with its electrical devices, a small traveling exhibit of miniature models was shown, covering the essential points of the care of the young child—his bathing, clothing, sleeping, and feeding. Most of the time was spent in examining the children and demonstrating methods (and results) of applying well-known principles of hygiene, within reach of every woman. At night meetings, using a simple acetylene equipment, slides were shown which, with a short informal talk, never failed to arouse interest.

Considering the sparcity of the population—many families not having a neighbor in sight—the attendance was most unexpected. Twenty-seven conferences were held with an average attendance of 78 at the white and 87 at the negro meetings. Twenty-two hundred and six rural persons were reached, exclusive of those attending the conferences at the county seat, and 162 children were examined.

As at the county seat, the audiences included all classes. There were represented the children of the prosperous planter, of his tenant, and of his day laborer. Many were brought by parents for advice in regard to feeding problems; others came with a physician who wished to confirm a diagnosis. At one meeting two adopted children were brought by their foster mother. On the way from a rural conference a father signalled the agents, as they drove past his house (apologizing, as he said, for "flagging the train") and begged their advice concerning his little lame boy who could not be brought to the conference. At a negro meeting, a colored elder who had come too late for the "scenery" (stereopticon slides) but in time for the talk, expressed his appreciation of the work being done for his race. In their enthusiasm the negro audiences often refused to be dismissed, and were left to discuss the new doctrine after the close of the meeting. Following one of these conferences, a mother and her two children who had missed the meeting the night before were found at the door the next morning waiting to have the children examined before the agents took an early train.

RESULTS OF THE CONFERENCES.

The results of the conference were seen on every side. Mothers were made more observant and more critical of their children and a general stock taking by the mothers of this section followed. A father who had brought a poorly developed child to the conference was heard to say several weeks later, "My wife couldn't go, but I went and took it all in, and we're raising our baby like the doctor said." Parents who had brought a child to one conference would often appear at a neighboring conference with a second or third child of their own or one of a neighbor's. Following the conference, many children received the attention of dentists and throat specialists; and others, whose needs had previously not been recognized, were brought into touch with their family physicians.

Many practical evidences of the work were seen in driving through the country. Babies heretofore kept indoors were found sleeping on the porch or out under the trees in homemade cribs. Mothers showed with pride their own or their husbands' modifications or adaptations of models seen in the exhibit. Playing pens, homemade toys, fireless cookers, iceless refrigerators, and flytraps were made by many. An ambitious teacher who was developing a domestic science department for mothers and young girls had reproduced in her school models seen in the exhibit.

The agents also indorsed the project of installing an incinerator at the county seat for the disposal of garbage and waste. The incinerator has now been in operation for over a year and is helping to convert an attractive town into one that is also healthful and sanitary.

During the conference of the Children's Bureau at the county seat the agents had an opportunity to join in an effort to crystallize public opinion upon the value of a visiting nurse. So convincing were the results of the first few weeks of this nurse's service, that after the negro conference the negro population secured pledges of almost the entire salary of a negro nurse, the white people supplementing the amount.

The response to the conferences in rural sections showed how eagerly the services of a public-health nurse for rural districts of the county would be welcomed. Such conferences as were held by the Children's Bureau, chiefly as demonstrations, might be held at intervals by a public-health nurse, as a part of her routine. Informal talks with the mothers at the conferences also revealed certain particular needs of the community which a public-health nurse would be able to meet, such as prenatal care and assistance at confinements, advice as to the care and feeding of the young child, examination of school children for physical defects with follow-up visits in the homes to make sure that the necessary treatment is secured, and the education of the community in the importance of hygiene and sanitation.

The children's health conferences proved a successful means of introducing the inquiry of the Children's Bureau in the State and secured the interest of various organizations to whose helpful cooperation the bureau is indebted for much of the material contained in this report.

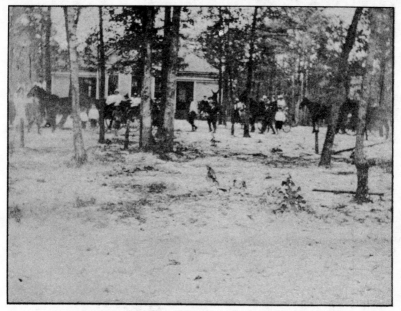

PLATE I.—AT THE CHILDREN'S HEALTH CONFERENCE.

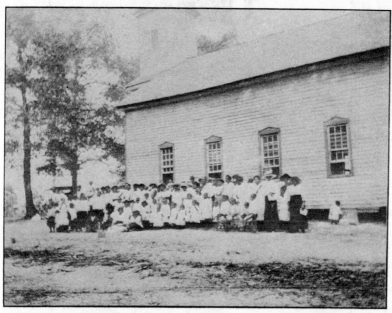

PLATE II.—A CHILDREN'S HEALTH CONFERENCE AT A NEGRO CHURCH.

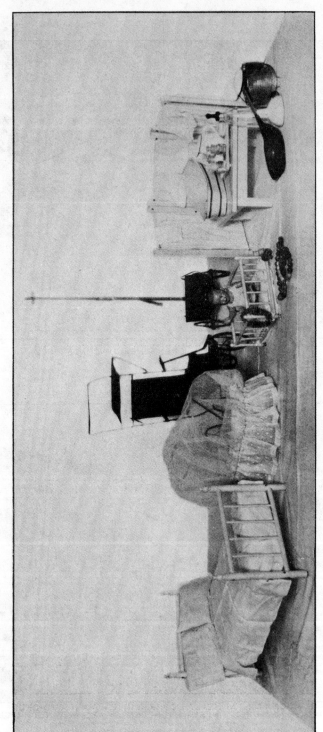

PLATE III.—THE INFANT-CARE EXHIBIT IS ALWAYS POPULAR.

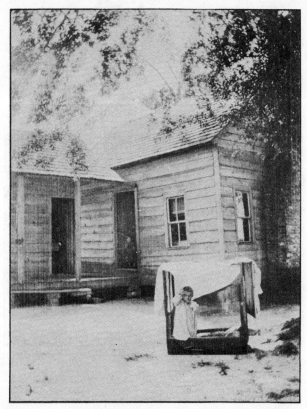

PLATE IV.—A HOMEMADE PLAYING PEN—COST, 40 CENTS.

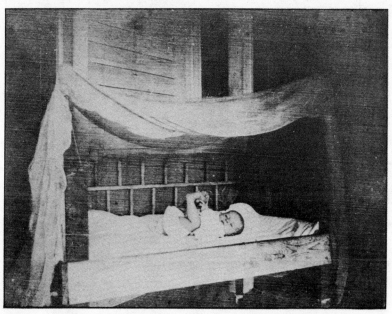

PLATE V.—OUT-OF-DOOR BABY IN A HOMEMADE CRIB.

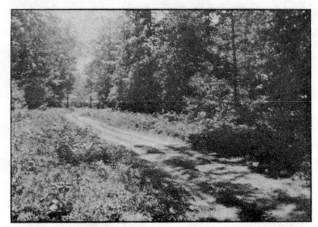

PLATE VI.—GOOD SAND-CLAY ROAD THROUGH THE PINE WOODS.

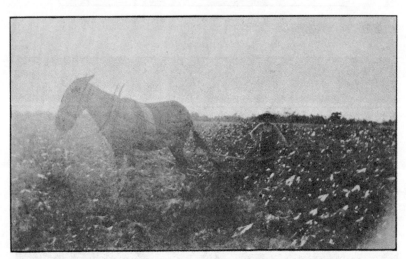

PLATE VII.—COTTON IS THE "MONEY CROP" IN THE LOWLANDS.

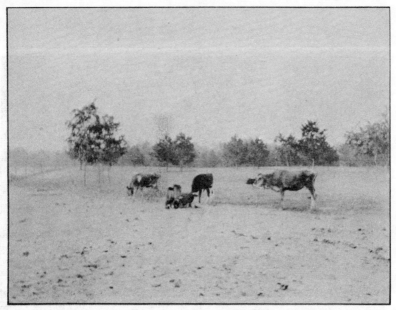

PLATE VIII.—SANDY PLAINS OF THE LOWLAND COUNTY.

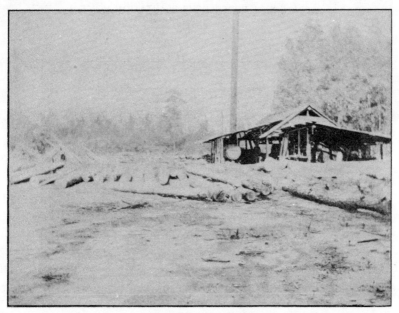

PLATE IX.—TIMBER LANDS ARE FAST DISAPPEARING.

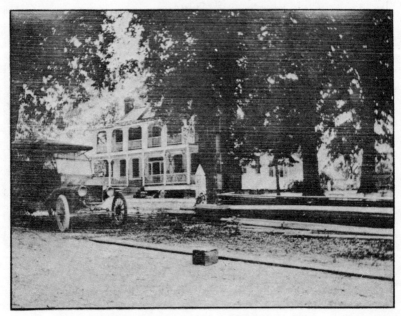

PLATE X.—A PROSPEROUS PLANTATION HOME.

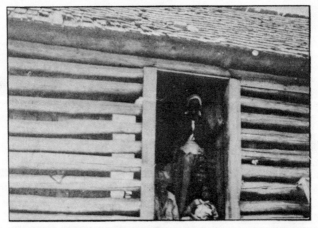

PLATE XI.—A NEGRO TENANT'S CABIN WITH DAYLIGHT SHOWING BETWEEN THE LOGS.

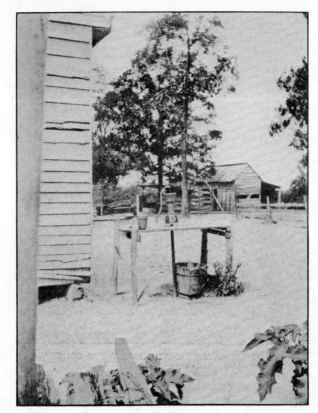

PLATE XII.—DRILLED WELL CONVENIENTLY NEAR THE HOUSE.

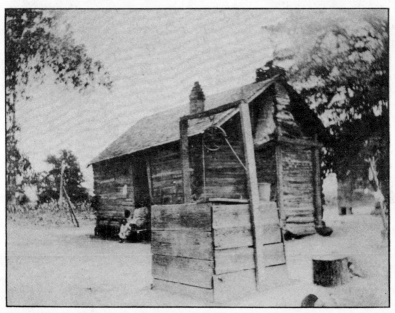

PLATE XIII.—THE DANGEROUS OPEN DUG WELL.

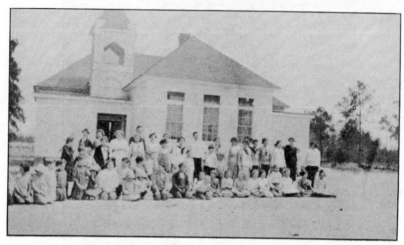

PLATE XIV.—A THREE-TEACHER WHITE SCHOOL.

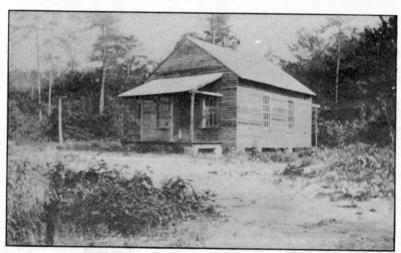

PLATE XV.—NEW ONE-TEACHER NEGRO SCHOOL.

PART II.

THE LOWLAND COUNTY SURVEY.

During the course of the rural conference local citizens were consulted in regard to the characteristics of the various townships of the county, and a township thought to be a typical rural section of the cotton belt was chosen for intensive study.

CHARACTERISTICS OF THE TOWNSHIP.

The township lies 6 to 14 miles from the county seat, which is the nearest town, and consists of open country along the bank of a broad swift stream. The land is low, level, and, except along the river bottom, is sandy and porous. The soil, debilitated by years of exclusive cotton growing, demands heavy and expensive fertilization in order to produce a good yield.

The climate is warm and humid, with the long summers especially adapted to cotton raising. The Weather Bureau records for the county seat, over a period of 28 years, show a mean temperature of 44° in January and 79° in July, with a minimum of −5° and a maximum of 103° for the year.

Farming is the chief industry and is pursued under a system of tenancy. Good water power is utilized only for small grist and saw mills. Great piles of sawdust mark the site of mills which have cut out most of the timber, and the forests have given way largely to farms.

The township has two main roads of sand-clay construction, maintained in good condition, which lead to the county seat. The other roads, however, are for the most part neglected; so also are the bridges, except one of steel construction. There are no railroads within the township. Rural free delivery of mail is available for all the families, and a few homes have telephone connections.

The history of the township dates back to the colonial period when the Cape Fear section was settled by Scotch Highlanders.[1] The Scotch strain and a preponderance of Scotch names have persisted in this section down to the present time. There has been practically no immigration of other nationalities and the population is uniformly native-born American, about evenly divided between the whites and

---

[1] McLean, J. P.: Scotch Highlanders in America, p. 102. Helman-Taylor Co., Cleveland; John Mackay, Glasgow, 1900.

negroes. The county has a rural population density of 27.9 persons to the square mile,[1] which also probably approximates the population density of the township. It is a considerably more thickly settled area than the average rural section in the United States, which has a density of 16.6 persons to the square mile,[2] but is more sparsely settled than the rural sections of the South Atlantic States for which the average rural density is 33.8.[2]

FINDINGS OF THE SURVEY.

ECONOMIC STATUS OF FAMILIES.

Land tenure.

The families in the neighborhoods visited fall roughly into three distinct social economic groups—landowners, white tenants, and negro tenants. Approximately three-fifths of the white families are owners of the land on which they live; of the negro farmers, only one in four is a landowner. Various systems of tenancy are found, the "half-share" basis being the most common. This is an arrangement by which the tenant and the landlord each gets half the crop; if the landlord supplies the stock, he and the tenant each furnish half the fertilizer; where the tenant supplies stock, the landlord furnishes all the fertilizer.

By far the majority of tenants are "croppers," rather than cash or standing rent tenants; an occasional family, however, pays rent outright—usually in cotton at the rate of one 450-pound bale of lint cotton for 12 acres of land under cultivation.

Crops and acreage.

The average farmer confines his operations to the raising of cotton and corn and a garden patch. Some also have a small acreage in tobacco, peas, small grain, peanuts, or sorghum cane. Cotton is the money crop and this section of the country, like other parts of the South, is suffering from an overcultivation of cotton at the expense of food and feed crops.

The country visited has a soil well adapted to cotton raising, except for a small area of sand hills. Cotton production per acre averaged seven-tenths of a bale on the white farms visited and three-fifths on negro farms.

Little produce is sold except cotton and cotton seed, and, rarely, tobacco, corn, stock, butter, chickens, and eggs. One of the most successful farmers of the township, however, makes it a rule to support his family on crops other than cotton, saving the profit on cotton always for enlarging his farm business. He finds it better to plant more corn, beans, etc., rather than cotton alone, which varies more in price than any other crop.

---

[1] Thirteenth Census of the United States, 1910, Vol. III, Population, p. 298.
[2] Thirteenth Census of the United States, 1910, Vol. I, Population, p. 55.

About half the white and over four-fifths of the negro farms of the township are "one-horse" farms, with approximately 25 acres in cultivation—often 15 in cotton and 10 in corn. With cotton production averaging well under a bale an acre, the limited one-horse crop is a poor dependence at best, even when operated by the farm owner who gets the whole of the crop made; when operated by a tenant on half shares, the family money income may dwindle to four or five bales of cotton, with a total cash value (at the time of the inquiry) of from $200 to $300.

Cost of cotton production.

Cotton is an expensive crop to produce; due to lack of a crop-rotation system, a good yield is impossible without heavily fertilizing the land. One ton to every 3 acres is the rule, which with fertilizer at $28 and $30 a ton at the time of the inquiry represents a considerable investment. Moreover, it is a handmade and not a machine-made crop, and labor is an appreciable item; help hired for "chopping" and picking cotton amounted to something like $6 or $7 a bale at the time of the inquiry. Ginning added another $2 a bale if ginned in town, $2.50 if at one of the neighborhood gins.

Credit systems.

The average farmer begins the season heavily in debt for his fertilizer which he buys "on time," payable in the fall of the year after the crop is made. Where a tenant is making a crop, the landlord gives his note for the fertilizer and the tenant settles with him at the end of the year; also, the average tenant family has to be "carried" by merchant or landlord for groceries and provisions used during the spring and summer. By the time the crop is gathered at the end of the season, its money value has been largely anticipated, and the clear profit remaining after the debts incurred during the farm season have been paid off leaves but a slim financial support for the family during the coming 12 months. "We feel rich after the crop is sold," one farm tenant expressed it; "rich till we get to the people we owe."

That the various systems of credit in the purchase of groceries and small goods are working to the detriment of the community is the opinion of many in the neighborhood. Some families, of course, pride themselves on always paying cash; others pay cash through the autumn and winter as long as the family income holds out and then buy "on time," payable with 6 per cent interest in the autumn after the crop is made. Chickens and eggs, and occasionally other produce, are traded at the country stores. The landlord usually keeps a commissary where such supplies as meat, corn meal, rice, sugar, sirup, coffee, snuff, and tobacco may be had and charged to the tenant at the same rate of interest he would pay at the country store. These accounts are long-time credits, payable in the fall of the year. Aside from the interest on the account, the time price is almost invariably higher than the cash price. A farmer who had bought "on time" last year is trying to pay cash this year, for from one-fourth to one-third is added to the price when he buys on time. For instance, he had bought a sack of "shipped stuff" on time for $2.50; on the same day at the same store his father bought a sack for $1.60 cash. Another farmer finds it cheaper to borrow money to carry him through the summer, about $50 at 10 per cent, than to buy "on time," paying 25 cents more on the dollar besides the 6 per cent interest when the bill is paid in the autumn. Sometimes a crop lien, or written contract with the crop as security, is required before the merchant will "run" a customer; often, however, the agreement is by word of mouth if the merchant feels reasonably sure of getting his pay. The negro farmer, more commonly than the white, buys on credit and suffers particularly from the high credit prices; a crop lien, too, is more likely to be required of him. One man explained that since the legal rate of interest is 6 per cent, only 6 per cent appears on the note, but, in addition, one pays about 10 cents on the dollar more for supplies bought on time. A negro woman who "owes out" about $20, pays 10 per cent—6 per cent interest and 4 or 5 per cent "what they call premery" (premium).

Another who had made 7 bales of cotton on half shares had no idea how much it brought, for the landlord took it all, including the seed, to square her debts. One negro family got supplies from the landlord's country store; they turned over all their cotton and seed to him; he settled with them in February and gave them $50 as their share of the crop (they had made 9½ bales of cotton on half shares and the landlord had supplied them with flour, sugar, "strip meat," and rice). "When fall comes, there's not much in it for you," said one tenant. The tenant family rarely keeps an account of its expenditures, depending upon the records in the landlord's books.

The installment plan, though in many ways filling a real need, also adds to the financial burden of many families because of the higher prices charged for installment purchases. Sewing machines are often bought in this way, also stoves, crayon portraits, books, and even medicines from the patent medicine man on his monthly rounds. A $25 sewing machine, at $2.50 down and $2 per month, costs the family $40 to $50. A mule is almost invariably bought on the installment plan; few families can afford the expense of paying outright the $250 to $300 cash price. Cooperative buying in this township, except in a few isolated cases, is practically unknown.

Crop disposal.

Cotton is usually marketed at the county seat, 6 to 14 miles away; tobacco is shipped to several points where it brings a better price than on the local market. Often the landlord buys his tenant's crop, almost invariably in the case of negro tenants. He can afford to hold his cotton for higher prices while the tenant must sell immediately to pay his debts.

Farm labor.

Among the tenant farmers, after a man has finished working his own crop, he, and sometimes his wife and children also, hire out for a few days at farm labor, to supplement their scant income. Farm labor, at the time of the inquiry, was poorly paid, 75 cents a day for a grown man, 50 cents for a grown woman, and 25 to 50 cents for children. Cotton picking is piecework, paid at the rate of 50 cents per 100 pounds picked, with 200 pounds per day as a good average.

HOME CONDITIONS.

Housing.

WHITE FAMILIES.—The children's home environment varies widely according to the social and economic status of the family. The typical home of the prosperous planter is a big, comfortable farmhouse, with a generous brick fireplace at each end—a traditional southern home, with its large cool rooms, deep verandas, fine trees, sturdy old scuppernong vines, and, in the distance, well-kept cotton fields.

The tenant's children are not so well provided for. The average tenant family occupies an unpainted, clapboarded cottage of four small rooms, ceiled inside but not plastered, often with no shade around the house—a hot, sandy little plat of ground. One family of tenants visited lived in a little rough shack in the midst of the woods, with insufficient cleared space around the house to admit any breeze. Flies, mosquitoes, and gnats were numerous though the family kept a bucket of pitch burning on the porch. Another tenant cottage—a rude shack of upright boards—is the home of father, mother, and five small children; the mother called it "shantying" and was anxious to move in the autumn. "The crop is too inconvenient, the water is bad (a dug well, open and unprotected, and only 12 feet from the house), the crib's too near, and there's a pond back there," summed up her objections to the place.

The farm tenant frequently moves from farm to farm in the hope of bettering his poverty-stricken condition, but usually not straying far from the neighborhood where he was born. The unstable nature of his tenancy and the lack of any permanent interest in his surroundings discourage any attempt on his part to improve his cottage or its grounds.

The sawmill hand is even more of a will-o'-the-wisp, moving constantly as the sawmill exhausts the surrounding timber. A mother whose husband "followed the sawmills" complained that "it was move every time the wind blows; if I was to say 36 times since I was married, I wouldn't miss it."

NEGRO FAMILIES.—Negro housing accommodations are almost uniformly poor. The commonest type of negro home is the old-fashioned log cabin of one, two, or three rooms, daylight showing between the logs. Such a house is hot and stuffy in summer with the sun beating in, while in winter it is almost impossible to heat it, even with the cracks chinked with mud and a roaring fire in the open fireplace. A cabin like this leaks in stormy weather and leaves the floor damp for a day or two afterwards. There is usually some attempt at decoration, gay-colored chromos, crayon portraits, and ornaments of various sorts within and flowers without on every side—four-o'clocks, sunflowers, weeping Mary, and tiger lilies. Rooms are incredibly small and stuffy, with low ceilings; often a cabin originally one-roomed has been cut up by thin partitions into two, three, or even four tiny rooms. Some cabins are windowless, many have windows without glass panes, heavy solid wood shutters taking their place. A number of negro homes were badly crowded for space; one-fourth of the families visited had five or more persons to a sleeping room. At one home, a small room, half the original room, with no window and absolutely dark, contained two beds where five persons slept. In another cabin an entire family of 12 slept in one large room with a curtain stretched from side to side.

Sanitation.

PRIVIES.—Sanitary conveniences are deplorably lacking at many white as well as negro homes. More than half the white families visited had no toilet of any description on their premises. One family of tenants explained that there had been a privy on the place when they came, but it was so filthy that it had to be torn down; another tenant, who upon moving into the present house had obtained a promise from the landlord to build a privy, had already lived there a year without one. More than one family frankly prefers to have no privy, disliking the idea of accumulated filth and not appreciating the dangers of soil pollution. Many families, however, recognize the importance of the privy in safeguarding the family health. Where a privy is present it is commonly of the open-in-back surface type, usually dependent upon the scavenging services of chickens and hogs, which have easy access through the open back; occasionally the privy is built on the side of a hill with the contents draining into the "branch." Some families, however, have the privy cleaned and the contents buried with reasonable frequency, and some attempt disinfection by the use of lime, dirt, sulphur, or wood ashes.

Four-fifths of the negro families visited were without a privy; often where there was one it was not in use, so little was its importance understood as a sanitary precaution against disease. "Yes'm," said a negro woman, "there's one there, but nobody uses it but company." One family "never fools with one; if you use it you have the bother of keeping it clean." A negro woman with higher standards, however, induced her husband to build one for her, though she was the only member of the family who desired it or ever used it.

WATER SUPPLY.—Although only one of the homes visited had a pump and sink inside the kitchen, white families were as a rule provided with a drilled well and iron pump within a few feet of the kitchen door. This type of well is usually satisfactory, the iron pipe protecting the water from contamination; occasionally a drilled well gives bad water because it has not been drilled to a sufficient depth.

Twenty-two of the 129 negro families and an occasional white family were dependent upon the dug well—not only open and unprotected from dust and dirt but also exposed to contamination from drainage, a particular risk in a neighborhood so lacking in sanitary conveniences. One tenant family carried water from the drilled schoolhouse well; they have an open well in the yard, but the water is not good. One negro woman had entire confidence in her own method of purification. "I put me a fish in the well and he cleanses the water," she said.

The State board of health, in its pamphlet on "Plans for Public Schoolhouses," comments upon the dangers of the open-topped well:

Open-topped wells are always dangerous and should never be used. During the course of a single year a tremendous amount of dirt, leaves, bugs, and other insanitary material gets in open-topped wells. Sometimes toads, lizards, snakes, and small domestic animals find their way into such wells. A good iron pump is infinitely safer than chains or ropes and buckets. In the case of open-topped wells the buckets, chains, and water in the well are very frequently polluted by dirty hands.[1]

Only an occasional family uses spring water, for springs are uncommon in this section of the country. A negro family carried water from a spring one-eighth of a mile away; it is not only far from the house but evidently unfit for use, being full of decaying matter and in no way protected from surface contamination. Another spring gets so low that it had to be walled in with boards to make the water rise high enough to be dipped with a pail. Rarely one finds the old-fashioned well sweep, picturesque but insanitary, with its "old oaken bucket."

FLIES AND MOSQUITOES.—Flies and mosquitoes in this neighborhood constitute a real pest during the summer months. Flies are numerous because of lack of toilets, open-in-back, exposed privies,

---

[1] Plans for Public Schoolhouses, p. 33, issued from the office of the State superintendent o f public instruction, Raleigh, N. C.

accumulations of manure, insanitary disposal of garbage and other refuse, and also because, in many cases, the stable and hogpen are located too near the house. Scattered ponds and some swamp lands are responsible for the prevalence of mosquitoes, which during the summer months make life almost unendurable after dark. Late in the afternoon a road through the woods can scarcely be traveled without a great branch as a weapon to beat off the mosquitoes.

The average family, white or negro, is without screens of any description. Only 19 of the white homes out of 127 visited, and no negro homes were adequately screened, i. e., with screens at both doors and windows. Several had screened the doors or the doors and kitchen windows. Fly paper and fly traps are used to some extent. Many families "smoke out" mosquitoes, using a bucket of smoking coals, pitch, or rags on the porch or doorstep.

DISPOSAL OF WASTE.—Garbage is fed to the hogs and chickens; other refuse is disposed of variously—burned by the more careful families, by others hauled off to the woods, thrown in the ditch, hauled to the swamp, swept out to the edge of the yard, thrown down an old well, hauled off to fill in low places, thrown in the thicket, burned around the iron pots used for boiling clothes, or thrown into a mill pond.

Manure is allowed to accumulate in the stables and constitutes a prolific breeding place for flies. "Most any day you can see the flies just a-weaving in that manure," said one mother; at this home every rain washes down into the manure pile, keeping it wet much of the time. It is usually removed only twice a year—spring and autumn— to be used as fertilizer for corn and potatoes. Aside from some half dozen farmers, who see to it that the manure pile is kept covered with straw, there is no effort at guarding against flies from this source. The State board of health in a leaflet on "Flies," for distribution in rural communities, advises having the manure hauled out and away from the stable regularly twice a week from April 15 to November 15, and once a week from November 15 to December 15, and from March 15 to April 15.

MATERNITY CARE.

The care of the mother during her pregnancy and confinement should be a matter of vital concern to any community. A recent bulletin of the Children's Bureau shows that in 1913 childbirth caused more deaths among women 15 to 44 years old than any disease except tuberculosis.[1] This bulletin further points out the close relation between the deaths of infants occurring in the first days and weeks of

---

[1] Meigs, Dr. Grace L. Maternal Mortality from all Conditions Connected with Childbirth in the United States and Certain Other Countries, pp. 7 and 9. U. S. Children's Bureau Publication No. 19, Miscellaneous Series No. 6, Washington, 1917.

life and the proper care of the mother before and at the birth of her baby; also the fact that each death at childbirth is a serious loss to the country, since the women who die from this cause are lost at the time of their greatest usefulness to the State and to their families. Moreover, the loss to the community occasioned by a failure to safeguard women at this time can be by no means adequately measured by the deaths occurring at childbirth. Many women endure a lifetime of ill health which they date from a particular confinement when for various reasons proper obstetrical and nursing care were lacking.

During the inquiry 79 white and 86 negro mothers—who had given birth to a child, live or stillborn, within five years previous to the agent's visit—were interviewed with especial reference to maternity care at their last confinement.

The early marriage age of the average rural woman of this section gives her a long childbearing period. Two-thirds of the white mothers visited had married at 22 years of age or younger, nearly half at 20 or younger; of the negro women, about three-fifths had married at 20 or younger—more than one-third at 18 or younger. Small families are uncommon in this section of the country, and it is the exceptional mother who has not borne a number of children. Approximately three-fourths (74 per cent) of the white mothers, married 10 years or more, and almost nine-tenths (89 per cent) of the negro mothers, had had six or more pregnancies.

The rural woman of this section has not yet realized that she is entitled to skilled attention in her confinement, and faces the perils of childbirth with undue serenity. Until the mother herself demands as her due (with her husband's recognition of the necessity for the expense) skilled medical and nursing care during pregnancy and confinement, there can be little hope of improved standards of maternity care for rural communities.

Lack of medical care was frequently mentioned as a serious drawback to country life. One young father wished "the Government would do something about it"; he thinks there should be at least one doctor in every township. That the Government should send medical experts through the country especially for women and children was the opinion of another who wanted to know why his wife has never been well since their second baby was born.

Although 27 physicians are resident in the county,[1] this is an inadequate medical service for a population of 33,719,[2] since it means an average of 1,249 persons to each physician, which is nearly twice the average—691 [3]—for the United States. Moreover, since 19 of the 27 physicians are concentrated at the county seat,

[1] American Medical Directory, 1916.
[2] Estimate of U. S. Bureau of the Census for 1916.
[3] Bulletin of the American Medical Association, Jan. 15, 1917, p. 114.

and the other 8 are scattered in small villages and through the rural sections, there is a decided lack of available medical service in various parts of the county. In the township covered by the survey no physician is resident, and the families are from 3 to 14 miles distant from the nearest doctor; not an excessive distance perhaps, but because of scant telephone connection and bad roads during part of the year the doctor is often inaccessible when sorel needed.

Facilities for medical, hospital, and nursing care.

The distance of the family from the physician is in many cases so great that medical assistance is called in only if the patient's condition is critical. Only 5 of the 127 white families visited and 15 of the 129 negro families were within 5 miles of a doctor; more than one-fourth were 10 miles or more from their nearest physician. Distance is not the only obstacle in obtaining a physician. A swift river, which must be crossed in a small bateau and which at times is impassable, forms a natural barrier, entirely cutting off the people of one community for part of the year from their nearest physician.

A strong county medical society has been in existence for some years and has been active in its support of public-health measures. Hospital facilities in the county are exceptional; there are two good general hospitals located at the county seat, one with 70 and the other with 25 beds. Each hospital maintains a training school for nurses.

A woman's club at the county seat is maintaining a public-health nurse, whose work at the county seat and in the surrounding mill villages has been so productive of results that a negro nurse for the negro population has recently been employed by that race. As yet, however, both nurses have confined themselves largely to the area adjacent to the county seat and little public-health nursing in rural neighborhoods has been attempted. The township of the survey is entirely beyond the territory covered by either nurse.

Maternal deaths.

The county had in 1916 an alarmingly high maternal mortality from causes connected with childbirth; 14 deaths (4 white and 10 negro) occurred during that year,[1] a rate of 41.5 per 100,000 population.[2] It is impossible to determine whether this rate is sporadic or usual, since mortality statistics for the State and its counties are not available earlier than 1916, when the State was admitted to the Census's area of death registration.

Moreover, in considering a small area and a small number of deaths, the rate is often misleading. However, with due allowance for error, mortality from causes connected with childbirth is exces-

---

[1] Information supplied by the bureau of vital statistics, North Carolina State Board of Health.
[2] Based on an estimate of the U. S. Bureau of the Census in 1916 of 33,719 for the county.

sively high. The rate in this county (41.5) is markedly higher than in the mountain county (21.9),[1] or in the State as a whole (24.7),[2] and is nearly three times as high as the 1915 rate (15.2) for the entire death registration area of the United States.[3]

Analysis of the county maternal mortality shows that though the rate for white women (17.3) is slightly higher than the average for the registration area of the United States (15.2),[3] the high total rate for the county is due to the abnormally high rate (93.9) among negro women. This higher rate of maternal mortality among negro women is in accord with the rates for the total area of death registration for which, in 1915, the death rate from causes pertaining to childbirth was 14.6 for white women as contrasted with 25.9 for negro women.[3] Puerperal septicæmia (childbed fever), a disease recognized years ago as largely preventable, caused the death of two of the negro women.

It is only recently in this country that public attention has been directed to the high mortality from childbirth and to a consideration of its underlying causes. A bulletin of the Children's Bureau on Maternal Mortality finds that the fundamental factors responsible for the lives of women lost in childbirth in this country are "first, general ignorance of the dangers connected with childbirth and the need of skilled care and proper hygiene in order to prevent them; second, * * * difficulties related to the provision of proper obstetrical care"[4]—a conclusion which is apparently true of this community as well as of the country as a whole.

Prenatal care.

The necessity for supervision and care of the mother before the birth of her child is becoming recognized in cities and towns; in this community, however, prenatal care is negligible.

A fair standard for adequate medical prenatal care would probably embrace the following points:[5]

1. A general physical examination, including an examination of the heart, lungs, and abdomen.

2. Measurement of the pelvis *in a first pregnancy* to determine whether there is any deformity which is likely to interfere with birth.

---

[1] See p. 68.

[2] Information supplied by bureau of vital statistics, North Carolina State Board of Health.

[3] Mortality Statistics, 1915, p. 59. U. S. Bureau of the Census, Washington, 1917. Sum of the rates there given for "puerperal fever" and "other puerperal affections."

[4] Meigs, Dr. Grace L.: Maternal Mortality from all Conditions Connected with Childbirth in the United States and Certain Other Countries, p. 24. U. S. Children's Bureau Publication No. 19, Miscellaneou Series No. 6. Washington, 1917.

[5] Outlined after consultation with Dr. J. Whitridge Williams, professor of obstetrics, Johns Hopkins University. See Maternal Mortality from all Conditions Connected with Childbirth in the United States and Certain Other Countries, pp. 12, 13. U. S. Children's Bureau Publication No. 19, Miscellaneous Series No. 6. Washington, 1917.

3. Continued supervision by the physician, at least through the last five months of pregnancy.

4. Monthly examination of the urine, at least during the last five months.

According to this standard, none of the mothers visited can be said to have had adequate prenatal care. Pelvic examinations were unknown, urinalyses rare, and in the majority of cases the physician knew nothing of the case until called to deliver the woman. Of the 79 white mothers for whom this information was obtained, 21, or less than one-third, saw a physician before confinement, and only 12 had urinalysis. Of the 86 negro mothers, 2 saw a physician before confinement and 1 reported urinalysis. When a negro midwife is to have the case, she occasionally stops in to see how the mother is progressing. Eight white mothers and 27 negro mothers had seen a midwife in this way, which can not, however, be considered prenatal care.[1]

Scant provision is made for the approach of childbirth. Commonly a physician or a midwife is notified through the husband, mother, or other messenger of the expected date of confinement. Many, however, fail even to make this provision, and, finding the doctor out on a call, much valuable time is lost hunting a substitute. The more prosperous families engage both a physician and a midwife—the midwife to serve as nurse and to come several days before confinement is expected, to be present in case of emergency.

Attendant at birth.

Two-thirds of the 79 white mothers were attended in confinement by a physician; that is, these mothers had engaged a physician, though in 10 cases he was late and arrived after the baby was born. The negro mothers were almost invariably dependent upon the midwife; only 5 of the 86 negro mothers had a physician, and in 1 of these cases the doctor was late. One had neither doctor nor midwife in attendance. Among the more ignorant of the negroes there was even some prejudice against doctors. "No'm," said one, "I had me a good woman every time."

Besides the difficulty in obtaining a physician because of distance, bad roads, and scarcity of telephones, cost is an important factor in determining the attendant engaged for confinement, many families considering the expense of a physician prohibitive. A midwife charges from $2 to $3, and, in addition to obstetrical services, renders other assistance, such as washing the clothing and bedding used, and cooking, cleaning, and helping in the care of the home and children.

Many experiences were reported by the mothers illustrative of the hazards of childbirth in a community where medical care is not always available.

---

[1] See p. 29.

A mother of three children, living on a comfortable farm of 150 acres, is 10 miles from the doctor. He has been engaged for every confinement but has always arrived too late. The first child was born unexpectedly and fell, striking its head on a chair; it had spasms before morning and died in three days.

Another mother became ill in the evening. A messenger crossed the river in the bateau for the doctor and found he had gone on another case. The doctor did not reach his patient until the next morning and delivery was delayed until he came, the mother suffering greatly. The baby was stillborn—a shoulder presentation.

In another instance, a child who, according to the mother's story, was alive when labor began was lost because the midwife was unable to manage the case and the doctor, who was out when called, could not be reached in time. When he arrived an hour after the delivery he found a stillborn child.

A mother, frightened at losing the previous baby when only 3 days old, sent for a doctor to attend her eighth confinement. He failed to arrive in time and the baby, prematurely born, died in three hours.

A mother of eight children, attended by a midwife at the first three confinements, decided to have a doctor thereafter. A doctor was engaged for each of the next three confinements but failed to reach her in time. When the last two children were born she had only neighbors present, though able and willing to pay for professional service.

A negro woman told of the long hard labor she had had, with the midwife unable to relieve the situation; the "white folks" for whom she and her husband worked sent for a doctor, but before he could get there from the county seat, a distance of 7 miles, the baby was born dead.

MIDWIVES.—Although according to tradition there were two white midwives in this section a number of years ago, to-day this service is drawn entirely from the negro race. Eight midwives were interviewed—7 women and 1 man—ranging in age from approximately 45 to 70 years. The practice of midwifery is often handed down from mother to daughter, as the profession of medicine is from father to son. Caste lines are sharply drawn among the midwives, two of the number doing the "quality" work.

Training for midwifery had in every case been limited to nursing for or assisting local physicians. Those interviewed had practiced from 6 to 26 years, all but two for over 15 years; only three of the eight interviewed were registered with the State board of health.[1] All are illiterate; one only can read and none can both read and write. In spite of illiteracy, however, some are women of good judgment and long experience, and with a certain amount of training gained through occasional nursing for physicians.

---

[1] See p. 104 for summary of law requiring registration of midwives.

Few of the midwives gave any prenatal care beyond dropping in for an occasional friendly call. None attempted a physical examination or urinalysis. Four reported that they advised the mother in case of any complications to apply to the doctor, though on general principles home remedies are recommended—salts, oil, "black draught," cream of tartar, and burdock for sluggish bowels; and peach-tree leaves, boneset, life everlasting, or mullein for sluggish kidneys. One midwife advises tea of "cidyus elder" to reduce the swelling of hands and feet. Some claim that single tansy is especially efficacious for threatened miscarriage.

Although the more prosperous families employ the midwife as a nurse, often having her in the house several days before confinement, in the majority of her cases she is the only attendant and is not called until the woman is in labor. Her preparation usually consists of washing her hands and putting on a clean apron. Two midwives claimed that they used bichloride tablets, though neither had any in the house at the time of the interview; one reported the use of creosol and carbolic acid, and one a kind of "lady powders," the name of which she could not remember. Three reported that they clipped and cleaned their nails. Four own bags or satchels also used for various purposes by other members of the household. None carry their own scissors and only one attempts sterilization of those found at the patient's home. Among the items reported in their equipment were ball thread, tansy, ergot, and half a dozen triturated tablets given one midwife by a doctor. For the most part they depend upon herbs and supplies found at the home of the patient.

The preparation of the mother for her confinement depends largely upon the circumstances of the family; one midwife insists upon a clean bed before and after confinement, though this was usually considered an unnecessary waste of linen. The proverbial old quilt is used by all but one, and one saves washing for her patient by using old rags with which she says she "can keep the bed clean for nine days."

The care of the mother consisted for the most part in copious drafts of tea from time to time, made of pepper, catnip, sweet fennel, mint, wormwood, or tansy. One midwife insists that she gives no medicines, that "if the woman needs medicine she needs a doctor." All admit two or more examinations during labor. One sees to it that all windows are kept closed, and another thinks it "against a woman to have too much air."

Prophylaxis of the new-born baby's eyes consists of washing with boracic acid by two, catnip tea by three, catnip tea and camphor by one, and plain water by two. No midwife had as part of her equipment the nitrate of silver furnished now on request by the State board of health. For sore eyes one washes them with breast milk, while another advises against its use, for in her opinion it poisons babies' eyes; two bind bruised house leak on sore eyes at night.

The cord is tied with twine or with various forms of cotton—ball, hank, or skein thread; one uses ravelings from a flour sack, and one silk.

The later care of a baby is usually left to the family, though five midwives indorse catnip tea, two soothing sirup, two whisky, four paregoric, and all give oil in some form. One especially recommends giving the baby a piece of fat meat to suck to clear the bowels. For sore mouth, sage tea, or honey and borax followed by a dose of oil, are advised.

Postnatal care.

The country doctor, serving a large area, finds it impossible to give his patients the same after care that is possible with the city physician. Moreover, the mothers commonly have not recognized the need for after care. In about half the cases attended by physicians, however, a visit had been made after the confinement, usually once only, though in eight cases the physician had made two or more postnatal visits. In 29 of the 56 cases (51 white and 5 negro) attended by a physician, obstetrical service was considered complete when the woman was delivered.

The midwife, if within walking distance, expects to see her patient two or three times, or until the baby's navel is healed. If, however, she lives at a distance, as often is the case, the care of the mother and child is left entirely in the hands of her family or neighbors. Of the 108 mothers attended by midwives (28 white and 80 negro), in 77 cases (almost three-fourths), the midwife either remained in the home a few days or returned at least once after confinement.

Nursing care in confinement.

Nursing care during confinement is almost invariably untrained. None of the mothers visited had had the services of a trained nurse; only two employed a "practical" nurse. In a number of families— 18 white and 15 negro—a midwife had been engaged to remain in the home after confinement to render nursing services. In a majority of cases, however, the mother was dependent upon untrained nursing, either by a member of the family, a relative who had come for that purpose, or by the neighbors, who are always ready to lend a helping hand. The neighbors were "mighty good," said one mother, "they never missed a day but five or six of them came in, and they were always ready to help cook a meal or do anything." One negro woman had as her only dependence her grandfather and her son of 14; another had only her husband at night, no one in the day time.

Rest before and after confinement.[1]

To some extent the amount of rest a mother can have before and after confinement is determined by the time of the year or by the stage of the cotton crop upon which depends the livelihood of the family If confinement occurs during the plowing and planting time, or while all hands are chopping or picking cotton, it is impossible for a woman to have the amount of rest she would be able to secure at a more opportune season.

Housework is commonly continued up to the date of confinement. Although, generally speaking, ordinary household duties may be pursued with advantage by many pregnant women, the lack of conveniences in rural districts makes the care of the household a real burden. The mother's share of "chores" (such as milking, churning, and taking care of the chickens and garden) and of field work is usually lightened, at least, and often is taken over entirely by other members of the family. A number of mothers—18 white and 49 negro women—in addition to their household duties continued with the usual chores and field work until they were confined, making no change in their toilsome daily program because of the approaching childbirth.

One mother had done a washing the day before her second baby was born; she is a regular field hand and chopped cotton all day, 5 days a week, up to the day before confinement. Another, a mother of five children, continued her housework, field work, and chores up to the date of confinement, and the morning of the day the baby was born picked 45 pounds of cotton and cooked a big dinner for her family of seven. A negro woman worked until that night, hoed potatoes, and had all her crop "right clean." Another, who had always kept on with her work up to the time of confinement, had had seven pregnancies, of which one resulted in stillbirth and five miscarriages (four to six months' term). "I went because I had it to do, but I wasn't able," said a negro mother of six children who continued field work until three days before confinement. Her baby was born in September and her daily work that autumn, in "cotton-picking time," included getting up before dawn to cook breakfast and dinner together (dinners are taken along to the field), and then a long day in the cotton field, picking cotton from "sun to sun."

It was uncommon to find women doing heavy farm work, and it is probably true that outside work in moderation is good for many pregnant women. Yet continued daily field work, in the glare and intense heat of this lowland country, in addition to housework, may not only add to the discomfort of pregnancy and the danger of confinement, but lessen the mother's ability to produce sound, vigorous children.

---

[1] See following section on "Mother's Usual Work."

Rest after confinement is equally uncertain, also depending somewhat upon the season of the year. Many of the white mothers reported nine days in bed and 27 were in bed for a longer period. Negro mothers were often up in three to five days; almost three-fifths were out of bed within a week. Housework is resumed soon after the mother is out of bed, chores more gradually. Among the white mothers field work is usually discontinued for the rest of the season. Negro women commonly return to the field in a month's time, leaving the baby at home with the older children, or occasionally taking the baby along to be deposited in a box of rags or on a pile of fertilizer bags at the edge of the field.

Mother's usual work.

Rural women of this section as a rule are burdened with a multitude of duties in the house and on the farm and only rarely have assistants other than the girls of the family. In addition to the cooking, cleaning, scrubbing, washing, ironing, sewing, milking, churning, care of chickens and garden, and canning and preserving the average woman also works side by side with her husband in the field helping to plant, cultivate, and harvest the crop.

Housework must usually be done without the services of hired help; only three of the women visited kept a servant regularly. In fact, indoor help is difficult to secure during the "chopping" season, while in "cotton picking time" it is practically impossible, since the negro women available for domestic service not only earn more money in the cotton field but also prefer field work with its greater opportunity for sociability.

An absence of household conveniences makes housework doubly hard. With the exception of sewing machines there are practically no conveniences for facilitating women's work. The majority of the homes have few of the modern improvements for cooking, which is done usually on a wood stove, with fuel provided from meal to meal.

Washing is commonly done in the open, the wash place consisting of a bench for the tubs and a big iron pot with a fire under it for boiling the clothes. Only six of the mothers visited used washing machines.

Old-fashioned implements are used for churning and butter making. Sweeping often is done with a homemade broom of short bunches of sedge grass for the house, or twigs for the yard, bound together with a hickory withe.

Carrying water is an arduous task. Only one of the homes visited had a pump and sink inside the kitchen, though white families are usually provided with a pump on the porch or within a few feet of the kitchen door. At a number of the homes, however, the water supply was at some distance from the house, which necessitated a considerable waste of the mother's time and strength.

One-fifth of the white families and over one-third of the negro families carried water over 50 feet; an occasional negro family carried water as far as a quarter of a mile. A number of tenants had no water on their immediate premises and had to carry it from the landlord's well. A mother who carried water something like 200 yards thought it was partly responsible for so weakening her that she lost her twin babies.

Field work, almost always on the "home farm," is general for both white and negro women. Of the 117 white married mothers, 90 had worked in the field before marriage (72 from early childhood) and 82 after marriage, though a number explained that since marriage their field work has been irregular, only occasional help in the busy season. Of the 89 negro mothers, 87 had done field work before marriage (74 from early childhood) and 85 after marriage. A grandmother, speaking for her married daughter insisted that "she picked cotton when she was 5 years old, she'd fill her little sack and empty it into mine."

Other forms of gainful work are uncommon among the women of this section. Before marriage some few had taught school or worked in the cotton-mills; after marriage some had helped in their husbands' stores; a few negro women had hired out for domestic service.

INFANT CARE.

Infant mortality.

By "infant mortality" is meant the deaths of infants under 1 year of age. An "infant mortality rate" as computed in the infant mortality studies of the Children's Bureau is the number of infants out of each 1,000 born alive within a given period who die during their first year of life. In this rural township, of the 520 white children live-born over one year before the agent's visit, 25 (1 child in 21) had died before reaching their first birthday, an infant mortality rate of 48.1; of the 528 live-born negro children, 34 (1 in 16) had died at less than one year, an infant mortality rate of 64.4.[1] The infant mortality rates for children of both white and negro mothers in this rural community are considerably lower, i. e., more favorable, than any found in the cities and towns which have been studied by the Children's Bureau; also much lower than in the mountain county which has a rate of 80.4.

---

[1] Computed on the basis of all children born alive at least one year previous to the agent's visit, it is obvious that children only a few months old at the time of the agent's visit could not be included, since some of these may have died afterwards before they were a year old.

A survey of a rural county of Kansas[1] shows a rate of 55 per 1,000, computed upon the same basis as the North Carolina rate. A comparison of the findings of these rural surveys with the findings of infant mortality studies in cities and towns, tends to confirm the impression that rural conditions are distinctly more favorable than urban conditions to infant life.

AGE AT DEATH AND MOTHER'S STATEMENT OF CAUSE OF DEATH.— The information obtained from the mothers as to the cause of the deaths of their babies was meager and unsatisfactory. Of the 25 white infant deaths, in 9 cases the mother did not know what had been the cause; of the 16 remaining, 7 had died of gastro-intestinal disorders, according to the mother, 4 of respiratory diseases, 2 were defective at birth. 1 had had an abscess of the liver, 1 measles, and 1 kidney trouble. Of the 34 negro infant deaths, in 13 cases the mother had not known the cause of death; of the 21 remaining, 6 had died of gastro-intestinal diseases, 4 of respiratory diseases, and 5 because of prematurity or congenital defect; the mother's ill health and mother's overwork were said to have caused the loss of 2, 2 were smothered in bed, 1 had fallen and broken its arm and leg, and 1 died during birth.

In this community, as in the cities and towns previously studied by the Children's Bureau, the greatest infant loss occurred within the early months of life. Of the 25 white infant deaths 16 had occurred within the first three months (9 within the first two weeks), 3 were between 3 and 6 months old, and 6 were over 6 months old at the time of death. The proportion of white infant deaths in these age groups approximates the average for the death registration area of the United States. Among the negroes there is a somewhat higher proportion of deaths in early infancy, i. e., within the first three months (24 out of 34, or 71 per cent), than the average for the death registration area (63 per cent).[2] Of the 34 negro infant deaths 24 occurred within the first three months (17 during the first two weeks), 3 were between 3 and 6 months old, and 7 from 6 months to 1 year.

STILLBIRTHS AND MISCARRIAGES.—Among the white mothers, 3.9 per cent of their pregnancies had resulted in stillborn children and 3.6 per cent in miscarriage. Negro mothers had lost 3.5 per cent of their children through stillbirths and 5.4 per cent by miscarriage. The percentage of stillborn children, both white and negro, in this community is considerably larger than in the rural county of Kansas studied by the Children's Bureau where only 1.8 per cent of the issues were stillbirths.[3] The white mothers of this community had

[1] Moore, Elizabeth: Maternity and Infant Care in a Rural County in Kansas, p. 41. U. S. Children's Bureau Publication No. 26, Rural Child Welfare Series No. 1. Washington. 1917.

[2] Mortality Statistics, 1915, p. 645. U. S. Bureau of the Census, Washington, 1917.

[3] Moore, Elizabeth: Maternity and Infant Care in a Rural County in Kansas, p. 30. U. S. Children's Bureau Publication No. 26, Rural Child-Welfare Series No. 1. Washington, 1917.

lost a slightly smaller proportion of children by miscarriages (3.6 per cent) than the mothers of the Kansas county (5 per cent). The number of negro miscarriages (5.4 per cent), however, was approximately the same as in Kansas.

A comparison with the rates of stillbirths and miscarriages found in the Children's Bureau inquiries in cities and towns [1] shows a slightly higher stillbirth rate for both white and negro mothers of this North Carolina township than was common in the cities and towns, and a slightly lower rate of miscarriages among the white mothers, but a somewhat higher rate among negro mothers.

Infant feeding.[2]

Methods of infant feeding in this community are largely a matter of tradition, the mothers depending upon the advice of neighbors and friends, since in the majority of cases it is impossible for the distant physician to supervise the feeding of his rural patients.

Breast feeding is universal. The rural mother as a rule is well able to nurse her child. Of the 78 white babies for whom feeding records were secured all were breast fed through the first 5 months; with the exception of 2 babies weaned, 1 at 6 months and 1 at 9 months, all were nursed during the entire first year. Of the 86 negro babies, all were breast fed during their first 2 months, all but 8 during their entire first year. Nursing is usually continued for 18 months, often until the child is 20 or 24 months old, or until another pregnancy interrupts lactation. Of the 35 white babies that had been weaned at the time the mother was visited, only 3 were 12 months or less at the time of weaning, 16 were between 13 and 18 months, 12 between 19 and 24 months, and 4 were 25 months or over. Forty negro babies had been weaned, 12 at 12 months or less; 16 at 13 to 18 months, inclusive; and 11 at 19 to 24 months (in 1 case the age of weaning was not known).

It was customary, however, among the majority of mothers, in addition to the breast milk, to feed their babies indiscriminately, in accordance with a popular supposition that a taste of everything the mother eats will protect him from colic. Seven white babies and 19 negro babies were given food in addition to breast milk from their

---

[1] Per cent of all issues resulting in stillbirth or miscarriage in cities and towns so far studied by the Children's Bureau have been as follows:

City or town.	Still-births.	Miscar-riages.	City or town.	Still-births.	Miscar-riages.
Johnstown, Pa.	4.5	3.3	Saginaw, Mich.	3.9	4.4
Manchester, N. H.	2.9	4.6	Akron, Ohio.	3.0	4.2
Waterbury, Conn.	3.4	6.8	Brockton, Mass.	2.6	5.3
New Bedford, Mass.	2.9	4.4			

[2] Feeding records covering the first year of the baby's life were obtained for the mother's last child under 5 years, a total of 78 records for white babies and 86 for negro babies.

first month of life. By the beginning of the fourth month 23 white and 45 negro babies were being fed. One mother fed her baby at 2 months because he was "hearty and wanted to eat." Another gave her babies a taste of almost everything she ate, especially in the spring, to prevent their having colic with every new vegetable. A negro mother, who reported that her baby had had nothing but the breast for the first seven months, upon reconsidering "reckoned he had had watermelon and the other children might have given him peaches and apples." Some few were fed "chewed rations" until the teeth arrived, i. e., the father or mother chewed the baby's food before giving it to him. "Sugar tits" of moistened bread, sugar, and a little butter, lard, or fat meat, tied in an old thin cloth, are common pacifiers. Fat meat is sometimes given as a purgative and, among the negroes, is a common substitute for oil. It is customary to give catnip tea until the mother's milk has come, often continuing the tea during the first few weeks.

PHYSICAL CONDITION OF CHILDREN FROM 1 TO 15 YEARS OF AGE.

General health.

The so-called "children's diseases"—measles, mumps, whooping cough, and chicken pox—have been widespread in this locality. Of other diseases, the most commonly reported were dysentery and stomach disorders of various sorts, pneumonia, malaria, "sore eyes," hookworm, tonsilitis, "worms," smallpox, and typhoid fever. Some half a dozen children among those visited have been considered by their families to be mentally defective.

It was shown a few years ago that the county was heavily infected with hookworm disease. During a campaign against hookworm, carried on in the county in 1911 by the Rockefeller Sanitary Commission (now the International Health Board of the Rockefeller Foundation) in cooperation with the State board of health, 3,301 persons were examined, of whom 1,839, or 55.7 per cent, were pronounced to be infected with hookworm. The campaign was apparently confined to the examination and treatment of individuals and did not include the erection of sanitary privies throughout the county which has been the important feature of the more recent hookworm campaigns in other counties of the State.

The International Health Board, in its report for 1915, describes the effect upon the population of a prevalence of hookworm disease:

In no country is the death rate ascribed directly to hookworm disease particularly high; this disease is never spectacular, like yellow fever or plague or pernicious malaria. It is the greater menace because it works subtly. Acute diseases sometimes tend to strengthen the race by killing off the weak; but hookworm disease working so insidiously as frequently to escape the attention even of its victims tends to weaken the race by sapping its vitality. Persons harboring this infection are more susceptible to such diseases as malaria, typhoid fever, pneumonia, and tuberculosis, which prey upon lowered vitality. But even more important than this indirect contribution to the death roll are the cumulative results—physical, intellectual, economic, and moral—which are handed down from generation to generation through long periods of time.[1]

Within recent years the county has been covered by a typhoid campaign also, during which free vaccination for typhoid was available for all persons of the county, through the cooperation of the State board of health with local authorities. In the course of the Children's Bureau survey an interesting story was told of the disastrous results that had followed the failure of one family to avail themselves of vaccination. The mother wanted them all to drive over to the schoolhouse and have it done, but the father thought it was not worth while; he had heard it made one sick and did not wish to risk losing time from work. In the midst of "cotton-picking time" the 15-year-old boy developed a bad case of typhoid; for weeks the mother and oldest brother had to give their entire attention to nursing the sick boy. This case of typhoid cost the family $50 for help hired to replace these three cotton pickers of the family and, in addition, a doctor's bill of $50.

Mortality of children from 1 to 15 years of age.

In the 127 white families visited there had been 17 deaths of children 1 to 5 years of age. According to the mothers' statements, 6 had occurred from intestinal disorders; 2 from meningitis; 2 from chills and fever; 1 each from pneumonia, measles, Bright's disease, "spinal disease," "stomachitis," and membranous croup; and in 1 case the cause was unknown. Between the ages of 6 and 15 only 1 death had occurred, and in this case the cause was not known.

Among the 129 negro families 25 children had died between the ages of 1 and 5 years—7 of intestinal disorders; 4 of respiratory diseases; 4 had been burned to death; 1 drowned; 1 strangled; 2 had died of typhoid; 1 each of scarlet fever, sunstroke, thresh, eczema, and congenital defects; and in one case the cause of death was unknown. There had been 5 deaths of negro children between the ages of 6 and 16—2 of tuberculosis, 1 of "worms," 1 had been shot, and 1 burned to death.

A striking proportion of deaths from accident was reported among the negro children—7 out of 25 deaths between the ages of 1 and 5 years and 2 out of 5 between 6 and 16.

Home remedies.

Distance from doctors and drug stores has usually resulted in the extensive use of home remedies and patent medicines. Many families keep a supply of drugs on hand, such as salts, camphor, oil, calomel, turpentine, paregoric, asafetida, and quinine.

---

[1] The Rockefeller Foundation, International Health Commission, Second Annual Report, 1915, pp. 11, 12.

A thriving business is conducted by a firm which maintains continuously an agent and a two-horse load of patent medicines in this section. Croup and cough "cures," liniments, soothing and teething sirups, remedies for women's diseases and for constipation are part of his stock and have a wide sale among his patrons. The remedies are usually put up in dollar packages with wrappers which make extravagant claims for their virtues.

The State board of health recommended to the legislature of 1917 the passage of a State law regulating the conditions of sales of trademark remedies as follows: (1) "The elimination of secrecy, requiring that the remedy publish its formula on the package," and (2) "a sufficient tax on the various brands of secret remedies on the market of this State to enable the State government to encourage and answer inquiries from the people regarding the action of any drug or combination of drugs."[1] Although the "secret remedies" law failed of passage, two important acts of the 1917 legislature concerning patent remedies provide (1) that the package or label of any drug product shall not contain any statement regarding the curative or therapeutic effect of such article which is not true[2] (in harmony with the Federal food and drugs act and copied by most of the States in their laws), and (2) that the sale is forbidden and the advertising unlawful of any proprietary medicine purporting to cure certain diseases, for which no cure has been found[3]—a law in harmony with advanced legislation upon this subject.

Negro mothers, in addition to a liberal patronage of patent medicines, also rely to a large extent upon homemade "teas" of native herbs, which they gather from early spring to late autumn. The majority of babies are given catnip tea from birth. For colds, favorite remedies are teas of pine tops, boneset, horehound, or pennyroyal. Purge grass is thought infallible for constipation. For diarrhea, the dollar weed is given, also sweet-gum leaves, queen's delight, or red raspberry tips; for "female troubles," red shank, slippery elm, burdock, and single or double tansy are in favor.

Diet.

Most of the families visited have gardens, though many, because the poor soil requires much fertilizer and labor, feel that they can not spare the expense or the time for a garden of any considerable size. The average family raises beans, tomatoes, field corn, sweet potatoes, Irish potatoes, cabbage, collards, turnips, okra, and field peas. The garden insures the family sufficient vegetables during the summer months, but for a good part of the year the diet is much more limited.

---

[1] Sixteenth Biennial Report of the North Carolina State Board of Health, 1915–1916, p. 58.
[2] Acts of 1907, ch. 368, as amended by Acts of 1917, ch. 19.
[3] Acts of 1917, ch. 27.

Few families conserve any variety of vegetables, usually depending upon sweet and Irish potatoes, collards, and turnips for winter use.

Although apples, peaches, plums, and cherries are scarce, blackberries, huckleberries, and scuppernong grapes are fine and plentiful. The more thrifty and enterprising housewives can, dry, and otherwise preserve fruit for winter use. The migratory life of the tenant family, however, offers small incentive to provide for the morrow.

Little stock is kept in this section, and a number of families are without milk and butter. The county makes but 3 pounds of butter to each person per year.[1] Poultry also is considerably below the usual quota in rural districts, and eggs are scarce. Few families keep sheep, though all have hogs, pork being almost the sole dependence for meat.

Corn is a staple article of diet, whether as "roasting ears," hominy grits, or ground into meal. Molasses, homemade from sorghum cane, is widely used for "sweetening" during the winter season.

The preparation of food, from the point of view of the needs of growing children, leaves much to be desired. This, of course, is not true of the more prosperous and intelligent families, but the children of the small tenant are given much of pork, fried food, and half-cooked starch in the form of hominy and of corn and wheat bread. This heavy diet of partly cooked starches, with an excess of fat and a deficiency of fruits and green vegetables (except in the summer), together with the custom of indulging children in the most undesirable habits of eating whenever and whatever they please, is doubtless a factor in the indigestion, which, according to the mothers, is one of their chief difficulties with the children. In many homes the child is allowed to go to the "safe" for leftovers whenever he can think of nothing else to do, with the result that he never knows the wholesome urge of a good healthy appetite, and his stomach knows no rest.

The rural mother has been at a great disadvantage; because of her remoteness and infrequent intercourse with her neighbors, she has had no standard of comparison by which to measure her methods and achievements. Now, however, the old order is rapidly changing, and every year brings her into closer touch with better and more modern methods of home economics and household management. The women of this township now have at their disposal the services of a county home demonstration agent, and are within a reasonable distance of community fairs, county fairs, and farmers' institutes, where lectures, demonstrations, and exhibits have been arranged for their benefit.

---

[1] Thirteenth Census of the United States, 1910, Vol. VII, Agriculture.

EDUCATION.
School law.

According to the school law, as amended in 1917, a North Carolina child must be in school between the ages of 8 and 14,[1] for four months of the school term each year. The 14-year age limit is a recent provision—a part of the important educational program enacted by the last session of the legislature and effective beginning September 1, 1917.[2] At the time of the inquiry, school attendance was compulsory only for children of 8, 9, 10, and 11 years. The law makes an exception in cases where the child is so physically or mentally handicapped as to make attendance impracticable; also where he lives 2½ miles or more from the schoolhouse; or where, because of extreme poverty, his services are necessary to his parents, or they are unable to provide him with suitable clothing or necessary books.[3] Since even under the terms of the new law, the child is assured of only 24 months schooling in preparation for his life work, the law is still obviously inadequate in its scope. Moreover, in this rural section at least, the "extreme poverty" exemption clause is liberally interpreted; and children are frequently kept at home to help on the farm during the busy seasons.

School term and attendance.

At the time of this inquiry, the school term in the neighborhoods visited covered five months, November to March, inclusive, with the exception of the largest school, which was in session six months (made possible by special local taxation). Not only is the term short, but attendance is irregular, the yearly average varying from 50 to 85 per cent of the total enrollment. Fewer children attend in November (cotton picking season) than at any other time during the term. In March, also, many of the older boys are kept at home to help with the spring plowing.

The majority of homes visited are within a reasonable distance of the school. Thirteen white and 27 negro families, however, with children of school age have no school nearer than 2½ miles, and, according to the school law, no child living that distance or farther is required to attend school.[3]

Although the majority of the children start to school at 6 years. over one-fourth had not been sent until they were 7 years or older, usually because the family lived at a distance from the school or the child was not as strong as the others. Occasionally a 5-year-old was sent along with the older children, not to have any share in the school work but "just to be going," as the mother said. Nineteen of the 257 white children of school age, and about the same propor-

---

[1] In Mitchell County school attendance between the ages of 8 and 15, and in Polk County between the ages of 7 and 15.

[2] Acts of 1913, ch. 173, sec. 1, as amended by Acts of 1917, ch. 208.

[3] Acts of 1913, ch. 173, sec. 2.

tion of negro children, had never attended school at all. One mother explained that her 9-year-old boy would have 3½ miles to travel to school—7 miles the round trip—the winters are hard and he has so many colds that she has not sent him.

It was gratifying to find so many of the older children of 15 to 20 years still in school, at least for the two or three winter months, ambitious to supplement in this way their inadequate schooling as young children. A child is usually well grown before he leaves school finally and as a rule has some good reason for leaving—he is needed on the farm or in the house, or he marries or goes off to work. A few were "tired of school," one did not like the teacher, one was "slow at books and ashamed to go," and one had left to join the Army. Poverty also is a frequent factor in poor attendance, particularly among the negro families. A negro mother lamented that her children could have gone more this year if they had had good shoes.

The short school term, together with irregular attendance, make it difficult for the child to progress rapidly in school. Ability to read and write is a minimum to be expected from him as a result of his contact with school; many, however, fail to achieve even this claim to education. In the families visited, approximately 1 white child out of 10, 1 negro child out of 3, between the ages of 10 and 20 years, had not yet learned to read and write.

Attitude of parents toward education.

As a rule the parents were interested in their children's school progress, though few ever visited the school or consulted the teacher. A proud mother told of her 10-year-old prize speller, who had missed only one word all last winter and not one the year before. One mother, who complained that the teacher let the children loiter and fight on the way home, was asked if she ever visited the school to talk things over with the teacher and admitted that she had never seen any one of their teachers. Although one out of six of the white mothers and one out of three of the negro mothers visited were themselves illiterate, the attitude often attributed to illiterate parents, that "what was good enough for us is good enough for our children," was not encountered in this community. On the contrary, it is often a consciousness of their own defective education that stimulates the parents to see to it that their children have better opportunities. A negro woman, who had attended school only four weeks in her whole life, explained that for that reason she is "pushing" the children—she wants them to get some "learning."

School facilities.

The township provides five schools for white children and four negro schools.

WHITE SCHOOLS.—The largest white school is a well-equipped, three-teacher school, with a course of study through the tenth grade; another is a two-room, two-teacher school. These two school districts have voted the special school tax (30 cents on the hundred dollars valuation of property and 90 cents on the poll tax), which is placed to the credit of the school district voting it. This amount may be used for various purposes, such as lengthening the school term, increasing the teacher's salary, building a new school, or getting an additional teacher. The three other white schools are old-fashioned, one-room, one-teacher schools, with a total enrollment of less than 30 children to the school. The township seems to offer an excellent opportunity for a consolidation of rural schools, in accordance with the newer standards for rural educational facilities.

County schools are supported almost entirely by county taxes, with the exception of limited grants from the meager State school fund and a special district school tax if agreed upon by a majority vote of the qualified voters of the district. The Progressive Farmer [1] urges the necessity for increased school funds:

The first thing and biggest thing we are going to say in this issue of The Progressive Farmer is this—that our folks in North Carolina, South Carolina, Virginia, and Georgia *ought to absolutely double their school taxes during the coming year.*

*   *   *   *   *   *   *

It is no use to say we can't afford it. With cotton at 20 to 25 cents a pound and tobacco and peanuts selling at corresponding figures, it is folly to say that we can't do more for our schools than we did when cotton was 6 to 10 cents and other crop prices in keeping with these. And we ought to be ashamed of ourselves if we don't do more. The time has come when any man ought to be ashamed when he leaves home if he can't say he lives in a local tax school district—and one in which the tax is adequate.

*   *   *   *   *   *   *

Look at the facts. The North Atlantic States spend $50.55 per year on schools per child; the South Atlantic States $18.91—not 40 per cent as much. The North Central States spend $44.15 per child; the South Central States $19.01—not half as much. North Dakota, a rural State, is spending $64 a year per child; wild Idaho $55, and even Mormon Utah $52, while Virginia spends $19, North Carolina only $12, South Carolina only $11, and Georgia $13. Nor can we say we are doing as well in proportion to wealth, for while North Dakota spends on schools 44 cents a year for each $100 of her wealth, Idaho 49, and Utah 51, Virginia and North Carolina spend only 28 cents a year per $100 of wealth, South Carolina 27 cents, and Georgia 29.

The Carolinas, Virginia, and Georgia therefore might double the amount they are spending for schools and even then not spend as much as some other States are spending.

The rural-school teacher of this section is poorly paid; five of the eight teachers of the township are paid from $45 to $75 per month, the other three only $40 per month for the five-month term—a meager yearly salary of $200. The average salary for the eight teachers of the township ($286) is, however, somewhat above the

---

[1] The Progressive Farmer, Saturday, June 30, 1917.

low State average of $243 for teachers in the public schools, but is scarcely more than half the average ($525) for the United States.[1]

Buildings and equipment.—All the school buildings are frame; three are in good repair, painted, and attractive, while two are unpainted and uninviting.

Each schoolhouse stands in a grove of trees, in most instances young oaks, but no attempt has been made in any case to beautify the grounds with shrubbery or flowers. All have plenty of play space, and the largest school is provided with a basket-ball court.

The larger schools are plastered and wainscoted, the one-teacher schools merely ceiled. All are heated by unjacketed wood stoves. The two larger schools are provided with cloakrooms; in the one-room schools the children hang their wraps on nails or hooks on the walls of the classroom. All the schools have new desks and chairs of graduated size, each accommodating two children, except at one school, which has individual seats. Blackboard space is inadequate—in one school only 12 feet—partly black cardboard and partly pine boards painted black. Aside from desks, chairs, and blackboards, little else in the way of equipment is furnished by the school authorities, and anything further must be added by the teacher or by interested school patrons. Two schools have pianos, only one has a dictionary, and three have no maps—which, as may be imagined, greatly hampers the teaching of geography. The children provide their own schoolbooks, paper, and pencils. An interested teacher of a one-teacher school had herself supplied her own primary, history, and geography "helps," desk copies of all textbooks used, material for county commencement exhibits, drawing paper, crayons, pencils when the children ran short, and had induced the local "community club" to contribute copy books.

School libraries at each of the schools are a source of enjoyment to the children during the school term.

Sanitation.—Drinking water is obtained from drilled wells on the school premises, except for one school, which used a near-by spring. There is usually a gourd or cup at the pump, but the teachers are making an effort to have at least each family of children bring a cup, which is a step toward the individual drinking cup.

Toilet facilities are inexcusably poor. Two schools have no toilet whatever, two have a toilet for girls only, while the largest has one for boys and one for girls.

School activities.—At some of the schools the children are eager and interested members of school clubs. An Audubon society is responsible for an enthusiasm for birds among small boys of that neighborhood; 12 bird houses were made by the boys of this school last year, exhibited at the county fair, and afterwards set up on the

---

[1] Compiled from Report of Commissioner of Education for year ending June 30, 1916, Vol. II, p. 30.

home farms. One mother whose boy has learned to know the birds and their notes confessed that it has made her notice the birds, too. A canning club, pig club, and corn club have headquarters at the schools and a remote one-teacher school has a "Robert E. Lee Society" which meets every Friday afternoon for debates or literary programs and has been found an excellent means of getting parents to visit the school. All the schools were well represented at the county commencement held in March at the county seat; a one-teacher school of this township was the winner of several prizes—for the best all around one-teacher school exhibit, for the best seventh-grade penmanship, for the best composition on the necessity for the protection of birds, and for the best beaten biscuit.

The township schools have not been used to any great extent for community purposes. Farmers' institutes are held yearly at the largest school, and the winter before the survey a "moonlight" school was also held there. Two other schoolhouses are used for meetings of the local community clubs, and at another a union Sunday school has its services on Sunday afternoons; occasionally political meetings also are held at the schools. For the most part the people have not yet accustomed themselves to the idea of a school as a social and community center, and the schoolhouse commonly stands idle and unused for over half the year.

NEGRO SCHOOLS.—The four negro schools of the township, like the average rural schools for negroes in the South, are poor.

The negro child of the township goes to school in a one-room, unpainted schoolhouse, and sits with several children in a row on a long homemade bench with no back except a rail and no place to hold his books and papers except on his lap. He "does his sums" on a homemade blackboard of three boards nailed together and painted black, and recites his lessons to a teacher (colored) who for five months draws a salary of $25 per month. His school term lasts 100 days, of which he misses no small share to help his father with the crop.

In two of the negro schools the course does not extend beyond the fourth grade; one has six grades, and the largest negro school of the township is of a better type, with classes up to the seventh grade and a teacher who draws a salary of $30 per month. At the negro county commencement this school was the winner of four prizes—more than any other negro school of the county.

Enrollment in the four negro schools varies from 44 to 96. All the teachers are overburdened by the number of pupils. It is plain one teacher's time divided among 96 children in seven grades can give each child only the merest smattering.

All the negro schools have undertaken industrial work of some description. The girls learn darning, buttonhole making, hemming, and embroidery. Lacking sewing machines at the school, the children cut, baste, and fit the garments there and take them home to sew. One teacher has attempted a weekly cooking demonstration at homes in the neighborhood. The boys make baskets and mats of corn shucks, mats of raveled tow sacks (in which cotton seed and fertilizer come), chair seats of splints, and maps which they color with crayons.

Two negro schools are using water from good drilled wells on the schoolhouse grounds, and another carries water from a drilled well at the nearest farm, 300 yards distant. One, however, still draws water from a dug well on the school premises—a shallow well only 12 feet below the surface, obviously subject to pollution by seepage, and also open and unprotected from dust and dirt. None of the four negro schools is provided with toilet facilities of any description.

HIGH SCHOOLS.—Besides the district schools the county public-school system provides at the county seat a good, well-equipped high school for white children and a normal school for colored. The colored "normal" is both boarding and day school and has a dormitory where, for a small sum, girls from the country round about may live during the school term, furnishing their own supplies and doing their own cooking and housework.

FARM-LIFE SCHOOLS.—There has been some discussion of a "farm-life" school for this county. This type of school, offering a course of study better adapted to rural conditions than the standardized school of the three R's, has proved its worth in other parts of the State and would be a distinct asset to this county.

The purpose of the farm-life school is to give to the boys and girls such preparation as the county public high schools give, and in addition to that to give the boys training in agricultural pursuits and farm life, and to prepare the girls for home making and home keeping.[1]

The course of study in a farm-life school (the State now has 21 such schools) includes such rural subjects as the following: Botany, agriculture, field crops, vegetable gardening, fruit culture, farm animals, feeding live stock, dairying, poultry raising, soils and fertilizer, rural economics, and farm equipment.

MOONLIGHT SCHOOLS.—This neighborhood has had a share in the State's campaign against illiteracy, holding a "moonlight school" at the largest school of the township. The "moonlight school," which originated in Kentucky and has been found effective there and in other States, is a night school for adult illiterates, conducted for short periods, usually at the public school by volunteer teachers, preferably on moonlight nights for the greater convenience of the

---

[1] Acts of 1911, ch. 84.

country people. The State department of public instruction is hoping by this means to reduce materially the illiteracy of white adults. North Carolina had in 1910 a higher rate of illiteracy (14 per cent of the male adult native white population) [1] than any other State.

CHILDREN'S FARM AND OTHER WORK. [2]

The effect of farm work on the development of the child is a practically unexplored field. It has probably been too often assumed, however, that a child's work on the farm is limited to morning and evening chores—all light work, with no tax on strength or endurance, and requiring only two or three hours a day. In this study the attempt was made to discover for this one rural township of the South the various farm occupations—both field work and chores—performed by children, the health hazards involved in each, ages and sex of the children, their working hours and their wages where the farm work is away from home.

A white family, living on a farm of 110 acres, with 30 acres in cultivation, consists of father, mother, and six children—two boys of 15 and 13, a girl of 10, boy of 8, girl of 6, and a 3-year-old baby. The two older boys plow, help set out the garden, hoe corn, strip fodder, gather corn, and chop and pick cotton; these boys also help take care of the stock and feed the hogs. The 10-year-old girl and 8-year-old boy drop corn and peas, hoe corn, chop and pick cotton, and pick peas; the little girl also helps her mother with the housework, and the boy takes the cow to the pasture and back and carries wood and water. The 6-year-old girl feeds the chickens, brings in stove wood, and helps irregularly with the cotton picking.

Chores.

Every farm child has a variety of chores to perform around the house and at the barn—the boys feed the mule, "tote" water, feed the chickens and hogs, chop wood and bring it in, "carry" the cow back and forth to the pasture, and weed the garden; the girls, besides their share of the housework, help with milking, churning, canning, and preserving. All these various odd jobs have been considered chores, as distinguished from regular field work with the crops.

Field work.

It was found that two-thirds of the white children and three-fourths of the negro children from 5 to 15 years old, in addition to chores and odd jobs, helped in the fields, cultivating and harvesting the crops. Children of all ages were at work in the fields; 51 were children under 8 (22 white and 29 negro); 120, of whom 47 were white and 73 negro children, were under 10 years.

---

[1] Thirteenth Census of the United States, 1910, Vol. I, Population, p. 1258.

[2] The discussion of children's farm and other work is limited in this inquiry to children from 5 to 15 years, inclusive, living at home at the time of the agent's visit, i. e., 219 white and 270 negro children, of whom 144 white children (88 boys and 56 girls) and 204 negro children (103 boys and 101 girls) worked in the fields.

Cotton is the leading crop, and in the cotton field a large proportion of the labor is performed by children of various ages, from the well-grown boy of 15 to the toddler of 5 or 6, who work along with the rest of the family in cotton-picking time.

Plowing, planting the cotton crop, and putting out fertilizer is usually considered a man's work, though sometimes done by the older boys. Thirty-eight white boys 9 to 15 years old and 53 negro children from 7 to 15 (51 boys and 2 girls) had helped with the plowing, using a one-horse plow. Cotton is planted with a "cotton planter" drawn by one mule. The boy's work consists in driving the mule and keeping to the top of the ridge—light work, for the soil has been plowed before. Some judgment and experience is required to manage the animal, keep him in a straight line, and hold the planter to the top of the ridge. Fertilizer is sometimes scattered by hand, but usually put out with a distributor drawn by one mule—light work that can be done by any boy who can plow.

The next process in the cotton crop is "chopping" the cotton, i. e., thinning it and weeding out the grass between the plants with a hoe (the grass between the rows is plowed under). On the first round the plants are "chopped out," leaving two stalks; on the second round only single plants are left, 12 to 15 inches apart. Numbers of children, of both sexes and all ages from 5 to 15 years, help with the chopping; for it requires little strength and no particular skill, except on the first round when there is danger of injuring the young plants. It is, however, very fatiguing in the hot sun of midsummer; and, because of the monotony of keeping the same position, the shoulders and arms ache from the muscular exertion, and the hands become cramped from holding the hoe. The chances are that any considerable amount of this sort of work is too severe for a young child. One hundred and two white children and 147 negro children had chopped cotton during the summer of the inquiry.

Cotton picking is the work of the entire family. One mother, when she puts "one at it," puts "them all at it." One hundred and forty-one white children and 204 negro children, of both sexes and all ages from 5 to 15 years, picked cotton. Many families take all the children to the field, even, as has been said, depositing the baby in a box under the trees at the end of the row. The cotton picker walks up and down between the rows, stooping over to pick the cotton and tossing it into a sack worn over the shoulder; when filled, the sack is emptied into a sheet spread out on the ground at the end of the row. Although cotton picking is light work requiring little strength, it has its bad features when the age of the children in the cotton fields is considered. There is exposure to sun and heat in the early part of the season; fatigue, due to long hours, monotony, and the stooping posture; and no small muscular strain from carrying the cotton—as much as 10, 15, or 20 pounds accumulates in the sack before it is emptied into the sheet. The pickers are also under some nervous strain, often racing one another to see who can pick the most in a day. Where they are working out for some one else, the pay is at piece rates—50 cents for every 100 pounds picked— which encourages speeding up.

Corn is usually planted with a planter drawn by one mule; in this case only the older boys who are "plow hands" would be called upon to help. Sometimes the old-fashioned method of "dropping" by hand is followed, and this is often done by the younger children. Hoeing corn is about the same process as "chopping" cotton and is done by children of the same ages.

Pulling or "stripping" fodder is considered harder work than hoeing corn and cotton, or picking cotton. Twenty-four white children and 52 negro children—boys and girls from 6 to 15 years of age— pulled fodder. The blades of the fodder are stripped from the cornstalks, tied in bunches to the stalks, and left to dry. It is doubtful whether any child who is not fairly well-grown should have this sort of work to do, since reaching the highest blades necessitates considerable muscular strain.

In the tobacco crop, as with cotton, children can be used at almost every step of the process. The plants are set out by hand, at intervals of about 18 inches. This is done by both boys and girls and is comparatively light work. The stooping posture would be trying if kept up for any length of time, but in two or three days a large crop can be set out.

A child of 8 or 9 can "top" tobacco; i. e., pinch off the small top leaves; he needs only to know how to count in order that he may leave the same number of leaves on all the plants. A week or so later the new sprouts are broken off; this is called "sprouting" or "priming." Young children go from plant to plant also, picking off the bugs.

Children can also "strip" tobacco, though some judgment is required for this; the large lower leaves are stripped from the plant, and care must be taken to gather only perfect leaves and to avoid breaking or crushing them. The next step is tying the leaves together in bunches of five or six, ready for curing—simple work and done by young children. Only the older boys and grown men can attend to the curing, which is a tedious process requiring judgment and experience.

Children under 16 have a share in various minor farm activities also, helping with the crops of peas, beans, and sweet potatoes, helping in the garden, and picking fruit and berries.

Working hours.

The hours of children regularly at work in the field vary, not only in the different families but also according to the season of the year. In spring and summer many work from "sun to sun"; others start to the field in the morning when the dew has dried, and work until about an hour before sunset. No work is done in the heat of the day; i. e., from 11 to 1 or from 12 to 2, unless the family is "pushed" with the crop.

In cotton-picking time the working day is from 7 or earlier until sundown with almost no time off for dinner; many families take their dinners to the field and eat as they go up and down the rows. "Some mornings the sun is an hour high and some it's not up yet before we're in the field," said one mother. One negro mother rouses her family at 4 o'clock; she was "raised that way"; her father and mother always ate their breakfast by candle light.

Wages when at work away from home.

Although most of the children work only on their own home farm, a number work out for the neighbors also a few odd days when their labor can be spared from their own crop. Chopping cotton is paid for by the day, girls between 12 and 15 making 40 cents a day and boys 50 cents. A 10-year-old boy was getting 40 cents and a boy of 8 years, 20 cents. Picking cotton is paid at piece rates—50 cents per 100 pounds—which encourages speeding up and accounts for a vast pride in the amount each child can pick. Children between 12 and 15 years of age pick from 125 to 200 pounds a day.

For the children to help with the crop is such a customary procedure that it is accepted as a matter of course. From instincts of thrift and industry, most parents wish their children to learn to work. It is by no means always a question of poverty, for children of well-to-do farmers are to be found in the field as well as those of poor tenants. A reasonable amount of farm work can hardly be injurious to the health of a sturdy, well-grown child, and early training in habits of industry will be of value to him later in life, yet there can be no doubt that interruption of the child's schooling in order to have him help with the crop seriously handicaps him. This can not be justified even in cases of poverty. Moreover, very young children should not be called upon to perform regular daily field labor with its accompaniment of long hours, exposure to the heat of the sun, monotony, and fatigue.

RECREATION AND SOCIAL LIFE.

Recreation, community interests, and the social aspects of country life are rather more developed in this township than in the average rural community where wholesome means of relaxation and diversion are too often lacking.

White families.

During the winter, social intercourse is largely confined to church-going, an occasional school entertainment, and now and then a visit to town on Saturday afternoons. In August, after the cotton is "made" (bolls formed and further cultivation impossible), there is leisure, before cotton picking, for visiting, entertaining, ice-cream suppers, picnics, and swimming parties at the picturesque mill ponds. A community club picnic has been the means of bringing together two or three neighborhoods every August. Speakers are invited, and an exhibit of home products is arranged, with prizes offered for the best bread, preserves, cake, flowers, and other home products. After a picnic dinner, athletic contests and a canning club demonstration occupy the afternoon.

Three church denominations are represented in the township, each with preaching services once a month. Two have Sunday school also every Sunday afternoon. Church rivalry—occasionally a source of discord in a small community—is remarkably lacking in this township, where the whole neighborhood attends services, ice-cream suppers, and "protracted meetings" at all three churches indiscriminately.

School entertainments of various sorts are given now and then such as Christmas celebrations, box suppers, "concerts," Easter-egg hunts, pound parties, ice-cream suppers, lectures on birds, and an occasional evening with a professional short-story teller. Sometimes admission is charged and the proceeds used to buy extra furnishing or equipment for the school. Thirty dollars, raised by the largest school last year, provided shades and curtains and basket-ball equipment, and paid the expenses of the school's share in "county commencement." A one-teacher school gave an interesting "measuring party" to which every person who came brought "a penny a foot and a penny for each inch over" of his height, and a prize was given to the tallest person present.

Athletic sports, unfortunately, arouse little interest. The township is without a single baseball team or tennis court. "Old Hundred"—something like baseball, but played with a soft ball—is popular among the school children at recess. One school has organized a basket-ball team for boys and one for girls. Swimming in the mill ponds or river is a favorite diversion with the boys, and the older boys and men occasionally fish and hunt for birds, squirrels, rabbits, and foxes. During shad season "fish fries" are popular with the young people.

Among the adults clubs and lodges are numerous, including Masons, Odd Fellows, Woodmen, two "community clubs," and various church societies. Farmers' institutes, held every year at the largest schoolhouse, are well attended by both men and women.

As an up-to-date farmer explained, "you can always get some new ideas; it got me in the notion of sowing clover." A farmers' union was organized a few years ago, but finally failed.

The community clubs (women's organizations under the leadership of the county home demonstration agent) are especially interesting and successful and are proving a definite force for progress in their neighborhoods. The programs at their monthly meetings embrace a variety of topics of interest to rural women, such as bread making, canning vegetables in the home, poultry raising, flower and vegetable gardening, and exterminating flies and mosquitoes.

A girl's "canning club," under the direction of the county home demonstration agent, has had two successful seasons. The girls plant and cultivate a garden of a tenth of an acre and can the products for home and market. Their demonstration of tomato canning is a popular feature of the annual canning club picnic.

A boys' corn club, discontinued the year of the inquiry, had made a good record the previous summer. A 15-year-old prize winner raised 101 bushels the first year and 106 the second, to the acre, which was three times his father's record of 30 to 35 bushels. The boy deep-plowed the soil and used more fertilizer, but his yield was out of all proportion to the additional expense. Another corn-club boy deposits in the bank the proceeds from his acre of corn. His father has him keep books and sell the corn himself, to teach him the business side of farming.

In three-fourths of the white homes of the township some sort of publication is taken regularly. A number of families are getting weekly rural editions of the county papers; several subscribe for semiweekly or triweekly Atlanta papers; and a number of farm papers are taken. Of magazines, however, there is surprising dearth; the so-called "woman's magazine" which so many women are finding helpful, with its pages on household management and the care of children, is seldom found in this section. Literary magazines, also, are rare.

Although the man of the house usually makes at least a monthly trip to town and in the fall of the year goes in almost every week, hauling cotton, going to town seems to be an arduous undertaking for his wife. She accomplishes it only about half a dozen times a year, when shopping is necessary or when the children clamor to be taken in for the county fair or county commencement. Often tenant families, lacking a conveyance, find the trip out of the question.

Migration from country to town is rare in this community. As the boys and girls grow up and marry, practically all settle in the same neighborhood where they were reared. A real contentment with country life is the rule; nearly every family expressed the firm conviction that "the country is the best place to raise children," some on moral grounds dreading the contaminating influence of town life and some on the grounds of health. One mother wished for better schools for the children, like the town schools, but thought the country the place to rear children, for, as she said, "there's more fresh air, and they can play about and are not as apt to catch contagious diseases as in town." A mother, reared in a mill town, objects to the long hours, hot sun, and loneliness of the farm. "In the mill town you weren't lonely, you could get up with somebody and talk and have a good time," she said. Another, however, was glad to get her little family away from the mill into the country, because it was easier to keep them from bad influences.

Negro families.

The negro is by nature gregarious and revels in social gatherings. Church is the most common meeting place and never lacks a good attendance. "The most we go," said one mother, "is to church, and that is so often that's all we can do." One takes her "little crowd" and goes to preaching, prayer meeting, and Sunday school not at one church but three—Falling Run, Brown Chapel, and Grays Creek all having her loyal support.

The negro school is often the scene of festivities; concerts are popular, with speaking, singing, and dialogues. A small one-teacher school has been provided with window curtains, a curtain to go across the "stage," and a large hanging lamp—all bought with the proceeds from an ice-cream supper given by the teacher.

There had also occurred recently a "farmers' dinner," a dime party, "pan cake tosses," an Easter barbecue, and a Fourth of July entertainment given by the Masons and the Eastern Star. Here and there a mother of a stricter turn of mind voiced her disapproval of anything of the sort, and merely allows her "children to go to church, or to a funeral, or to a sickness, or something like that, and straight home again." More than one negro mother prided herself upon her severity with her children. "I don't let mine stroll about to learn more devilment," one explained. Negro boys were only slightly interested in athletic sports, swimming, fishing, hunting for birds, squirrels, and rabbits; some few played baseball. One negro family rejoices in a cheap little graphophone which the mother had seen advertised in the papers as a good way to keep the boys home at night.

Clubs and "societies" have a fascination for the negro; most of them are organizations paying a benefit in case of sickness or death. "Society" dues, ranging from 10 to 50 cents a month, are a heavy drain on the poverty-stricken negro family, though payment is kept up even at a real sacrifice, spurred by the dread of sickness or of death and pauper burial. Usually a disproportionately larger amount has to be paid into the organization funds than is ever recovered by benefits. Moreover, it is a rule of the orders that no benefit can be claimed if there has been any lapse in payment.

Trips to town are rare, for the negro family is usually without a mule and has to "chance it" with the neighbors or sometimes on the landlord's farm wagon.

Two-thirds of the negro homes are without a newspaper or magazine of any sort, though one mother explained that they sometimes see a paper in the neighborhood, and she thinks "it makes your mind feel better" to read the paper. Another family brought out three mail-order catalogues which constituted the family reading matter for the year.

Among the negro families the consensus of opinion seems to be that "for a regular stay place, country is the best"—a sentiment almost universally expressed but with interesting variations: "I'd rather live in my smokehouse than stay in town"; the country "becomes poor folks better"; in the country "you're not all scroughed up."

Some strongly disapprove of town with its "racket and foolishness" and are convinced that it is well for children to be reared far from such contaminating influences. "Country children always have to work; town children just play and learn badness." Another mother thinks her children are better off in the country where it is more open and the children have room for play.

One knows the country is healthier; there are more odors in town; when she goes in on Saturdays she comes home with a sick headache every time. "There's more pure fresh air in the country," said one, "and folks in town have to eat canned goods. The country's free and easy; you can raise anything you need." Food and fuel are a consideration with the negro family. One said: "The country is best for me, where I can get my living better, and when I get cold I can get me a piece of wood and make me a fire and when I get ready to go somewhere I can go without stepping in somebody's door." Another woman likes the country where she can get her own wood and light, and raise her own "something to eat."

On the other hand, some would rather live in town. "We have to work so hard for something to eat out here we don't want it when we get it," was the verdict of one. Another has a first cousin in town and likes town best, for "everything is handy and you can run out and get what you want." Two negro women wanted to move to town because of hard work on the farm; "it's a heap harder with the sun burning your back up" than work in town. A woman who had come from town where it was "right good and lively" complained that "here you hardly see anyone pass only about twice a month." Another thinks, however, "there's no call to get lonesome in the country; there's always plenty of work to do."

It is only recently that public attention has been directed to the recreation and social life of rural communities. Certain nation-wide developments, such as the movement for "the school as social center," indicate a marked interest at present, in this phase of rural life. An act of the last session of the legislature of this State "to impove the social and educational conditions in rural communities"[1] is in accord with present-day efforts for more widespread opportunities for wholesome means of entertainment and diversion in rural sections of the country.

---

[1] See p. 109.

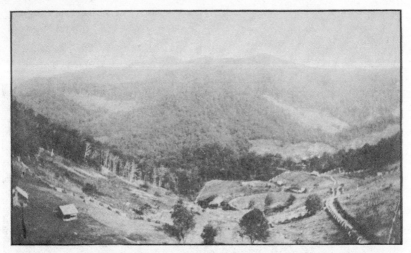

PLATE XVI.—MOUNTAIN COUNTRY OF THE SOUTHERN APPALACHIANS.

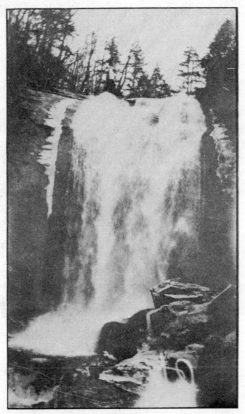

PLATE XVII.—FALLS OF THE TUCKASEEGEE ("SUNNING TURTLE").

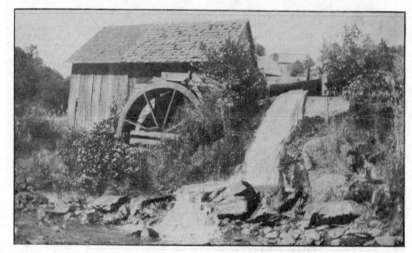

PLATE XVIII.—A MOUNTAIN GRIST MILL.

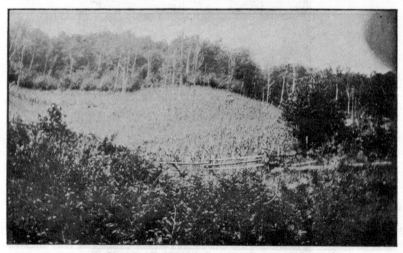

PLATE XIX.—A HILLSIDE CORNFIELD.

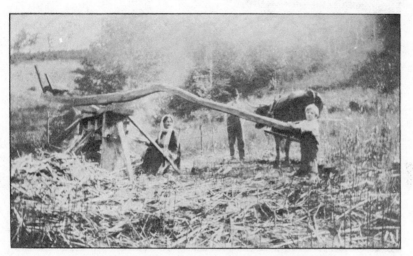

PLATE XX.—GRINDING SORGHUM CANE FOR MOLASSES.

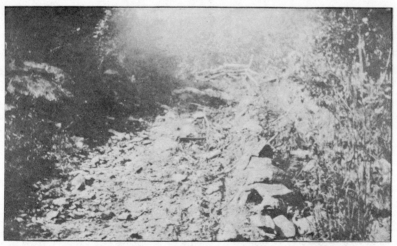

PLATE XXI.—BAD ROADS—AN OBSTACLE TO PROGRESS.

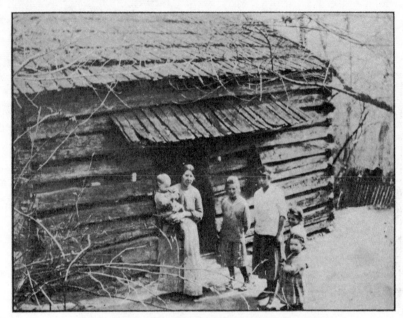

PLATE XXII.—A LOG CABIN IN THE MOUNTAINS.

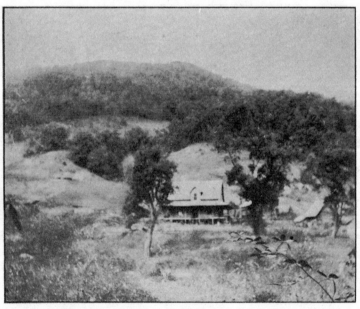

PLATE XXIII.—A MORE COMFORTABLE MOUNTAIN FARMHOUSE.

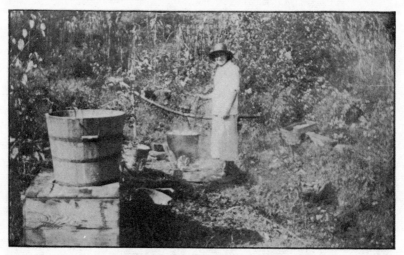

PLATE XXIV.—A MOUNTAIN WASH PLACE.

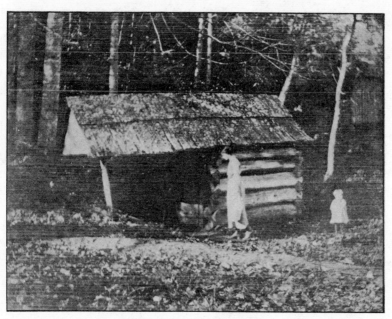

PLATE XXV.—AT THE SPRING.

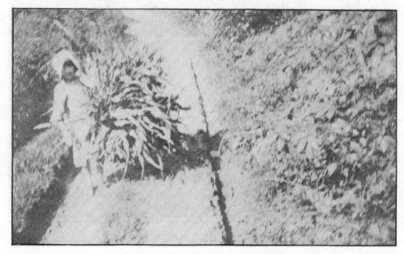

PLATE XXVI.—"TOTING" FODDER.

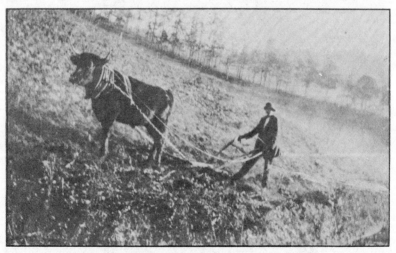

PLATE XXVII.—PLOWING FOR WINTER WHEAT.

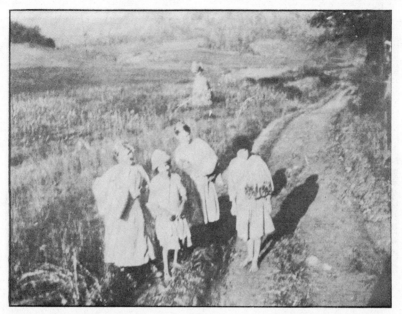

PLATE XXVIII.—ON THE WAY TO SCHOOL, CARRYING CORN TO THE MILL.

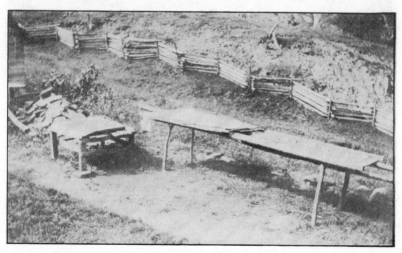

PLATE XXIX.—FRUIT DRYING IN THE SUN FOR WINTER USE.

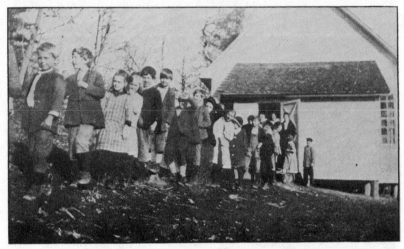

PLATE XXX.—STURDY CHILDREN OF A MOUNTAIN SCHOOL.

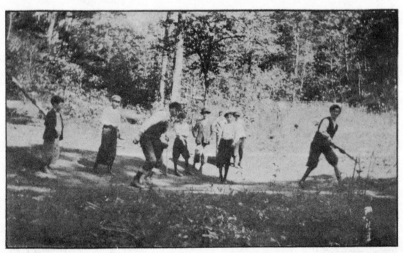

PLATE XXXI.—A SCHOOL "NINE" WITH HOMEMADE BALL AND BAT.

PART III.

THE MOUNTAIN COUNTY SURVEY.

After consulting with various authorities, and after visiting several counties in the western and mountainous sections of the State, a county was chosen for the survey which is thought to be representative of the highland region from topographical, industrial, and economic points of view. It was decided to make the house-to-house study in three distinctly rural townships with a combined population equal to that of the township chosen in the cotton country. The selected areas, while not representative of the most prosperous farming districts of the mountains, are not, on the other hand, an extreme of isolation, but are thought to be fairly typical, embodying many customs and characteristics of the mountain section. From the fact that in the mountain townships chosen, as well as in the lowland county township, all families having children under 16—and not selected families—were visited, we may infer that this is a fair cross section of the rural child population of the mountain country. The survey covered 231 families and included 697 children under 16.

CHARACTERISTICS OF THE TOWNSHIPS.

The selected townships are at the nearest point 4 miles and at the farthest point 25 miles from the county seat, which is their nearest town. It is a rough and rugged country with mountains ranging from 3,500 to 6,000 feet closing in the district on all sides except along the main highway. The broad, rich valley at the county seat becomes more narrow as the roads wind through the mountains and along the noisy streams. Beautiful natural scenery, blue-misted peaks, laurel-bordered streams, and charming waterfalls are characteristic of the mountain country. The bracing and invigorating climate has become famous for its healthfulness and in near-by counties has attracted large numbers of tourists. The summer is short and a rigorous winter closes in early, contributing doubtless to the hardiness of the people. The records of the Weather Bureau over a period of 6 years show a mean temperature of 39° in December to 73° in July and August: a minimum of −9° and a maximum of 96°.

Except for the main highways, the county roads are rough, precipitous, and, in winter, almost impassable. The result is that the mountain family is economically handicapped by the difficulties of

59

crop disposal and is also cut off from social life within the neighborhood, and from the stimulating intercourse with other communities which makes for progress.

Even the main highways are impassable to automobiles for any distance from the county seat except during the summer months; other roads can not be traveled by automobiles at any season of the year; many, as they ascend into the hills, becoming trails which none but a sure-footed horse or pedestrain would attempt. Occasionally the road ends abruptly at a swift mountain stream, and only a good guesser can tell whether to ford up stream or down to find its continuation. Often the road follows the creek and is subject to fierce storms and freshets which wash out the road, leaving gaps, ruts, and bowlders to impede travel.

There is no railway communication, the townships lying 4 to 25 miles distant from the railroad, but scant telephone service (none whatever in one of the townships), and only a "star route" delivery of mail along the main road between post offices.

A large and varied stand of timber is giving way before the logging camps and sawmills, which are gradually pushing into the more distant mountains. Dilapidated flumes down the mountain sides mark the passing of this industry, or rather the exhaustion of the supply. However, the leading industry of the section is still the conversion of timber into various products, and "nowhere else in the temperate zone," according to Kephart, "is there such a variety of merchantable timber as in western Carolina and the Tennessee front of the Unaka system."[1] Quantities of bark and wood of chestnut-oak and other oaks, hemlock, pine, etc., are sold to the tanneries at the county seat. "Pins"—strips of wood used by the telegraph and telephone companies to hold insulators to the poles—are also sold in quantities.

Unlimited water power is found in this section, utilized mainly for running sawmills and the many small gristmills along the mountain streams, where a certain proportion of the grain ground is charged as toll. Grinding by water power in the primitive but picturesque mountain mill is a slow process; a favorite story is told of a bird that flew into the bin for food but starved while waiting for the trickling stream of meal.

Small mica mines are scattered through the mountains; they are owned and worked by families or groups of interested men and furnish an occupation for odd times. The output is bought by agents who travel through the country representing electrical, automobile, and stove manufactories.

---

[1] Kephart, Horace: Our Southern Highlanders, p. 54.

The mountain region is said to be a "natural apple-growing section"; also designed by nature for grass growing, cattle raising, dairy farming, and cheese and butter making.[1]

Farming, on account of the topography of the land, is fraught with many difficulties. Bad roads and distance from market also constitute real obstacles, with the result that, while nearly every man considers himself a farmer, his farming is on a small scale, his object being to raise sufficient food for his family rather than to produce a crop for market.

The early settlers of the mountain country were Scotch-Irish who, after a sojourn in western Pennsylvania, reached the southern highlands by migrating southward through the mountains. These Scotch-Irish along with some Irish and some Pennsylvania Dutch, as Kephart points out in Our Southern Highlanders, "formed the vanguard westward into Kentucky, Tennessee, Missouri, and so onward until there was no longer a West to conquer. Some of their descendants remained behind in the fastnesses of the Alleghenies, the Blue Ridge, and the Unakas and became, in turn, the progenitors of that race which by an absurd pleonasm, is now commonly known as the 'mountain whites,' but properly Southern Highlanders." [2]

The townships chosen for the inquiry are populated wholly by native white Americans, usually of Scotch-Irish descent. This county, like the lowland county, is considerably more thickly settled than the average rural area of the United States. The population density per square mile is 26.3 as compared with 16.6 for the rural area of the entire United States.[3]

FINDINGS OF THE SURVEY.

ECONOMIC STATUS OF FAMILIES.

Mountain homes are scattered along the valleys of the streams and follow the "coves" or depressions in the hillside worn by the swift creeks in their courses down the mountain.

Farm acreage.

Little farming is done except on the "bottom land" along the rivers, where the soil is fertile and yields a rich harvest of grain or potatoes, without being fertilized. The mountain sides are cultivated with difficulty; each family has a garden, a hillside of corn, usually also winter wheat, a small plot of tobacco for home use, sorghum for sirup, and ordinarily keeps bees. The average so-called farmer, cultivating only 6 or 7 acres of corn and still less of wheat, usually raises enough foodstuffs to supply his own family, but has no

---

[1] University of North Carolina Record, No. 140, p. 29.
[2] Kephart, Horace: Our Southern Highlanders, pp. 151, 152.
[3] Thirteenth Census of the United States, 1910, Vol. I, Population, p. 55.

crops to offer for sale. His farm occupies from 50 to 100 acres, only from 10 to 25 acres of which is improved land.

Farming methods in the mountains are primitive. Stolid oxen are commonly the beasts of burden, not only because their cost is less than that of horses or mules but also because they need not be stabled and their strength and endurance particularly adapt them to the mountain country.

Land tenure.

Although a few families of "renters" were found, home and farm ownership are the rule, and farm tenancy is relatively small as compared with the cotton country. When a young couple marry they usually move into a little house on the old home place, "make a crop" of their own, and live there rent free until the land is divided at the father's death, and the portion on which they are living finally becomes theirs. Five-sixths of the families in the three townships either owned their own farms or lived with the grandparents on their land. The neighborhoods visited included a few families of "renters," usually on the most remote and undesirable farms, often on the mountain tops with no road other than a sledge trail of mud. Some renters' families make their crop on two-thirds shares, furnishing the stock and two-thirds of the fertilizer and getting two-thirds of the crop; others "get what they make" in return for various improvements or services performed, such as clearing the land, building the new house, tending stock, etc.

Family income.

Farming in the mountain country does not produce a living, and the mountain family must derive its small income from a variety of sources. After the crop is laid by, the farmer and his boys turn their attention to the timberlands, where they peel bark, make pins, and cut acid wood and cord wood to be hauled to "the railroad" and sold for cash. Bark (used for tanning hides at the county-seat factory) is peeled from black, white, and chestnut oaks and from hemlock; and at the time of the survey was sold by the cord at $11 for the chestnut oak, $8 and $9 for black and white, and $9 for hemlock. Often the farmer hires it hauled to town, paying half what the load brings. Pins for telegraph and telephone poles sell for $4 per 1,000— extremely poor pay when one considers that it takes a man and a boy two days to make that many pins and two days more to haul them to town. If the farmer hires them hauled, it costs him $2, one-half the price of the load. Acid wood brings $5 a load and telegraph poles $3 apiece. Mica mining adds to the family income in some cases. The mines are small excavations in the hillsides, often manned only by the father and the boys of one family, sometimes with four or five neighbors hired to help at $1.25 per day. Many of the men and grown sons go off on what is locally called "public works" during the winter, i. e., at the sawmill, kaolin mine, or lumber camp, where wages at the time of the survey were from $1.50 to $2 a day. A few days' farm labor—helping the neighbors after their own crop is made—adds a few dollars more to the credit of the family. Farm work is paid at the rate of $1 per day for men, 50 cents for women, and 35 cents for children.

A typical family of father, mother, and five children had 15 acres of land in corn; they raised none for sale, in fact had to buy corn for their own use before the season was over. In the course of 12 months they had sold a steer in the "settlement" for $20 and had traded at the country store about $15 worth of chickens and eggs, in addition to 3 bushels of beans at $3 per bushel and 3 bushels of dried fruit at 5 cents a pound; the "men folks" had peeled 5 cords of bark which they hired hauled to town at a profit of $25 and had made and taken to town 6 loads of "pins" at $4 a load. The father of the family "went off to public works" for two months in the autumn as a hand at the sawmill, earning $1.50 per day—a total family cash income from all sources of $167, which must support a family of seven, covering every expenditure, for a 12-month period.

Even with no expenditure for rent or fuel, and very little for food, the meager cash income of the average mountain family is insufficient for its support in any reasonable degree of comfort. Among the families visited, 3 out of 5 had a net cash income of less than $200; 4 out of 5 lived on less than $300; and 9 out of 10 on less than $500.

Farm expenditures.

Although the farm income is low, farm expenses are also low; commercial fertilizer is rarely used for corn and not to any extent for wheat, the average family buying only 4 or 5 sacks at $2 a sack for winter wheat. Hired help is negligible, an occasional day's work is "swapped," and sometimes during the busy season the neighbors help for a few days at a time at $1 per day.

Methods of purchasing.

The average mountain family scorns debt and prides itself on paying cash for everything bought. The long-time accounts, credit systems, crop liens, etc., so common in the cotton country, are non-existent in these neighborhoods. Except for such provisions as soda, snuff, coffee, sugar, soap, and kerosene, usually purchased at the country store, it is customary to send to town for food, clothing, and other supplies to be purchased for cash with the proceeds from the sale of a load of bark or pins. Mail-order purchasing is practically unknown. When something is needed between trips to town, the woman of the house trades a chicken or two at the country store. Eggs, dried fruit, butter, etc., are also disposed of in this way.

Disposal of crops and other produce.

Most of the small amount of farm produce sold is disposed of in the "settlement," i. e., among the neighbors. Corn, potatoes, wheat, sirup, stock, hogs, and sheep are usually marketed in this way. Meats, butter, apples, beans, and cabbages are often hauled to town; sometimes corn and potatoes also. Marketing produce in the rough mountain country is a difficult problem. In some neighborhoods visited the haul to market is from 15 to 25 miles over rough roads—at least an all-day trip and often requiring a day each way. Some few farmers haul their produce to the mill towns of South Carolina—a four to six day trip in "prairie schooners," camping out by the roadside at night.

HOME CONDITIONS.

Housing.

The average mountain home is picturesque rather than comfortable. With his own hands the early settler built for his family a one-room cabin of rough-hewn logs with a deep-sloping shingled roof; no windows, no porches, a door at each side, and a fireplace of rough field stone chinked with mud. So substantial were these early homes that many are still occupied, still attractive, the weathered logs in perfect harmony with the surrounding hills. The log cabin, however, is no longer built; it has been largely supplanted by two other types of homes—the rough shack of undressed upright boards, and the more comfortable modern clapboarded cottage of at least four rooms, with porches, often an upper story, and usually ceiled. Sometimes the old and new exist side by side, with a clapboarded wing, porches, and windows added to the original log cabin.

The interior of a mountain cabin is often unusually interesting; its walls and rafters darkened from the smoke of the open fire in the rough-stone fireplace; stubby little split-bottomed chairs drawn up before the fire; deep feather beds spread with gay patchwork quilts; clean flour sacks of dried beans and apples stowed away in every corner; and festoons of red pepper, strips of pumpkin, and drying herbs hanging from the rafters. A spinning wheel often occupies the place of honor on the front porch, and hanks of snowy wool hang from the rafters waiting to be knit into wool socks for winter wear. On the hillside back of the house one finds a colony of bee-hives locally known as "bee gums," commonly of black gum logs hollowed out and capped with a square piece of board.

In a typical log house of one room, shed, kitchen, and loft—a quarter of a mile up a steep mountain trail from the nearest neighbor—a father and mother are rearing their six children. Asters and cosmos, towering head high, almost obscured the house from view; a little creek dashes past, 50 feet below. Trays of apples and beans were drying in the sun. Inside, the house was not ceiled and the mother had papered the walls with newspapers which, she said, "turned the wind" and kept them warmer and more comfortable, though not so warm as a "tight" (sheathed or plastered) house would.

A little two-room cottage, almost hidden from the road by a dense intervening wilderness of laurel and rhododendron, is the home of a family of father and mother and five children; the house, of upright boards, ceiled inside, was immaculately clean and in perfect order at 8 o'clock in the morning. Snowy hand-woven counterpanes covered the three homemade beds. The open fireplace held an iron pot of beans cooking for dinner. The porch was piled high with wool drying in the sun, and the yard was clean and bright with flowers.

An occasional painted two-story farm dwelling shelters the members of a family who have prospered at farming and on "public works" until they are the owners of a considerable tract of land and are leaders of the settlement in which they live. Comfortable house furnishings, two fireplaces, porches—front and back—a capacious barn, good spring house, and well-built privy all testify to a prosperity above the average.

The common type of mountain home, however, is lacking in certain essentials of a comfortable dwelling place, the most frequent defects being insufficient space, which necessitates overcrowding; insufficient light, due to the small number and size of windows; and the difficulty of heating when the house is a loosely constructed log cabin or unceiled cottage.

A majority of mountain homes in the townships visited were small in spite of the abundance of timber in the vicinity; over one-third are one- or two-room houses; less than one-fifth have more than four rooms. Limited house space coupled with families above the average in size (in over half the homes visited there were six or more persons in the family) results in overcrowding within the house, often quite as serious as in the congested sections of cities. In one-fourth of the homes there were five or more persons to each sleeping room; 38 families of two to nine persons were housed in one-room cabins, cooking, eating, and sleeping in one small room.

At one home a grandmother, a great-grandmother, and three boys— 8, 15, and 21—all sleep in one room. A family of father, mother, and 10 children were living in a cabin of two rooms and loft. At another home the father, 19-year-old son, and two young daughters slept, lived, and ate in one room, cooking in the fireplace.

Keeping the house warm in winter is a difficult problem with most families. Many houses are unceiled, with cracks between the logs or undressed boards. Even with these cracks chinked up with mud and good fires in the open fireplaces and in the cookstove, the house is far from comfortable.

Sanitation.

WATER SUPPLY.—Almost every mountain family draws its drinking water from a clear sparkling spring, which is counted as one of the family's choicest possessions. "It's good water," said one mother, "everybody says it's the best water in this country." Another woman, who had just returned from a visit to her daughter in town, "could hardly drink the town water." She would "drink and drink and then wasn't satisfied."

That there is a real danger lurking in the use of spring water in a locality where insanitary conditions prevail is as yet unrecognized. Many springs are below the house and in a position to receive the house drainage. Lack of privies greatly increases the danger of contaminated water.

Of the 10 wells in the neighborhoods visited, only 3 are of the drilled type—usually considered the safest form of water supply for rural households. One family has had a well drilled through solid rock from top to bottom; the top is cemented, and the well is provided with a good pump. At one home, an open well had been in use until three years ago when, after a case of typhoid fever at the next house, the county physician condemned the well and had the family sink a new one, which is closed in with a tight board platform and has an iron pump.

Another family uses "branch" water through the winter; the spring is so far away that carrying water such a distance in rough weather would be a great hardship. In this case, though there is no house above the family on the "branch," there is no reason to believe the branch water would be free from pollution, for the settlement is not remote, and there is considerable passing back and forth over the mountain.

PRIVIES.—Sanitation falls far short of present-day standards for rural communities. Privies are extremely rare, only 1 family in 10 having a toilet of any description. It is not uncommon to find a considerable prejudice against them, many families disliking, as do some families of the cotton country, the idea of filth accumulated in one place. Where a toilet is present at all it is usually for reasons of privacy; i. e., where the house fronts a frequently traveled road, with no woodland in the immediate vicinity. The intimate relation between good sanitation and good health is little understood. The few privies in the neighborhood—25 among the 231 families visited— are almost invariably built far out over the "branch," the contents washing down the swiftly moving stream. The State board of health is constantly emphasizing the importance of improved rural sanitation and pointing out the direct connection between lack of privies and the transmission of such diseases as typhoid, hookworm, and the diarrheal diseases.

DISPOSAL OF REFUSE.—Garbage is commonly fed to the hogs; other refuse is either burned or thrown, with small idea of a sanitary disposal, into a hollow down the hill, into the branch, raked away from the house, or thrown into the woods.

Manure accumulates in the stable to be used as a fertilizer twice a year, for spring corn and winter wheat. No attempt is made to treat it in such a way as to guard against flies. It is quite common, however, for the barn to be located at some distance from the house, often 100 or 200 yards away, or "on the other side of the hill." Where this is the case, the fly nuisance is less objectionable, but by no means negligible.

FLIES.—Flies are numerous because of the primitive, insanitary conditions prevailing; mosquitoes, however, are rarely if ever seen. No one of the homes visited was adequately screened; some few have screen doors or screens at doors and kitchen windows, but it is only in rare cases that any attempt at screening has been made.

MATERNITY CARE.[1]

During the inquiry 160 mothers, who had given birth to a child—live or stillborn—within five years previous to the agent's visit, were interviewed with especial reference to their maternity care at their last confinement.

Large families are common in the mountains; the women marry early and bear children at frequent intervals. Slightly over two-thirds of the mothers had married at 20 years or younger and nearly half at 18 years or younger. Of 103 women visited, who had been married 10 years or more, 90 (87 per cent) had had 6 or more issues.

Facilities for medical, hospital, and nursing care.

Facilities for the care and treatment of sickness are strikingly lacking in this county. Only five physicians [2]—four at the county seat and one in a village where a normal school is located—overburdened almost to the breaking point, are the dependence for medical service of a population of 13,718.[3] This is an average of 2,744 persons to a physician, which is over four times as many as the average (691) for the United States.[4] The concentration of physicians at the county seat is to be expected, for social and financial reasons; but, because of rough roads, at times almost impassable, and an absence of telephone communication, also because of the prohibitive expense of a day's trip from physician to patient, the greater

---

[1] See discussion of general need for maternity care as given for the lowland county, p. 26.
[2] American Medical Directory of 1916, pp. 1153, 1163.
[3] Estimated for 1916 by the U. S. Bureau of the Census.
[4] American Medical Association Bulletin, Jan. 15, 1917, p. 99.

part of the county is practically cut off from medical service. There
is no physician resident in either of the three townships of the survey,
and the families live from 3 to 25 miles from the nearest doctor.

The county has no hospital, the nearest being located at the county
seat of the adjacent county, reached once a day by mail stage across
the roughest of mountain roads. No trained nurses are resident in
the county, and patients are entirely dependent upon the well-
meaning but untrained services of neighbors and relatives.

Maternal deaths.

The maternal mortality of the county indicates a need for consideration of the problems of prenatal and obstetrical care. During
1916 there were three deaths in the county from causes connected
with childbirth,[1] a rate of 21.9 per 100,000 population.[2] Here, as in
the lowland county, it is impossible to determine whether this rate
is sporadic or usual, since mortality statistics for the State and its
counties are not available earlier than 1916, when the State was admitted to the area of death registration; also, a rate is often misleading when the area is small and a small number of deaths are
considered. However, it is significant that this rate is higher than
the rate (17.3) among the white population of the lowland county,
approximately the same as the rate (21.1) for the white population
of the State as a whole, and distinctly higher than the average for
the death registration area of the United States in 1915 (15.2).[3]

Prenatal care.

Prenatal care of mothers in the mountain country, as in rural
sections of the lowlands,[4] is practically nonexistent; even mothers
living within 6 or 8 miles of a physician rarely consulting him during
their pregnancy, content usually with notifying him of the expected
confinement. Even this precaution is often omitted and valuable
time is lost hunting a substitute when the family physician is away
on a call. No one of the 160 mothers visited can be said to have
had the supervision which has been described as constituting "adequate" prenatal care.[5] Of the 160 mothers, 124, or more than
three-fourths, had had no advice or supervision whatever during
their pregnancy, and no prenatal care of any sort; only 7 had seen a
physician previous to confinement; and only 1 had had urinalysis.
Twenty-eight mothers had been visited by the midwife before confinement—visits, however, usually social rather than professional
in character and not involving a physical examination of the mother.

---

[1] Information furnished by the bureau of vital statistics of the State board of health.
[2] Based on the U. S. Census's estimated population of 13,718 for the county in 1916.
[3] See Mortality Statistics, 1915, p. 59. U. S. Bureau of the Census, Washington, 1917. Sum of the rates
there given for "puerperal fever" and "other puerperal affections."
[4] See p. 29.
[5] See p. 30.

Attendant at birth.

Because of the inaccessibility of physicians,[1] the midwife has necessarily been employed to a large extent for obstetrical work.

The more prosperous and intelligent families called a physician to attend the mother in confinement; 68 of the 160 mothers had been attended by a physician at their last confinement; the others, with the exception of 2 where a relative assisted and 1 where there was no attendant whatever, depended upon neighborhood midwives. In 5 cases at the last confinement and many times in previous confinements the doctor had been late, not arriving until after the birth of the child. Several families who had intended to employ a physician failed altogether in their efforts to reach him.

This inability to secure adequate medical attention at childbirth had often resulted disastrously. A mother in a remote little cabin far up on a mountain trail was very miserable during pregnancy. Twice a week for the last two months her husband went down the mountain to the nearest store and telephoned to the doctor in an effort to keep him informed as to her condition. When labor came on, however, it was impossible to get the doctor, and the mother suffered all night before he arrived and delivered her. One of her twins died at birth.

The doctor was sent for one night to attend a woman in confinement, but the country was "all frozen up" and he said that he could not make the 8-mile trip until the next day. A midwife was called in; the mother's health has been poor ever since this confinement.

A mother whose baby died at birth is confident the child would have lived if they could have got the doctor there in time.

One woman had twins several hours apart; the doctor was late and the mother thinks that without the assistance of a midwife she and the second baby would have died. After this experience she engaged both doctor and midwife for each confinement. The doctor was late also when her last child was born.

Another family tried all night to get a doctor, but the baby strangled before he reached them, though it was born alive.

At one home a midwife was engaged, but when summoned had gone to a "union meeting" at the church and failed to arrive until three hours after the baby was born.

A mother who has lost two of her five children in stillbirth does not know the cause; the babies were both alive when labor began, but the mother always has had a long tedious labor. She never has had a doctor.

A mother of nine children, too isolated in her home at the end of the trail for a doctor to reach her without excessive delay, has never had a doctor in attendance at confinement. On two occasions a midwife

---

[1] See p. 67.

was engaged, but the mother's experience has led her to feel slight confidence in midwifery, and she now prefers to manage for herself, with the aid of her husband and what information she can get from the woman's page of their farm paper. When her first child was born, the midwife came four days before; this made extra cooking for the mother who, in additon, had to carry wood and water. When it was found to be a case of breech presentation, the midwife did not know what to do, and became so excited that she had to be sent away because she was disturbing the mother.

MIDWIVES.—All the 11 midwives liv ng n the district studied were interviewed, also 2 from an adjoining township who are sometimes engaged by women of this section. Eleven are white and 2 negro, ranging in age from 39 to 65 years. Five can read and write and 2 state that they can read but not write; only 3, according to their reports, are licensed by the State board of health. The experience of these 13 women in midwifery had extended over periods of from 5 to 25 years.

Charges ranged from $2 to $5, $3 being the common price. Services rendered included delivery and from one to three postpartum visits if within walking distance. If desired, they stayed from two to seven days, assisting in the work of the household after the mother and baby had been made comfortable. In this case, an extra charge of $2 per week was made.

None of the midwives report any supervision of pregnancy, physical examination of the mother, or urinalysis. With the exception of one who recommends that her patients use sulphur freely to regulate the bowels, no prenatal advice of any sort is given.

In preparation for their cases two midwives use carbolic or antiseptic (bichlorid) tablets; four merely wash their hands. One midwife owns a bag and carries carbolic acid, antiseptic tablets, and spirits of ammonia. Three attempt no preparation of the patient. Ten prepare the bed if they arrive in time. All use old quilts, though four have clean linen before and after confinement, if possible. Quinine, black-pepper tea, red-raspberry, lady-slipper, and other teas are commonly given to hasten confinement. Other remedies are sweet apple bark, cinnamon, garden sage, black gum, star root, hemp, and bead wood.

From one to three examinations of the mother are usually made during labor; three midwives make no examination, one because she believes in letting nature take its course. Another makes no examination so long as the patient seems to be doing well. One makes an immediate examination, for she wishes to be honest with the patient and with herself, and if the child is not "properly placed" wishes the doctor called at once.

Nine have never called a doctor, though a few would do so if the patient were not doing well—that is, if there were a prolonged labor (24 hours or more), a "preternatural present," rigors, or nervousness.

Postnatal care.

Usually the doctor makes no return visit to the mother after the birth of the child; of the 68 mothers attended by physicians only 9 had had any medical supervision after childbirth. The distance from the physician, the almost prohibitive cost of his visits, and the lack of recognition by the mothers of the importance of after care are generally the deterrent factors.

The midwife, if living any considerable distance away, stays sometimes several hours, occasionally for two or three days; where she is a near neighbor it is customary for her to "drop in" every day or so in passing. Of the 89 mothers attended by midwives, in 7 cases the midwife had remained in the home; in 40 she had made one or more postnatal visits. Even the mothers attended by midwives, however, in many cases were left entirely to their own resources after the child's birth.

Nursing care in confinement.

Trained nursing in confinement is wholly lacking. No one of the mothers visited had had the benefit of either a trained or "practical" nurse during confinement; 11 had been nursed by the attending midwives. Of the 160 mothers, 148 were dependent upon untrained nursing—that is, members of the household, relatives, neighbors, or friends.

Rest before and after confinement.

Though not under the strain of helping make a crop for market as in the eastern county, much of the burden of providing for the family falls upon the mother, who often feels that she can not spare the time either for sufficient rest before or a reasonable convalescence afterwards.

As a rule, however, during this period, other members of the family take over the heavier part of the mother's work—washing, milking, and field work; for the last three months of pregnancy, at least, the average mother stops helping with the field work. Thirty-five of the one hundred and sixty mothers, about one-fifth, had continued their field work beyond three months before confinement, this depending largely upon the season of the year in which confinements occurred. Certain weeks of summer and autumn are the busy seasons with the crop, when all possible help is needed in the field.

In this section the mother's period of rest in bed after confinement is usually limited to from 7 to 10 days. About one-third of the mothers visited were in bed two weeks or more, though in a few exceptional cases they were up and about their work in three or four days. A strong wholesome-looking mother of seven children told the agent that everybody wonders that she does not break down and get old; she thinks it is because she is careful to rest sufficiently after

her children are born. She works up to the last minute, for she feels
stronger when carrying her children than after confinement; afterwards, however, she rests for a month, which she thinks is "every
woman's entitlement."

Mother's work.

The work of the mountain mother is burdensome and she bears
more than her share of responsibilities of the household. Her housework includes washing, ironing, cooking, cleaning, sewing, and often
spinning and knitting for the family. Handicapped by lack of modern conveniences, her task involves undue hardship. In most of the
homes cooking is done on a small wood stove, with none of the modern conveniences; often the only implements are iron kettles, pots,
and ovens which may be used interchangeably on the stove or in the
fireplace; the latter is still preferred by many for baking corn bread
and sweet potatoes. A scant allowance of fuel is provided from
meal to meal. During a rainy spell, or when the father is away or
sick, or the children off at school, the mother may be left without
fuel, though wood grows at her very door.

Carrying water, a toilsome journey up and down hill several times a
day, usually falls to the lot of mother and children. No one of the
families visited had water in the house or on the porch, and only 1
out of 5 within 50 feet of the house. Twenty families carried water
over 500 feet and 8 families were from an eighth to a quarter of a
mile distant from their springs.

The wash place, consisting of tubs on a bench and a great iron wash
pot in which the clothes are boiled, is usually close by the spring.
Much straining and lifting and undue fatigue are involved in this outdoor laundry. Sometimes even a washboard is a luxury, substituted
by a paddle with which the clothes are pounded clean on a bench or a
smooth cut stump.

Much of the family bedding is homemade, the work of the women
and girls in their leisure hours, after the crops are laid by or in the
evening by the fireside. Besides the time-honored "log cabin" pat-
tern, their collections of patch-work quilts include such quaint and
intricate designs as "Tree of Life," "Orange Peel," and "Lady of
the White House." Many a mountain home has its spinning wheel
still in use and occasionally one finds an old-fashioned hand loom.
Some homes display a collection of coverlids and blankets, handmade
at every step of the process. The wool was grown on the home farm;
sheared from the sheep; washed, carded, and spun by the women
and girls of the family; dyed, sometimes with homemade madder,
indigo and walnut dyes; and woven on the loom into coverlids and
blankets. Even the designs are often original or variations of old
favorites, like the "Whig Rose," "Federal City," and "High Creek's
Delight by Day and Night."

The other duties of the mother are largely seasonal. From December to August the children are home from school and she has their help. Together they make the garden; help plant the corn and peas for winter; gather them when ripe; pull fodder and dig potatoes; feed the stock; and perform the usual farm chores of milking, churning, and carrying water. In many homes the mother may be found doing chores which are usually considered a man's work, unduly prolonging her working hours and exposing herself to more stress and strain than is compatible with her own health or that of the children she is bearing.

It is uncommon for help to be hired in the home, except occasionally for a few days during confinements. Moreover, with the exception of sewing machines, household conveniences are totally lacking. Hard-working women complained that the men have planters, drillers, spreaders, and all kinds of "newfangled help," but that nothing had been done to make women's work easier.

Practically all the mothers visited, besides their housework and chores, had helped in the fields more or less—hoeing corn, pulling fodder, and so forth. Of 212 mothers, 188, almost nine-tenths, had worked in the field before marriage; 167 since childhood; and 166, or three-fourths of the mothers visited, had helped in the field after marriage.

A woman's field work in the mountain country is not so extensive or fatiguing as in the lowlands where the cotton crop requires the constant labor of the entire family many hours a day during a long summer and autumn. In the mountains, little farming is done, the average family raising no appreciable farm produce for sale. The woman helps plant and hoe the corn and in the autumn helps harvest the crops—stripping fodder, carrying it to the barn, making sirup from sorghum cane, picking beans, gathering apples, and digging potatoes. Her field work is not arduous in itself, but only because it is undertaken in addition to her already numerous duties—caring for the children, housework, sewing, canning, and chores.

INFANT CARE.

Infant mortality.

These townships of the mountain country have a considerably higher—that is, less favorable—infant mortality rate than any of the rural sections so far studied by the Children's Bureau. Of 1,107 children born alive, whose birth occurred at least one year before the family was visited, 89 had failed to survive their first year, an infant mortality rate of 80.4 or a loss of one child in 12. This rate (80.4) is almost twice as high as among the white children of the lowland county (48), and considerably higher than the infant mortality rate in the county studied in Kansas, computed on this same basis, which

was 55 per 1,000 live-born children.   Kephart[1] mentions the high
infant mortality among the mountain children:

> Mountain women marry young, many of them at 14, 15, and nearly all before they
> are 20.   Large families are the rule; 7 to 10 children being considered normal and 15 is
> not an uncommon number; but the infant mortality is high.

The infant mortality rate shows a considerable variation with the
age of the mother, being least favorable where the mother is under
20 and most favorable between the ages of 25 and 29.[2]

AGE AT DEATH AND MOTHER'S STATEMENT OF CAUSE OF DEATH.—
A proportionately greater loss of infant life occurred within the first
two weeks than at any other time within the year, as repeatedly
shown in previous studies of infant mortality.   Of the 89 infant
deaths, 38, nearly half, had occurred within the first two weeks;
7 were deaths of babies 2 weeks, but less than a month old; 17 were
1 month, but less than 3; 8 were between 3 and 6 months; and 19
were 6 months, but less than 1 year.   The proportion of infant
deaths occurring in the last half of the year is considerably higher
than is common and may be attributed about equally to feeding
disorders and to disturbances of the respiratory tract.

Prematurity was the most important cause of infant loss in these
communities.   Of the children that failed to survive their first year,
one in four (22 out of 89) had been prematurely born.   "Bold hives"
is a term encountered throughout the mountains, used loosely to
designate infant ills of various sorts, particularly gastro-intestinal
disturbances and croup.   Seventeen babies, according to the statement of the mothers, had died of the "bold hives."   Ten infant deaths
from gastro-intestinal causes and 14 from respiratory causes were
reported, besides those which may have been included in the blanket
term "bold hives."   There were 2 deaths from measles and 2 from
whooping cough.   Eight were due to the following causes: 1,
"scrofula"; 1, "eczema"; 1 was "found dead in the morning"; 1
was "always sickly"; 1 "took fits"; 1 was "malformed"; 1 "died
all at once"; and 1 was "drowned."   In 14 cases the cause of death
was not reported.

---

[1] Kephart, Horace: Our Southern Highlanders, pp. 258, 259.
[2] The rates are as follows:

Age of mother.	Infant mortality rate.
All ages	80.4
Under 20	133.9
20–24	94.3
25–29	60.0
30–34	60.9
35–39	84.6

(40 and over not shown because such a small number of births occurred at this age.)

STILLBIRTHS AND MISCARRIAGES.—The proportion of children still-born (2.3 per cent) is slightly less than in the lowland county for either white (3.9 per cent) or negro (3.5 per cent) mothers. A somewhat larger percentage of pregnancies had, however, terminated in mis-carriages, 5.5 per cent, as contrasted with 3.6 per cent for white mothers and 5.4 per cent for negro mothers in the lowland county.

Infant feeding.

Feeding records, covering the history of the baby's feedings during the first year of life, were obtained for the last child under 5 years and included 160 children.

As in many rural districts, infant feeding follows traditional methods. Distance from the physician is so great that his super-vision of feeding is out of the question, and books and magazines with articles on infant care are extremely rare. The result is that the mother relies wholly upon the advice of relatives and neighbors and her own experience.

Breast feeding is universal. Every one of the 157 babies for whom records were secured had had some breast feeding from birth up to the ninth month. Weaning is commonly left to the inclination of the baby itself; of the 67 babies weaned by the time of the agent's visit, only 10 were weaned before reaching their first birthday. Commonly they were 13 to 18 months old (33), while 17 were 19 months to 2 years, and 4 were over 2 years at the time of weaning.

In addition to the breast milk the average baby is given from an early age a taste of everything the mother eats. As a rule hunger is the only recognized cause for crying, and the mother's indulgence knows no bounds when it comes to feeding her baby. That the child's stomach is overloaded by indiscriminate and unwise feeding is due not at all to indifference but to her determination that he shall not go hungry.

Catnip, ground ivy, or red alder teas are commonly given in the early months—almost universally for the first three days. Usually after three or four months the child is "fed" tastes of solid food. One mother fed her children after three weeks. "When I went to the table they went with me," she said. Another had fed her last baby catnip tea, coffee, and sweetened milk during the first three days, then sugar and milk to the second month, and after that everything she ate. Her babies "mighty near live on sugar till they are big enough to eat." Often it is the children who "spoil" the baby and begin his irregular habits of eating.

Many, of course, are more careful with the baby's diet. "It doesn't do them much good if you keep burning them up with strong meat and vegetables," had been the experience of one mother. Another had fed her first and second child from birth, but is convinced that she made a mistake, and therefore gave the third and fourth noth-ing but the breast.

PHYSICAL CONDITION OF CHILDREN FROM 1 TO 15 YEARS OF AGE.

General health.

Without a physical examination it is, of course, impossible to make any but the most general statements as to the health of the children visited. The most common illnesses, according to the mothers, are associated with the gastro-intestinal tract—colic, diarrhea, dysentery, and cholera infantum being reported in many cases. Next in frequency came the complications of the respiratory tract, locally designated as "phthisicy" conditions, which were found in numerous households. The child would "choke up" with cold, and be "wheezy," and so forth. "Pneumonia fever" and pleurisy were terms loosely used, but were recognized as being illnesses of serious import.

Contagious diseases, especially measles and whooping cough, were common in spite of the remoteness of the homes. With no public health protection, at the time of the inquiry, in the forms of quarantine, placarding, reporting, and no medical inspection of schools, the children were continually at the mercy of such diseases. Diphtheria and typhoid have also been fairly common. A number of cases suggestive of meningitis were reported and six known cases of infantile paralysis were found (occurring previous to 1916), besides others which it was impossibe to verify. Unlike the lowland county, malaria is rare in this region.

Hookworm or "dew poison" is common, almost universal, among the barefoot children of the mountains. A hookworm campaign was conducted in the county in 1913 by the Rockefeller Sanitary Commission, now the International Health Board of the Rockefeller Foundation. During the campaign 1,202 persons were examined, of whom 774 or 64.4 per cent were found to be infected. This campaign, like that in the lowland county, was confined to the examination and treatment of individuals and did not include the erection of privies throughout the county, which has been the important feature of the more recent campaigns. The efficacy of hookworm treatment is now recognized in this county, but only continued educative work along sanitary lines and a widespread provision of sanitary privies can make such a campaign effectual. When even the schools are not equipped with privies of any description, the public can not be expected to take very seriously the menace of soil pollution.

An interesting disease peculiar to this mountain region and to parts of New Mexico and Tennessee is the milk sickness, or "milk sick," as it is persistently called. This affects all ages alike and is often urged as a reason for substituting other foods for milk for young children. It is said that one or two men of the county claim to be specialists in the disease, which is, however, almost invariably fatal; and not only the public but also the skilled and experienced medical profession of this vicinity have a wholesome dread of "milk sick." The disease is thought locally to have occurred only where the cow has been pasturing in certain shady coves of rich vegetation and usually in the spring of the year. It is said that as these coves are cleared of their dense vegetation milk sickness disappears.

According to Rosenau,[1] milk sickness—

was once very prevalent throughout the central part of the United States, and was one of the dangers our pioneering forefathers had to contend with. In some localities the disease was so prevalent and fatal that whole communities migrated from the milk-sick sections to parts where the disease did not occur.

We are told by Col. Henry Watterson that Nancy Hanks, the mother of Abraham Lincoln, died from this disease in 1818 after an illness of a week. In the words of Col. Watterson, "the dreaded milk sickness stalked abroad smiting equally human beings and cattle." * * * It is an acute, nonfebrile disease due to the ingestion of milk or the flesh of animals suffering from a disease known as "trembles." The affection is characterized by great depression, persistent vomiting, obstinate constipation, and a high mortality * * * there is no known cure or prevention except the elimination of the disease in cattle, which fortunately is rapidly taking place.

Neglect of the teeth, eyes, and ears is particularly noticeable in these communities and affords common cause of distress and disability. The average child is in serious need of dental attention; several cases of "sore eyes" and of trachoma were found; running or "bealing" ears was a common occurrence, a number of children having defective hearing due to lack of suitable attention.

Mortality and mother's statement of causes of death.

Forty-six deaths of children from 1 to 5 years of age had occurred, of which the largest number, according to the mother's testimony, were due to respiratory diseases—4 of pneumonia, 3 of croup, 1 of diphtheria, 4 of whooping cough, and 1 of "lung trouble." Seven children were said to have died of meningitis, 4 of flux, 2 of cholera infantum, 2 of typhoid, and 2 had been burned to death. According to the mother's testimony, in other cases death had resulted from scrofula, bold hives, spinal disease, paralysis, drowning, stomach trouble, diarrhea, "rising" of head and throat, scarlet fever, fever, inflammation of stomach and spine, teething, and 1 "because it was a blue baby." Ten children had died between the ages of 6 and 16 years, of meningitis (2), diphtheria, pneumonia, Bright's disease, worms, typhoid, scarlet fever, 1 from drowning, and 1 of whose death the mother could not give the cause.

Medical care.

The rural child of the mountains, just as was the case with the rural child of the lowland county, instead of being immune from the ills of the city child, is subject to the same diseases and, in addition, is seriously handicapped by the lack of available medical service.

---

[1] Rosenau, M. J.: The Milk Question, pp. 129, 130. Houghton-Mifflin Co., Boston and New York, 1912.

The area studied was from 4 to 25 miles from a licensed physician. The nearest substitutes were two men supposed to be specialists in the treatment of "milk sickness," an Indian doctor living somewhere in the mountains who was said to be an expert in "summer complaint" and skin eruptions, and medical students or traveling practitioners who sometimes pass through the country. The five licensed practitioners of medicine resident in the county,[1] even working to the limit of physical endurance, find it quite impossible to reach the whole countryside. It is unavoidable that the children should suffer from this lack of medical or public-health supervision.

One home is 20 miles distant from the nearest doctor—a day and a half's journey unless one travels by night. Once, 10 years ago, the family sent for the doctor, but he was unable to get a horse, so failed to arrive. The mother in this home is exceptional. She has 11 fine, robust children, all of whom are living, and has amassed a fund of common-sense methods which she applies in rearing her family single-handed, as she must, being completely cut off from medical advice.

This mother "begins with their diet"; she sees to it that they have plenty of fruit, vegetables, milk, and eggs the year round. The baby's milk has her particular attention; she is careful to keep it perfectly clean and has a big box over the spring where the milk can be kept cool and good. She has the children bathe regularly, change their clothes often, and sleep in fresh air summer and winter. She says "the boys are in the river most all summer." When the children appear ill she sends them to bed without supper—only a drink of water, keeps something hot at their feet, gives them salts, and takes care that they are clean "inside and out." Due to the mother's skilled nursing, the whole family weathered even smallpox without a doctor.

Home remedies.

The mountains are full of fragrant herbs noted for their medicinal qualities. Every home, however small, has its stock of herbs, gathered by the housewife each in its proper season and stage of development. The most commonly used were catnip, pennyroyal, and ground ivy for colds and grippe and "to break out the hives"; boneset for coughs and fever; life everlasting, lady slipper, and red raspberry for colds or fever, stomach trouble, or headache, and to "quiet the nerves and make a body rest"; red alder for hives; goldenseal for colic, stomach trouble, sore throat, fever, and as a tonic; partridge vine (also known as wallink, pheasant berry, one berry, and mouse-ears) to break out the hives; black-snake root for cramps, colic, colds, and fever; camomile for stomach trouble; ginseng for colic, stomach trouble, hives, sore throat·or mouth; and gulver root for the

---

[1] See p. 67.

liver. "All sorts of teas" was one mother's explanation of her habits of doctoring. On the other hand, with some families teas are not in favor; one mother "hardly ever uses teas any more"; and another "never could see that teas and such do much good."

Homemade salves, poultices, and liniments are numerous. For sores a salve of heart leaves, carpenter leaves, or balm of gilead, rosin, and fresh butter stewed down; for rheumatism a liniment of kerosene, turpentine, camphor, and apple vinegar in equal parts, with salt; for coughs, a sirup of catnip, horehound, Indian turnip, and honey; and for cuts, bruises, and sores "tincture of lobelia," made by chopping the whole plant and making a strong extract, then adding whisky and straining.

In addition to teas, oil, salts, turpentine, paregoric, sulphur for sores, a patent "pneumonia cure," and various forms of cordials and "drops" (soothing sirups) are popular. Patent medicines are not patronized to any great extent.

Diet.

With the excellent climate and soil of this section a variety of diet is possible. The average family raises in small quantities cabbage, potatoes, beans, beets, onions, tomatoes, corn, sweet potatoes, and pumpkins; occasionally peppers, kershaws (a species of squash), cucumbers, parsnips, and turnips. Fruits are limited to apples, which are raised in abundance, wild grapes, and occasionally peaches. Cereals, milk, and eggs are more common than in the lowland county, and besides the pork—the main dependence of the families in the lowland county—there are also poultry, beef, and mutton.

From spring to autumn may be seen the systematic preparation for winter. Aside from the storing of grain, potatoes, and apples, each yard has its stretchers of drying peas, beans, sliced sweet potatoes, and apples; poles strung with great orange rings of pumpkins, bunches of tawny tobacco and fragrant herbs. Porches are hung with festoons of peppers, onions, and leather breeches (beans strung in the pod). When dried, these stores are neatly packed in "pokes" (flour sacks) and stored for winter.

Much fruit is canned—apples, berries, peaches, etc.—in boiling water without sugar. Jars are packed with wild grapes and filled with boiling sirup; jam, jelly, fruit butter, and pickles of all kinds are made. Apples are "bleached" in great quantities—a process which keeps them white, moist, and juicy like fresh apples, but requires no sugar nor cooking. The apples are peeled, sliced, and turned into a covered barrel or cask with a perforated bottom through which fumes of sulphur are allowed to percolate. The receptacle is kept covered by only a heavy cloth, and apples are added from time to time, and subjected to the same process. Kegs of kraut are made and gallons of beets and beans similarly packed. In fact, if all housewives showed the same thrift, economy, and ingenuity characteristic of the mountain woman, this country would produce enough food and to spare.

The mothers are earnest and hard working in their efforts to do their best for their children, but they lack an understanding of the needs of the growing child. This was shown in the unsystematic, promiscuous feeding, in the preparation of underdone starches, in excess of fats, and in a too hearty diet. Three heavy meals a day are served and food ad libitum between times—potatoes, beans, peas, meat, and big doughy biscuits, or partially cooked corn bread.

This county has no home demonstration agent, no farmers' institutes with their sessions for women—in fact no organized means for an exchange of stimulating ideas and improved methods of household management.

EDUCATION.

In spite of the compulsory-attendance law, the mountain child in the townships visited is not getting his just educational rights. He attends school during the five months' term in a hit-or-miss fashion for a few years, then stops altogether, at an early age, usually under 16 years, before he has acquired even the first essentials of an education. "They have it here now so the children have to go to school," said one mother approvingly of the school law. Another, however, thinks the State has no right to compel children to go to school and then fail to provide good roads and transportation; her children are obliged to cross a deep and very swift creek; the uncertain foot bridge is often out of place; and the children often come home wet to the waist after fording the stream.

School term and attendance.

The school term, at the time of the inquiry, covered from four to five months, usually beginning the first of August and extending to the middle of December. The midwinter school term, customary in most parts of the country, is impossible in this section because of the rough weather, bad roads, and distance of the children from the school; in the spring the children are needed at home to help with the planting.

For one reason or another schooling is continually interrupted, the most common causes being farm work—particularly "fodder pulling" in the fall of the year—and bad weather. In one family the children missed two months out of the five-months' term; they have to "stop out and help a lot" and besides "when it gets too cold and rough they can't travel this mountain." Such irregular schooling discourages even the most ambitious. For example, a 16-year-old boy who has gone a while every year but has had to stop to gather fodder, plow, sow wheat, etc., is so "disheartened" at falling behind his classes that he threatens not to go any more.

A number of homes have no school within a reasonable distance; one-third of the families visited are 2 miles or more from the school; in 39 families children of school age are not compelled to attend at all, since there is no school within 2½ miles of their home, which is the greatest distance they can be compelled by law to travel. An unusually bright, alert 11-year-old boy has only 11 months schooling to his credit; he wants to be in school, but the family lives on a remote mountain top and the 6-mile round trip to the school would be too much for him. The mother of a 9-year-old "teaches him at home." "He's so young and it's so far to walk, and school is confining on a young one," she says. At the home of a family of "renters" living 3½ miles from the schoolhouse, the father is distressed because his three children—aged 10, 12, and 14—are having no schooling; it is impossible for them to go such a distance, especially since they have to travel a steep trail straight up the mountain. He has been hoping for a school nearer in order that the children may attend regularly. "There wouldn't be any day so cold but that we could wrap them up and send them, then," said he. The children's mother thinks "it looks like a renter's children ought to have a chance as well as anybody's." One of the schools attended by the children visited is badly located on the summit of one of the highest mountains in the whole system. A strong, robust adult would find the long climb up the mountainside a trying ordeal. For little children it is almost impossible, and irregular attendance is the result.

Although the majority of children begin school at 6 years of age, over one-fourth are not sent until they are 7 or older because of the distance they would have to travel and the rough weather to which they would be exposed. As a rule a child has stopped school before he is 16.

The short school term and irregular attendance are probably responsible for the slow progress made by many of the children. It was surprising to find that over one-third of the children 10 to 20 years old in the three townships visited were unable to read and write.

Attitude of parents toward education.

At a number of homes, instead of making school a serious business, there seemed to be a tendency on the part of parents to humor the children in their whims. Three children—aged 6, 8, and 10—who did not like the teacher, were allowed to stay home whenever they pleased. Another teacher is severe with the children and the father is afraid to make his boys attend against their will "for fear something will go wrong." One mother "never sends hers until they want

to go; children never study to do good until they take the notion,"
she said.   Another thinks if you send them at 6 they "get a disgust
at school and want to quit." In one family the oldest child, aged 14,
is sickly; "he couldn't go and we kept home the other one (13 years)
to humor him," said the mother.

Many parents, however, in spite of the hard struggle to make a bare
living on the mountain hillsides, with "fighting blood" aroused are
trying to give their children every possible opportunity for schooling.   A mother who herself had to work from early childhood has
always sent all her children to school with a grim determination
to give them a "grand education"; she cheerfully shoulders the farm
work, pulling fodder, cutting tops, etc., in the field all day that the
children may be kept in school.   In another mountain home there
hangs a framed certificate showing that a 9-year-old girl, the youngest
in the family of 10, was neither absent nor tardy during the entire
school term last year.   A girl of 14, another "youngest child," has
gone to seven "schools" (school terms) and has never missed a day
or been late.   One mother, herself illiterate, "wants her children to
be well-educated so they can read the Bible."

A large family in a poverty-stricken little home at the foot of a
high mountain, many miles from the nearest town, has had all kinds
of bad luck, and if it had not been for the mother's ambition for
them the children could not have had a chance.   Once when there
was an unusually good teacher at the subscription school, and the
family could not afford to send the children, the mother went to the
teacher and asked him if he would accept the heaviest pair of wool
blankets she could weave instead of tuition.   He agreed.   She later
made the same arrangement with one or two other teachers.   When
the time came to send the two oldest girls to the town school, the
mother and the oldest boy took a cane mill over the mountains,
making sirup on shares, wherever people raised cane.   They sold sirup
and made enough to start the girls, borrowing the rest with the understanding that the girls would pay it all back the first year they taught.
At the town school the girls made gratifyingly high records in scholar-
ship.   The mother is a splendid type of woman, desperately anxious
that the children shall "learn and get ahead."

It is customary in this county for the teacher to take the school
census before the term begins, a plan which gives her, often a stranger
in the neighborhood, an excellent opportunity to visit and get ac-
quainted with the children's parents.   During the term, however,
little visiting is done; occasionally the teacher goes home with one
of the children for the night and occasionally a mother or father
visits the school to explain why their children must stay at home and
help with the crops.   Nothing like the parent-teachers' associations
of the cities has ever been organized and there seems to be little coop-

eration between the parents and teachers in planning together for the best welfare of the children.

Need for medical inspection of schools.

Several children are missing school because of physical defects, some of which might easily be corrected; with medical inspection of school children and the "follow-up" visits of a public health nurse, much of this absence could be avoided. A 9-year-old boy has been in school for two years, but could not learn anything, so his father took him out last year at Christmas; his eyes were bad and everything blurred when he tried to read. No efforts have been made to have his eyes examined and he will probably be out of school indefinitely. A 12-year-old crippled child will have but little schooling, though a special shoe might remedy the difficulty. The school is only an eighth of a mile away, but the road is rough and slippery, crossing a creek by a foot log, through a boggy meadow, and up a steep rocky hill.

School facilities.

Seven district schools are available for children of the three townships visited; only two of the seven are one-teacher schools. In one school the children can advance as far as the eighth grade; in three, to the seventh; and in the others no higher than the sixth. The schools have not adapted themselves to farm life; none is equipped for domestic science; none is emphasizing improved methods of farming.

Teachers' salaries are low; of the 13 teachers in three townships, 8 were paid at the rate of $40 per month, a total of $200 for the five months' term; 5 received only $30 a month, or $150 for the entire school year.

The schools are well built, ceiled, painted, and in good repair. It was interesting to learn, however, that in order to build the two newest schoolhouses, no school was held for a two-year period in these two school districts, this being the only way funds could be diverted for that purpose.

School equipment is meager and antiquated. Only three of the seven schools have desks and chairs of graduated size, each accommodating two children. The other four manage as best they can with long, old-fashioned, homemade benches, which are uncomfortable, can not be adjusted to the size of the individual child, and afford no desk space. Books, papers, etc., must be held on the lap, which makes it particularly difficult for the children to learn to write. Blackboard space is insufficient, and two of the schools have neither a map nor a globe. Schoolbooks are another of the teacher's problems, the law requiring them to be furnished by the parents, who are often unable, sometimes unwilling, to provide a complete set. In a remote one-teacher school only two boys were supplied with the full collection of books used in their classes. At another school, the teacher reports, they scarcely average two books to a class.

All the schools are heated by unjacketed wood stoves. The older boys keep the stove supplied with wood, chopping it during school hours; the boys work in relays for a week at a time, losing most of the morning lessons during their "turns."

Only two of the seven schools have libraries, in spite of the ease with which one can be secured. The State school law provides for the establishment of permanent school libraries at rural schools, on condition that the local district raises $10; $10 is then added by the county and $10 by the State, and the fund of $30 used to purchase books from a list approved by the State superintendent. The State library commission at Raleigh also has available for loan a traveling library which costs the borrowers only the freight both ways.

Sanitation.

Sanitary conveniences are lacking. One only of the seven schools is provided with a privy for the girls. The other schools have no toilets whatever—a particularly dangerous condition in a country where the spring, so easily polluted, is the common source of drinking water. All the schools obtain their drinking water from springs. A State bulletin [1] stresses the importance of privies at the public school as follows:

In a few sections of our State it is a regrettable fact that at some schoolhouses no provision whatever is made for the proper care or disposal of this excrement. Near-by woods and undergrowth form the only means of privacy. As a matter of fact, it is really more essential that a school be provided with at least two good privies than that it have desks or even a stove. There is absolutely no argument in favor of not having good privies. The absence of such sanitary precaution jeopardizes the lives and health of the teacher, children, and community. Many typhoid fever outbreaks are spread directly by this means.

The school and the community.

The mountain schools are not availing themselves of their opportunity to build up a community spirit and a well-knit community life in their districts. The school building is all too rarely used for purposes other than the school session. Where the church has no building of its own, the schoolhouse is used for church services; also for an occasional political meeting. Two schools have special Friday afternoon programs with recitations or a spelling match; in another there is a fairly well-organized literary society, which meets once a week. The fact that this is attended by the whole neighborhood emphasizes the need of social diversion. One teacher had once arranged a Thanksgiving celebration; another had an entertainment in October; and usually "school closing" is observed by some sort of special program. Aside from these few efforts, the schools contribute nothing to the social life of the neighborhood.

Plans for Public Schoolhouses and School Grounds, pp. 69, 70. Issued from the office of the State superintendent of public instruction, 1914.

CHILDREN'S FARM AND OTHER WORK.

Field work.

The mountain child, as well as the child of the cotton country, does his liberal share of the field work, besides his regular chores at the house and barn. Over nine-tenths of the children visited, 8 to 15 years old, and 11 younger than 8 years, worked in the fields along with their parents, helping to sow and harvest the crops; a number also helped in the timberland after the crops were laid by.

In a typical mountain family, the two boys of 11 and 14 help with the plowing and the planting of corn, dropping and covering the corn by hand, also helping to plant beans and potatoes. Through the summer they hoe corn, and in the autumn pull fodder, gather corn, pick beans, gather apples, dig potatoes, and help make sirup. Their two little sisters of 8 and 9 hoe corn irregularly through the summer and in the autumn pick beans, gather fruit, and help their mother dry the apples and beans for the winter. The children attend to most of the chores also—the boys cut the wood, see that the fires are kept up, and feed the stock; the little girls assist in the home work and help bring in wood and water.

Plowing in preparation for the crops, usually with a one-horse plow, is the work of the men and the older boys. Eighty boys from 9 to 15 years old were "regular plow hands."

Corn is usually dropped by hand; planters are rarely used, partly because of the expense and partly because they are less satisfactory on the steep hillsides. A father of eight children was asked why he had not bought a corn planter. "I already have eight," said he. Forty-two children, boys and girls, "dropped" corn.

Hoeing corn requires the services of the entire family. Practically all the children who did field work of any kind (234 out of 240), hoed corn—children of all ages from 5 to 15 and both boys and girls. Fatigue and some muscular soreness result from the constant striking with the hoe and from maintaining the same slightly stooping posture, grasping the hoe handle in the same position. As a rule, however, in the mountain country the corn field is a mere "patch" and the labor involved is spasmodic, a few days at a time or a few hours a day, unless the family is hard pressed with work after wet weather. In a family of 10 children, the 15-year-old "dropped and the others covered corn; and all who were large enough hoed corn." These children work from 8 in the morning until "just time to go after the cows."

Many children miss school for two or three weeks during the fall of the year to help with fodder pulling.[1] Two hundred children, 132 boys and 68 girls, pulled fodder; 33 were young children 6 to 10 years old, 82 were children under 12 years.

---

[1] For description of fodder pulling, see p. 51.

Children also help bring in the fodder. If it has been tied to the stalks to dry, the stalks are cut by hand, loaded into a wagon or sled, hauled to the barn, and stored away. This can be done only by the men and older boys. Where the fodder has been stacked in loose bundles, even a young child can shoulder and "tote a bundle or two of fodder" to the barn. The fodder is not heavy but rough to handle; it cuts and chafes the skin. Some farmers cut and shock the corn. When this method is followed, only the older children help. The stalks of corn and fodder are gathered, stacked lengthwise about a single stalk, and bound around with a blade of fodder— an operation involving some muscular strain and requiring strength, height, and arm reach, since the corn is tall and the stack large around.

Men and older boys also gather the corn and haul it in. The ears are broken from the stalk, tossed into a wagon or sled, and hauled to the barn. One hundred and four of the older children helped gather corn.

Wheat—a winter crop in this section—is commonly sown broadcast, usually by a full-grown man, sometimes by the older boys, who must be skilled and experienced in order to get the seed scattered evenly. Wheat is sown in the autumn and harvested the next summer. Cradling is the work of a grown man; the boys and girls help in raking, binding, gathering, shocking, and hauling the wheat.

"Grass," or hay, is cut by the men and older boys; mowing machines are occasionally used on "bottom land," but the old-fashioned scythe is necessary on the hillsides. Strength and muscular force are required to swing the heavy blade. In making hay, men and older boys rake the hay from the ground, toss it onto a wagon or sled, and haul it to a corner of the field, where it is forked off and built into one or more stacks, according to the size of the crop. A boy doing this kind of work must have strength enough to toss the hay onto the stack, and strength and height enough to handle the fork.

Tobacco curing, in the mountains, far from being the elaborate process found in eastern North Carolina, consists simply in hanging the leaves out somewhere in the open air to dry, under a shed or on the porch. When the leaves have been stripped from the stalk, they are tied in bunches and suspended from a pole to dry, then done up into twists by the children.

Making sirup from sorghum cane utilizes the labor of every member of the family. Eighty-seven children helped with the sirup making. The older boys help cut the cane and carry it over their shoulders to the cane mill or load it on a sledge drawn by a steer, and bring it down the hill. At the mill a child of 12 can feed the cane between the revolving cylinders, which crush the cane and extract the juice. A younger child often drives the horse, mule, or steer which furnishes the power to run the mill. After the juice has been extracted from the cane, it is strained once or twice through cloth—"a flour poke"—into a long deep vat, in which it boils for from two to three hours. Women and older girls do the straining. While it boils, the thick scum which continually rises must be kept skimmed off, always the work of the older people; toward the end one of the grown women of the family must be on hand to judge when the proper consistency has been reached; after the sirup is taken from the fire it is strained once more; here again the older children help.

Chores.

The mountain child also has a variety of chores about the house and barn. The boys cut wood and bring it in, carry water to the house, take water and dinners to the men in the field, drive the cows, feed the stock, carry slops, run errands, and "go to mill" with corn, while the girls help with the cooking and sewing; cleaning, milking, and churning; drying beans; drying, bleaching, and canning fruit; and taking care of the chickens.

The boys' share in getting in the wood lies in cutting it into lengths with an ax or crosscut saw. Only a few days' supply is made ready at a time, and wood is cut all through midwinter in all kinds of weather. It is hard, fatiguing work, and involves the danger of injury with the saw or ax. Various odd jobs fall to the lot of the older boys, such as clearing ground, cutting briers, chopping weeds, and building fences; that is, simple rail fences, the common type in the mountain country.

If a child is undeveloped, he is spared the usual chores and occasional field work of the average country child.

Lumbering.

After the crops are laid by, the older boys help their father in the timberland, supplementing the scant family income by hauling to town a few loads of bark or pins. In the spring when the sap rises is the time for stripping the bark. After the tree has been cut down, a steel wedge is slipped between the bark and trunk, forcing the bark off in strips—the work of a grown man, sometimes done by a boy of 15 or 16 if large and well grown. The boy's share of the work usually is to pile the bark out of the way as it is stripped, for drying. In late summer the boys help load it on the sled or wagon. Boys also assist in guiding the sled, drawn by a steer, down the mountain to the wagon road; the bark is then ready to be loaded on the wagon and hauled to town. Working with the bark requires considerable strength and muscular force, and fatigue and muscular soreness result from such heavy work. Thirty-six boys from 8 to 15 years and two girls had helped peel bark and pile it out of the way.

Pins formerly were made of locust and brought a good price but, owing to the scarcity of that wood, the industry is no longer profitable and is reserved for odd times. Oak is now used. The tree, after being felled, is sawed with a crosscut saw into 14 to 16 inch lengths; a boy 10 years old can take one end of the saw, his father taking the other. Twenty-five boys and two girls, from 10 to 15 years of age, helped make pins. The actual making of the pins requires two persons, one with an ax and wedge, the other with a maul—home-made of tough, fine-grained hickory. The first worker dents the timber with his ax, then inserts the wedge and holds it in place, while the second deals the wedge a blow with the heavy maul, splitting the timber. The boy usually holds the wedge while the older man wields the maul; occasionally they change about to "spell" each other. As a rule, only a rather well-grown boy over 12 would help make pins, since he must have bodily strength and muscular power sufficient to handle the heavy maul and crosscut saw.

Usually only older boys are sent to town with a load of bark or pins, though two boys—11 and 13—have been making the 12-mile trip alone for three years, driving a double team of horses, mules, or steers. It is usually an all-day trip; the roads are bad, with deep mud holes, bowlders, etc., and are so narrow that considerable maneu-vering is necessary in order to pass another team. The boy must have strength, muscular power, and size enough to hold back a double team down the steep hills; also alertness, for the main roads to town are traveled by cars as well as teams. The trip involves fatigue and muscular and nervous strain. Bark is driven to the acid factory at the county seat and unloaded by the driver; the factory buyer weighs it and pays by the cord, standard prices, according to whether it is chestnut oak, white oak, black oak, or hemlock. Pins are hauled to the railroad and sell as a rule for $4 per 1,000.

Working hours.

Working hours on the mountain farm are irregular. So little land is cultivated that farm work is not continuous; on some days a few hours during the day, on others nothing but chores. During the busy seasons all hands put in a full day's work in the field; but these seasons are concentrated into a few weeks—during spring and autumn plowing, in the summer after wet weather, and at harvest time. Although each family has its own custom, usually a workday begins about 6 in the spring and summer, 7 or 8 in the autumn, and ends at sundown, with an hour off for dinner. Some families prefer to "lie late" in the morning to avoid the heavy dew, and then work until dark instead. The children of one family work from "dawn to dark" when not in school; they are up before dawn, do the chores, feed stock, gather fruit, carry slops, do the milking, then go to the field.

Wages when at work away from home.

As a rule, the children doing farm work, work only on the home farm, helping their own family. A few of the older children, usually over 12, also work out for wages, often for relatives, a day or two at a time and not more than two or three weeks during the season, when work on their own crop permits. Some instances were found of younger children working out. A 10-year-old boy hoed corn about 10 days last summer, making 50 cents a day for a 10-hour day. A boy of 11 hoed corn for his uncle during the past two summers, five or six days each summer, at 25 cents for the regulation 10-hour day. Two boys of 8 and 10 hoed corn and helped with the fodder at 25 cents per day. A boy of 11 plowed, hoed, helped with the hay, corn, and sirup for a few days at 40 cents a day.

RECREATION AND SOCIAL LIFE.

Social life in the mountains is extremely limited, in most neighborhoods resolving itself into attendance at "preaching" once a month, Sunday school "rally," and county fair once a year, and visiting among the neighbors in the immediate vicinity.

Even church is often inaccessible and out of the question in rough weather. A mother of a poor tenant family high up on a mountain top laments that her children never get to Sunday school or "preaching"; on Sunday she reads the Bible to them and has the blessing, and "that's the best I can do," she said. Another mother takes her children to church once a month and to Sunday school occasionally. They have no way to go, however, unless they walk and it is "much too worrisome a trip with children." A family, out of reach of church in any direction, explained that they used to have preaching over across the mountain, but not enough people went, so the preacher refused to come any more.

Where the children can get to Sunday school their enjoyment of it is intense. A little 10-year-old girl has kept all her Sunday school cards from last year and this, and has them pasted on a piece of cardboard and tacked up on the wall. The annual Sunday school "rally" is one of the few community gatherings to which all the families take their children and their dinners, and spend Saturday and Sunday at the church, singing and visiting and listening to the "circuit rider." Elaborate preparations are made; hogs and beef are butchered, chickens killed, all the best jellies and preserves are brought out, and bread and cake baked in abundance for the picnic dinner spread beneath the trees.

The schools, as has been said, are used very little for social purposes. One school until last autumn had never had an entertainment as far back as anyone could remember, another had planned for one last year, but it rained. At a more enterprising school, however, was found an interesting and flourishing literary society, so successful that it is filling the schoolhouse at its Friday night meetings. At one of the meetings, after several recitations by the younger children, six of the older boys debated cleverly on "*Resolved*, That Washington deserves more credit for defending America than Columbus for discovering it."

Lack of organization, of community interests, and of "teamwork" have long been characteristic of the mountain people. Aside from the few men who maintain membership and a lukewarm interest in the Masons, Odd Fellows, or "Juniors," there are no clubs of any sort in the neighborhoods visited. In less than one-tenth of the families was there any member of the family belonging to a social organization.

Books are seldom bought and, as a rule, only from traveling agents; a very miscellaneous collection of reading matter is secured in this way. Newspapers and magazines are rarely found in mountain homes. Over half the families visited take no periodical of any sort. The county paper is subscribed to most frequently; about one-fourth of the families were taking farm papers. Only 9 of the 231 families visited had subscribed to any of the woman's magazines.

One father would take a newspaper, but can not spare the time to make the 11-mile round trip to the post office across the mountains—almost a day's journey. A magazine, particularly if illustrated, is treasured highly. A 14-year-old boy is "so fond of reading that when he has a book or paper he won't go to bed until he has read it."

The smaller children, as well as the older ones, are in need of means for recreation. The play spirit is conspicuously absent. Toys are uncommon; the few dolls of the neighborhood are too highly prized for common use as playthings. A little crippled girl has two Christmas dolls, still in the boxes in which they came two or three years ago, tacked up against the wall.

The isolation of the mountain people, particularly the women and children, their lack of intercourse with their neighbors, with the townspeople, and with the outside world can not fail to impress the visitor. Bad roads and lack of conveyances, together with scarcity of telephones and absence of mail service close at hand, are largely responsible for cutting off the family from outside communication. The rural free delivery has not yet penetrated to the neighborhoods visited. They have instead the "star route" system by which the mail carrier travels only the main roads between post offices. Families living at a distance from the post office find it difficult to make the journey for their mail with any regularity. One family, at the end of a steep mountain trail, visited September 5, had not been to the post office for mail since July.

Trips to town are infrequent.   Town shopping for the whole family is largely intrusted to the "men folks," and their many natural
blunders in selections of feminine apparel are accepted with stoical
fortitude.   "There's no call for me to go to town," said one woman.
In a probably typical family the father goes to town every week or
two, the mother once or twice a year, and the older children about as
often as the mother, though they "are like their father and would go
every week if they had a chance."

Often it is the difficulty of taking young children that keeps the
family so closely at home.   A mother, who has not been to town for
three years, "likes to go, but with such a crowd of children (seven)
she can't figure how to take them all along."   A mother at the end of
a lonely trail has never been to town in her life; she has not been to
the country store—5 miles away—since her oldest girl (now 15) was
a baby, but "aims to go next spring if she lives and nothing happens,
and do her own trading again."   A mother who leads a lonely life,
with her husband off on "public works" and the children at school,
has never been to a fair or a show in her life and never gets away
from home at all except to her nearest neighbors, a quarter of a mile
down the mountain.   A bad trail, merely a sledge road straight up
the mountain, leads to their cabin, the last of that cove; it is rarely
that anyone comes along that way.   Another has never seen a railway train in her life; she went to the county seat once with her husband—15 years ago, the day after she was married—but the train
was late, and it was so cold that they could not wait and had to come
back to the mountains without seeing it.   Her husband gets to town
two or three times a year.   None of the children has ever gone
except the oldest, who went last year to "show the doctor her ton-
sillitis."

Few families have a conveyance of any sort; aside from three sur-
reys in the neighborhoods visited, travel must be performed in a farm
wagon or, more commonly, afoot.   Sometimes the wagon, loaded
with pins or bark, drawn by a pair of oxen, is accompanied to town
by various members of the family who, though walking, can easily
keep pace with the slow-moving oxen.   One family that seldom leaves
the neighborhood had "planned on going" to the county fair this
year, but could not get room in the neighbor's wagon and owned no
team.

Few of the families visited expressed any desire to move to town.
A mother of 13 children was proud of the fact that "not one of my
children wants to go to town to live."   Of one man strongly averse
to town it was said "the quickest he can get away is too long for him."

Some of the mountain families visited had lived elsewhere and
returned to the mountains.   A family consisting of father, mother,
and four children are all glad to get back from the mill village.

The mother thought she could not endure spending her life there where she had to put each child to work as soon as possible. She had been so sorry for the country people who had sold out before going to the mill and had no home to come back to. Another family had tried the mills for three years but were glad to get back to the mountains, "where there is freedom and enough to eat and burn." In another family the children all liked the mill town better than the mountains, and the family would have stayed there, but contracted measles; one boy died, and the grandfather was ill for four or five months. Another mother has no use for a cotton mill, "you burn up in there with no air; the children never got to sit down from the time they went in in the morning till they came out at night, 11 hours."

On the other hand, the hardships of the mountains have so impressed themselves upon the lives of the people that some are anxious to leave for the sake of the children, if not for themselves. A mother in a lonely cabin on the mountain top does not like the mountains, but "a poor man can't buy a river farm." She "wants to move down lower because of schooling and preaching."

Another woman on one of the best farms in the country, who was herself reared in town, wishes to move back to town next year that the children may be near good schools and get to church and Sunday school and have the doctor at hand. Also, she misses the fresh meat and the good things one can buy in town. One mother complains that "a body has to work mighty hard to live and hardly can live in this country." Another "would rather live in a smoother place than in this steep country, but not in a city; it's too binding in"; she wants to "make her own beans and roasting ears."

One family is divided among itself; the father has no use for towns, the mother would not live there unless she could have her garden and chickens; she "would rather live on a farm if she had a real farm, but gets tired of these mountains where you can't raise anything." The two oldest girls are not satisfied with the old cabin on the creek and want to move to town, and the boys, too, "want to go where they can see more."

Rural communities such as have been described in this mountain county, where isolation and a lack of community spirit are characteristic, are especially in need of such plans as the State superintendent of public instruction and the executive secretary of the State bureau of community service are developing in connection with a recent act of the legislature to provide for the incorporation of rural communities.[1]

_____

[1] See p. 109.

PART IV.

SUMMARY AND CONCLUSIONS.

The findings of these surveys of child care in a typical lowland or cotton-raising county and in a typical mountain county of North Carolina are significant not only for the counties studied, but also for rural areas in many of the southern States.

The population of the areas studied is uniformly native-born American of native parentage—in the lowland county about evenly divided between the whites and negroes, and in the mountains exclusively white. In the lowland county, farming is pursued largely under a system of tenancy, two-fifths of the white and three-fourths of the negro farmers visited being tenants. Farm acreage is small; about half the white and over four-fifths of the negro farms visited are "one-horse" farms; that is, worked with one horse or mule, and with only approximtaely 25 acres in cultivation. Cotton is the "money crop" and is an expensive crop to produce. The small tenant operates his farm under the heavy handicap of the crop lien system.

In the mountain county, farming, on account of the topography of the land, is attended with difficulties. Although nearly every man considers himself a farmer, he farms on a small scale, with the object of raising sufficient food for his family rather than producing a crop for market. The average farm occupies some 50 to 100 acres with only 10 to 25 acres of improved land. The scant income derived from farming must be supplemented by the sale of timber products at the county seat, by mica mining, and by "public works" at the sawmill, kaolin mine, or lumber camp. Although there were a few families of "renters," tenancy is not nearly so common as in the cotton country, and the majority of families own their homes and the land on which they live.

The children's home environment in the lowland county families visited varies widely according to the economic circumstances of the family, the children of the landowners having more comfortable as as well as more healthful surroundings than the tenant's children. Lack of sufficient house room at many tenant homes is perhaps the most serious housing defect, resulting in overcrowding, particularly of sleeping quarters. Sanitation is a serious problem; more than half the homes of white families and four-fifths of the negro homes have no privy of any kind; at a number of homes, drinking water is obtained from a dug well—obviously an unsafe source of supply, particularly in a district where soil pollution is widespread.

The typical mountain home is picturesque rather than comfortable. Certain housing defects are common; notably lack of sufficient house space, which results in overcrowding, especially of the sleeping rooms; insufficient light, many of the older cabins having no windows other than heavy wooden shutters, which, when closed, leave the room quite dark; and the difficulty of heating loosely constructed cabins and rough board houses during the severe winter weather. Sanitation is primitive. Nine families in 10 have no toilet of any description. The spring, the common water supply, is dangerously subject to pollution because of the absence of privies.

Both counties have a strikingly high maternal death rate from causes pertaining to childbirth—in the lowland county, 41.5, and in the mountain county, 21.9 per 100,000 population, as compared with the rate, 15.2, for the entire area of death registration.[1] In the lowland county, though the rate for white women, 17.3, is somewhat higher than the rate for the death registration area, the high total death rate is due to an alarmingly high rate, 93.9, among negro women.

An urgent need for provision for maternity care was one of the most important findings of the survey; facilities for guarding the health and life of the mother at childbirth are totally inadequate in the rural communities visited. In the lowland county, though two-thirds of the white mothers were attended in childbirth by a physician, one-third of the white mothers and over nine-tenths of the negro mothers had employed a negro midwife. A physician was often out of the question for various reasons such as cost, distance, scarcity of telephones, and bad roads during part of the year. It was evident from the testimony of the mothers that the midwife was a precarious dependence when complications had arisen. Ample facilities for hospital care are available at the county seat, from 4 to 14 miles distant, where two hospitals are located. This county has also made an excellent beginning in public-health nursing, with a nurse for white and one for negro women; their time, however, is so largely occupied at the county seat and in the surrounding mill villages that they are unable to render any appreciable amount of nursing service in the rural districts of the county. Few of the mothers visited had had any prenatal advice or attention. Nursing care at confinement, except in a few families who had engaged a midwife as nurse in addition to the doctor, consisted of the untrained services of relatives and neighbors; none of the mothers had engaged

---

[1] Mortality Statistics, 1915, p. 59. U. S. Bureau of the Census, Washington, 1917. Sum of the rates there given for "puerperal fever" and "other puerperal affections."

a trained nurse, and only two a "practical" nurse. The majority of the mothers also failed to receive adequate supervision during their convalescence after childbirth.

In the mountain county no physician is resident in any of the three townships of the survey, and the families live from 4 to 25 miles from the nearest doctor. There is no hospital within the county, the nearest being located at the county seat of the adjacent county, reached once a day by mail stage across the roughest of mountain roads. There are no trained nurses in the county, and patients are dependent upon the well-meaning but untrained services of relatives and neighbors. Trained nursing in confinement was wholly lacking. No one of the mothers visited had had the services of either a trained or "practical" nurse during confinement; some few had been nursed by attending midwives; the others, by relatives, neighbors, or friends. Prenatal care is practically nonexistent; more than three-fourths of the mothers visited had had no advice or supervision whatever during their pregnancy. Over half the mothers were attended in confinement by a neighborhood midwife. Inability to secure medical attention at childbirth had sometimes resulted disastrously, according to the testimony of the mothers. Postnatal visits are rarely made by the physician, but where a midwife lives close by, which is often the case, it is customary for her to "drop in" every day or so in passing.

The Children's Bureau, in a publication on Maternal Mortality,[1] suggests that the following plan is essential in order to secure adequate medical and nursing care for mothers and babies in a rural county:

1. A rural nursing service, centering at the county seat, with nurses especially equipped to discern the danger signs of pregnancy. The establishment of such a service would undoubtedly be the most economical first step in creating the network of agencies which will assure proper care for both normal and abnormal cases. In the rural counties in the United States which already have established nurses, the growth of this work will be watched with the greatest interest.

2. An accessible county center for maternal and infant welfare at which mothers may obtain simple information as to the proper care of themselves during pregnancy as well as of their babies.

3. A county maternity hospital, or beds in a general hospital, for the proper care of abnormal cases and for the care of normal cases when it is convenient for the women to leave their homes for confinement. Such a hospital necessarily would be accessible to all parts of the county.

4. Skilled attendance at confinement obtainable by each woman in the county.

In the lowland county, the most immediate need in respect to maternal care seems to be for the employment of a rural nurse for the white and one for the negro women of the rural sections of the

[1] Meigs, Dr. Grace L.: Maternal Mortality from all Conditions Connected with Childbirth in the United States and Certain Other Countries, p. 27. U. S. Children's Bureau Publication No. 19. Washington, 1917.

county, which are now out of reach of the public-health nurses at the county seat. Prenatal care and assistance at confinement, also postnatal supervision and advice as to the care of the young baby, would be important phases of the work of the rural nurse. In the mountain county, a cottage hospital at the county seat would prove of value to the mothers within a radius of a few miles; while roads continue to be as poor as at present, however, any facilities at the county seat will be inaccessible to the greater part of the county's rural population. There is an obvious and immediate need for rural nurses, to visit the mothers in their own homes. This county at present, unlike the lowland county, has no public-health nurse. The ways in which a nurse could be of help to mothers in this district have been indicated.

Although even one public-health nurse in a county can accomplish much along educational lines as to the proper maternity and infant care and the care of the school child, on account of the territory to be covered, one nurse alone obviously can not meet all the needs of the rural mother and child. The ideal which has been attained in a few counties is the division of the county into smaller districts with a county nursing service and community nurses; in a small district the nurse can do bedside nursing and nursing at the time of confinement, as well as more general educational work. Methods of initiating a rural nursing service on the county plan are described in a recent publication of the Children's Bureau [1] as follows:

In certain counties the work was established at first through private subscriptions; enough money was raised in this way to support a nurse for a period of 6 to 12 months; after the value of the work had been demonstrated the county authorities appropriated money to continue it. This was in recognition of the fact that public-health nursing is not a charity but is a measure for health protection to which all the people of the community have a right. In one county in a Middle Western State a federation of women was formed which included all the organizations of women in the county—women's clubs, ladies' aid societies, and parent-teacher associations, as well as small neighborhood groups of rural women. Largely through the efforts of this federation a tax was levied by referendum vote and a large sum of money provided for health work. Two nurses are now employed by this county.

In many counties the nursing service has been established through the employment of a nurse for the rural schools, and this method has proved very successful. In other counties the nurse has begun her work as a tuberculosis nurse; in others as an assistant to the county health officer. Whatever the beginning of the work, the nurse soon finds that the assistance which she can give to mothers in the care of themselves and of their babies is one of its most important developments.

In planning a rural nursing service two things are essential:

1. Every effort should be made to get the right nurse. The nurse employed should have had training in public-health or visiting nursing such as is given now in many training courses, and should also have practical experience. Nurses who have had hospital training only are not fitted to carry out public-health nursing successfully.

2. Ample provision must be made for transportation through the county.

---

[1] Moore, Elizabeth: Maternity and Infant Care in a Rural County in Kansas, pp. 49, 50. U. S. Children's Bureau Publication No. 26. Washington, 1917.

The communities visited in the lowland county have a low rate of infant mortality—48 per 1,000 live-born white children, a loss of 1 child in 20, and 64 per 1,000 live-born negro children, a loss of 1 child in 16. The considerably higher death rate among negro infants, as well as the previously mentioned higher maternal death rate among negro mothers, indicates a need for further efforts directed toward prenatal, maternal, and infant care for the negro population. The mountain townships visited have a considerably higher—that is, less favorable—rate of infant mortality than either of the rural sections so far studied by the Children's Bureau. Of 1,107 children born alive at least one year before the agent's visit, 89 had failed to survive their first year—an infant mortality rate of 80.4, a loss of 1 child in 13 as compared with a rate of 55 in a Kansas county studied by the bureau,[1] and 48 in the lowland county of this survey. Even in the mountain county, however, the rate of infant mortality is low as compared with the rate in cities and towns.

In the mountain county, prematurity was the most important cause of infant loss. One child in four that failed to survive its first year had been prematurely born. Moreover, nearly half the infant deaths had occurred within the first two weeks. This is additional evidence of the urgency of prenatal care for the mother, additional evidence also of the need for a rural nurse who as one of her duties would advise the mother as to prenatal and infant care.

It is significant that the comparatively low rate of infant mortality of the rural communities visited, in both the lowland and the mountain county, is coincident with universal breast feeding of infants. In the lowland county, all the 78 white babies for whom feeding histories were secured had been nursed during the first five months; of the 86 negro babies, all were breast fed during their first two months; in the mountain county, every one of the 115 babies for whom feeding histories were secured had been nursed from birth up to at least the ninth month of age. In both counties nursing is usually continued well into the second year. In addition to breast feeding, however, the babies are often indulged from an early age in tastes of family diet.

The interest shown by the mothers in having their children examined at the children's health conferences held by the Children's Bureau in the lowland county, suggests the desirability of a periodic examination of infants with opportunities for informal advice to the mothers as to infant care. Such examinations might be held by physicians, with a public-health nurse in attendance, at accessible centers scattered through the rural sections of the county. The nurse might also establish her headquarters at these centers where

---

[1] Maternity and Infant Care in a Rural County in Kansas, p. 41.

she could be available for consultation with mothers who need her advice and from which centers she would visit homes and schools of that district.

The rural child is subject to the common diseases of the city child and is handicapped by the lack of medical care in sickness. In the absence of a physician within a reasonable distance, and of a county nursing service, the mother is thrust upon her own resources in case of sickness, and must rely largely upon home remedies. In the low-land county, patent remedies, especially croup and cough "cures," liniments, soothing and teething sirups, remedies for women's diseases, and for constipation have a widespread sale. A recent "secret remedies" bill recommended to the State legislature of 1917, by the State board of health, failed of passage. In the mountain families, and in some of the white and most of the negro families of the lowland county, "doctoring" with native herbs is customary. A periodic physical examination of the school children, as proposed by the State board of health, should be an important step in the checking of disease.

Family diet from the point of view of the growing child leaves much to be desired; it is probable that the heavy diet of the average family, with an excess of fat and partly cooked starch, and a deficiency of fruit and vegetables except during the summer months, together with the custom of indulging children in promiscuous habits of eating, is a factor in the indigestion which according to the mothers is one of their chief difficulties. Diet is more varied in the mountain than in the lowland county, but is still scarcely adapted to the needs of the child.

There is a very obvious need in these rural communities for increased attention to educational opportunities for the children. Under the terms of the school law, attendance is compulsory for children between 8 and 14 years for only four months of the school term, but even this is practically unenforced. The school term is short—commonly five months for white and four months for negro schools—and this, together with irregular, spasmodic attendance makes progress difficult. The rough roads, bad weather, and need for help with the farm work are responsible for the irregular attendance. Between the ages of 10 and 20, approximately 1 white child out of 10 and 1 negro out of 3, in the lowland county, had not learned even to read and write; in the mountain families, this rate was approximately 1 out of 3.

In the lowland county communities, two of the white school districts have voted the special school tax and have well-built, well-equipped schoolhouses. Three of the white schools, however, and all the negro schools are one-room, one-teacher schools. School sanitation is notably deficient. Only one of the five white schools has one toilet for boys and one for girls; two have one for the girls only, while two of the white schools and all four negro schools have no toilet facilities whatever. In the mountain townships visited, most of the seven school districts have new buildings, painted and in good repair; school equipment, however, is meager and antiquated. Sanitary conveniences are lacking. Only one of the seven schools is provided with a privy for the girls, and the other schools have no toilets whatever, a particularly dangerous condition since the spring is the source of drinking water.

The children of the family performed a considerable share of the farm labor on their home farms, working in the fields along with their parents, helping to sow and harvest the crops, a number in the mountains also helping in the timberland after the crops were laid by. In the lowland-county communities, two-thirds of the white children and three-fourths of the negro children 5 to 15 years old, in addition to doing a variety of chores, helped in the fields, cultivating and harvesting the crops, particularly chopping and picking cotton and hoeing corn. In the mountain country, farm work is irregular, since little farming is done, and usually the busy seasons with all hands putting in a full day's work are concentrated into a few weeks.

Although early training in habits of industry is desirable, and though a reasonable amount of farm work would scarcely injure a healthy child of sufficient size and strength, children's work on the farm, such as is described in this report, has certain objectionable features, the most serious of which are the undue strain upon the strength of the child, the interruption of his schooling, and, in the lowland county, the ill effects upon his health of prolonged exposure to the heat of the sun.

In the lowland-county township, opportunities for recreation and social intercourse are more numerous than in many rural communities. School entertainments are given occasionally, and other means of social diversion are popular, such as picnics, ice-cream suppers, swimming parties, individual entertaining and visiting, and Saturday trips to town. Clubs and lodges of various sorts are found. Three-fourths of the white families subscribe regularly for some sort of publication, usually weekly rural editions of the county papers. Migration from country to town is rare, and the average family is satisfied with country life.

Negro families also have ample means of social intercourse. Church is their common meeting place and frequent services are held. The schools occasionally arrange an entertainment to raise money for some needed article of equipment. Clubs and societies are common among the adult negroes, and are usually organizations which pay a benefit in case of sickness. Trips to town are infrequent, due to a lack of mules and conveyances. The negro family also is genuinely content with country life.

In the mountains facilities for recreation are extremely limited and badly needed. Social intercourse consists largely of attending "preaching" once a month, county fair once a year, and an occasional visit to the neighbors in the immediate vicinity. There is a marked lack of community interests and of social organizations of any sort. Books, newspapers, or magazines are seldom found in mountain homes. Few families have a conveyance of any sort, hence trips to town are rare, especially for the women and children. Here, as in the lowland county, few families expressed a desire to move to town. Some, however, were eager to leave for the children's sake—to be more convenient to school, church, and doctor.

PART V. APPENDIX.

THE STATE AND ITS RELATION TO CHILD WELFARE.

STATE BOARD OF HEALTH.

Through an exceptionally effective, progressive-minded State board of health, alive to the needs of the rural population, which constitutes a large portion of the inhabitants of the State, much is being accomplished along the lines of public health and sanitation.

ORGANIZATION.

With an original annual appropriation of $100 in 1877, the State board of health soon made itself a necessary factor in the welfare of the State. In 1909 the services of a full-time health officer were secured. Since then public health work has developed into a well-organized department with an executive office, State laboratory of hygiene, State sanatorium and bureau of tuberculosis, and bureau of engineering and education, vital statistics, rural sanitation, soil pollution, and accounting. In 1916 the State ranked twentieth in per capita expenditure for public-health work, $0.026, the expenditures of the other States ranging from $0.0073 in Tennessee to $0.1521 in Florida, according to compilations by Dr. Charles V. Chapin, for the American Medical Association.[1]

BIRTH REGISTRATION.

The "model law" for birth registration went into effect in North Carolina July 1, 1913. Its enforcement has been particularly difficult in this State because of the rural character of the population, and also because of the large proportion of births attended by midwives. In June, 1916, registration of deaths was considered complete enough to warrant the inclusion of North Carolina in the death registration area of the Bureau of the Census. Recently (December, 1917), the inclusion of the State in the census area of birth registration marks the culmination of the effective efforts of the State board of health toward improved statistics.

As a test of birth registration in the areas covered by the survey, all births which had occurred in 1915 (found by house-to-house visits during the course of the inquiry) were checked back to the

---

[1] Sixteenth Biennial Report of the North Carolina State Board of Health, 1915-1916, p. 17.

records at the county seat. Of the 61 births occurring in that year in the township of the lowland county, 48, or 79 per cent, had been registered. In one of the mountain townships, none of the 21 births occurring in 1915 was registered; the registrar appointed for the township had refused to serve and the office was allowed to remain vacant during the entire year. Another mountain township had registered 21 out of 23 births, and the third, a small, remote township 20 miles from the county seat, had registered every one of its 13 births.

EDUCATIONAL CAMPAIGNS.

To interest the general public in hygiene and sanitation, the board of health has in constant use a portable motion-picture outfit suitable for work in rural districts, a series of illustrated stock lectures, traveling exhibits, and an extensive press service. The motion-picture health films reach, among others, a large class of people who read very little, and these films present to them in simple form the principles of sanitation and disease prevention. The picture show makes the rounds of rural schools in an automobile, which carries an extra engine to run the lights and furnish power for the pictures. A "Charlie Chaplin" movie lends variety to the health films and a victrola furnishes music during the changing of reels.

Outfits of lectures on health subjects, illustrated by a set of lantern slides with a stereopticon lantern, are furnished free of charge to Y. M. C. A. workers, teachers, preachers, and others interested in public health. The traveling exhibit presents the more important health problems by means of charts and models, usually accompanied by a demonstrator. The press service sends out to newspapers of the State a daily article of from 200 to 300 words, publishes a monthly bulletin, and issues special pamphlets.

HOOKWORM, TYPHOID, AND PELLAGRA CAMPAIGNS.

In a five-year campaign ending May, 1915, the Rockefeller Sanitary Commission, now the International Health Commission, examined 267,999 citizens of the State for hookworm infection, and treated 95,618 infected citizens, also improving 1,796 privies.[1]

The State bureau of rural sanitation has reached 21 counties with its typhoid vaccinations and given three complete vaccinations to 100,000 people, vaccinating an average of 4,761 persons in each county—from 16 to 20 per cent of the population of the counties.[2]

A pellagra campaign in one county has been fruitful of lasting results, convincing the public of the value of a more varied dietary.

[1] Sixteenth Biennial Report of the North Carolina State Board of Health, 1915–1916, p. 61.
[2] Sixteenth Biennial Report of the North Carolina State Board of Health, 1915–1916, p. 45.

SOIL POLLUTION WORK.

This work, which has for its object the control of diseases spread through pollution of the soil, is a recent development and so far has been conducted in only one county. The method followed, as described in the annual report of the State board of health is "to visit each and every home in the county and demonstrate to the people the ways in which this class of diseases is spread and to interest them in providing sanitary privies as a preventive measure. Also, an important part of the campaign is to examine and give treatments for hookworm disease and vaccinations to prevent typhoid fever." [1]

POSTGRADUATE CLINICS.

One of the most interesting features of the State board of health program has been the development through the cooperation of the State board of health and the State University of a home postgraduate course in children's diseases for the doctors of the State. The fundamental principle consists in bringing the teacher to the class instead of sending the class to the teacher. The plan was initiated in 1916 in two counties. Two experts were obtained to bring a six-weeks' course to 80 rural physicians, the expense of from $2,000 to $2,500 being shared by them. The amount which each physician paid was about $30, whereas, had he gone to any of the large hospital centers for such a course the expense would have amounted to from $300 to $400, including travel, lodging, and the loss of income during absence. The course consisted of a lecture and clinic one day a week in each of six towns of the counties selected. Physicians were allowed to bring their own patients for consultation, and so urgent was the demand for the clinics that they will doubtless be repeated another year, the subject to be chosen by the subscribing physicians. [2]

PUBLIC-HEALTH NURSING.

The State sanatorium and bureau of tuberculosis of the State board of health has been instrumental in securing a director of public-health nursing for the State, in cooperation with the Metropolitan Life Insurance Co., which pays one-half her salary and expenses. The Metropolitan company has also cooperated in local nursing activities, awarding five scholarships in public-health nursing in the University of Cincinnati. In 1916 a three-days' conference of the 35 public-health nurses of the State was held at the State sanatorium; one result of this conference was a great stimulation throughout the State of interest in public-health nursing. By February, 1918, there were in North Carolina 65 public-health nurses [3] (more, it is reported,

[1] Sixteenth Biennial Report of the North Carolina State Board of Health, 1915–1916, p. 46.
[2] Sixteenth Biennial Report of the North Carolina State Board of Health, 1915–1916, p. 28.
[3] The University of North Carolina News Letter, Vol. IV, No. 13, Feb. 20, 1918.

than in any other southern State). They were supported by public funds, mill companies, women's clubs, philanthropic groups, churches, and lodges, aided by the Metropolitan Life Insurance Co. The demand for public-health nurses is greater than the supply. To meet this demand, the State board of health, in cooperation with the University of North Carolina, is planning a training school for public-health nurses.

REGISTRATION OF MIDWIVES.

A recent act to prevent blindness in infancy,[1] passed by the State legislature of 1917, requires the registration of midwives with the State board of health "in order that the prophylactic solution and necessary instructions may be furnished them." A penalty of from $10 to $50 is prescribed for midwives failing to register. Although this is an important step in the right direction, as yet no provision has been made for an examination or supervision of midwives.

PREVENTION OF BLINDNESS IN INFANCY.

An act of the legislature of 1917[2] makes it "unlawful for any physician or midwife practicing midwifery in the State of North Carolina to neglect or otherwise fail to instill or have instilled, immediately upon its birth, in the eyes of the new-born babe two drops of a solution prescribed or furnished by the North Carolina State Board of Health."

QUARANTINE FOR INFECTIOUS DISEASES.

The reporting of infectious diseases to the State board of health was made compulsory by an act of the legislature of 1917,[3] which also provides means for control and supervision of such diseases. By the terms of this act, it is the "duty of every physician to notify the county quarantine officer of the name and address, including the name of the school district, of any person living or residing, permanently or temporarily, in the county about whom such physician is consulted professionally and whom he has reason to suspect of being afflicted with whooping cough, measles, diphtheria, scarlet fever, smallpox, infantile paralysis, typhoid fever, typhus fever, Asiatic cholera, bubonic plague, yellow fever, or other diseases declared by the North Carolina State Board of Health to be infectious and contagious, within 24 hours after obtaining reasonable evidence for believing that such person is suffering from one of the aforesaid diseases." In cases where the patient is unattended by a physician, the duty of notifying the quarantine officer falls upon the parent, guardian, or householder in the order named. It is the duty of the

---

[1] Acts of 1917, ch. 257, sec. 8.   [2] Acts of 1917, ch. 257, sec. 3.   [3] Acts of 1917, ch. 263, sec. 7.

county quarantine officer to report cases of the above-mentioned diseases to the State board of health within 24 hours after the disease has been reported to him. The State board of health is empowered to make such rules and regulations as may be necessary for the supervision and control of these diseases. Persons willfully violating the law or the rules and regulations adopted by the board of health are guilty of a misdemeanor and subject to fine or imprisonment.

PHYSICAL EXAMINATION OF SCHOOL CHILDREN.

Considerable attention is now being directed to the care of the rural school child. Many localities have developed a complete program for supervision of the child's health and physical development during his years of schooling, with medical inspection of the children periodically, and a school nurse who visits in the homes and sees to it that the child receives the treatment which has been recommended. It has been proved that school medical inspection needs a school nurse to make it effective.

In this State the board of health has developed a "unit of school inspection" which so far has been carried on in six counties. The bureau of rural sanitation in the first 19 months of its existence inspected 206 schools, examined 15,751 children, found 7,390— almost half—to be physically defective in some respect and has been instrumental in having 10 per cent treated.[1] The value of this plan lies chiefly in arousing local interest through demonstration; it does not meet the need for permanent periodic examination of the children or for a permanent school nurse. Recently a unique compulsory State-wide plan has been devised by the board of health and enacted into law by the legislature[2] for the physical examination of school children at a minimum of expense. The teachers themselves will make the examinations according to a manual of instructions prepared by the State board of health and State superintendent of public instruction with the assistance of the United States Public Health Service. A record of each examination will be made on cards provided by the State board of health and transmitted to a physician in each county designated by the State board of health, who will notify the parent or guardian of any child with serious physical defects as defined by the State board of health to bring the child before him for a thorough physical examination.

According to the law it is compulsory for a parent so notified to bring his child before the physician. The physician will be compensated by the county commissioners for the examinations. Parents are then notified of any defect discovered and advised as to the treatment which the child should receive. Arrangements will be

---

[1] Sixteenth Biennial Report of the North Carolina State Board of Health, 1915–1916, pp. 45, 46.
[2] Acts of 1917, ch. 244.

made by the State board of health and State superintendent of public instruction with physicians and dentists of the county to treat school patients at a reduced cost, 20 per cent of which may be paid by the State board of health, provided the county commissioners will pay 20 per cent. This leaves only 60 per cent of the cost to be borne by the parents, besides securing for them a reduced rate for their children's treatment. The law provides that every school child shall be examined at least once every three years, and that the work shall be so planned by the State board of health and State superintendent of public instruction as to cover the entire State once in every three years.

"COUNTY UNITS."

Much of the work of the State board of health is carried on by State board of health agents in each county under the "county unit" system, by which the State and county share the expense of educational health work. Under this system school inspection "units" have been conducted, and typhoid, hookworm, pellagra, etc., have been dealt with.

Recently the State board of health, in cooperation with the International Health Board of the Rockefeller Foundation, has contracted with 10 counties of the State for a three-year program of health work in those counties. The program agreed upon is to consist, in each county, of units devoted to soil pollution, quarantine and disinfection, school inspection, life extension, and infant hygiene—all under the direction of a full-time health officer, and at an average yearly cost to the county of between $3,000 and $4,500. Definite contracts have been agreed upon and signed by the State board of health and representatives of the cooperating counties.

Public-health activities have reached a high degree of development in this State and are carefully and efficiently organized under the State board of health. The next step might well be the organization of a division of child hygiene; no doubt this important feature of the health program will be developed shortly by this State just as it has become an important part of the State boards of health in New York, Kansas, New Jersey, Ohio, and Montana. Such a bureau correlates the various health problems of childhood, such as the reduction of infant mortality, prenatal and infant care, medical inspection of schools, health of children in State institutions, and activities of children's conferences and clinics.

AGRICULTURAL ACTIVITIES.

Under the joint leadership of the State and Federal Departments of Agriculture, according to the terms of the Smith-Lever Act,[1] various organizations throughout the State are stimulating an interest in higher standards of farming and farm life.

---

[1] 38 U. S. Stat. L., Pt. I, p. 372 (act of May 8. 1914).

COUNTY AND HOME DEMONSTRATION AGENTS.

Ninety-six counties of the State, including the lowland county at the time of this survey and the mountain county recently, have a county agent who by demonstration and other methods interests the farmers of his county along the lines of improved methods of agriculture, farm management, marketing, purchase of supplies, and so forth.

Home demonstration agents to interest farm women in modern household economics are present in 58 counties, including the lowland county of the survey.

BOYS' AND GIRLS' CLUBS.

Clubs, open to boys and girls between the ages of 10 and 18, are proving an effective means of reaching the rural community through the child. These clubs are supervised by State agents, assisted by county agents, usually cooperating with school officials and rural teachers.

Boys' corn clubs were the first organization of this type. The corn-club boys raise an acre of corn, usually on their fathers' farms, and prizes are offered for the most successful corn-club member— based on the largest production at the lowest cost, with the best exhibit of 10 ears and the best essay on the year's work.

Boys' pig clubs are arousing interest in pork production, and are teaching the boys profitable methods of feeding, the value of the best breeds, and the home production of meat for the family.

Boys' and girls' poultry clubs are demonstrating poultry raising, handling, and marketing, the value of uniform product of high class for cooperative marketing, better care of poultry and eggs, and the increased revenue derived from better breeding and management.

Girls' canning-club work has developed into one of the most important features of the State relations service. The girls plant and cultivate a garden of a tenth of an acre, and can the products for home and market. Prizes are awarded on the basis of the quality and quantity of the canned product, the profit shown by cost accounting, and a written account of how the crop was made.

FARMERS' INSTITUTES.

Farmers' institutes with lectures and demonstrations by experts, for both farmers and farm women, had been held in many counties during 1916, including the lowland county of this study.

This lowland county has been well organized for rural progress, with its county agent and home demonstration agent; its well-established corn, pig, poultry, and canning clubs for the boys and girls; a flourishing and stimulating county fair with an infant-welfare section; and, for some years past, sessions of the farmers' institutes.

The mountain county, on the other hand, at the time of the survey showed a total lack of community organization of agricultural activities—no county agent, no demonstration agent, no boys' and girls' clubs, no farmers' institutes throughout the county. The county fair is the only stimulus to improved farming and farm life,' and even at the county fair the exhibit of farm products is meager and almost overshadowed by the cheap commercial amusements offered. The recent employment of a county agent is an important beginning toward an improved agricultural program for the county.

RURAL CREDITS AND FARM LOAN ASSOCIATIONS.

Ample facilities for extending credits to the farmer, thus combating the "crop-lien" and high-interest evils, have been organized and a variety of systems, State and Federal, devised by which the farmer can borrow money for land purchase or improvement.

The Federal farm loan act,[1] which affords an opportunity to secure long-time credit (from 5 to 40 years) at a rate of interest not to exceed 6 per cent, should not only help the farmer to secure capital, but, because the money will be borrowed through a local farm-loan association, should also stimulate cooperative enterprise.

The McRae rural credits bill,[2] passed by the 1915 legislature, provides for the organization of credit unions for short-time credit under the supervision of the State board of agriculture. Loans by the credit unions under this law can be made to members for the purpose of raising crops only and are loaned upon the name of the farmer. The rate of interest is limited to 6 per cent. In the autumn of 1917 there were 14 rural credit unions in the State—more, it is said, than in any other State.

COUNTY FAIRS.

The majority of the counties of the State, including the two counties visited, held county fairs in 1916. The county fair has won an assured place for itself in the activities for rural progress, affording as it does an opportunity for the farmer to compare his results with the best achievements of the county, and with the produce of his neighbors who face the same problems and surmount the same obstacles that he must reckon with. Farm women also benefit by exhibits of household products—jellies, jams, preserved fruits and vegetables, cakes, bread, needlework, and knitting.

In this State, as elsewhere, the county fair has also been found an excellent opportunity for presenting to the mothers the newer ideals in child care and giving them the advantage of expert advice as to the physical development of their children. A number of counties have

---

[1] Farm Loan Act, act of July 17, 1916. 39 U. S. Stat. L., p. 360.
[2] Acts of 1915, ch. 115.

introduced baby conferences of various types as a feature of the fair with a growing tendency to abolish, or at least to minimize, the competitive element, which was a prominent feature of the earlier baby contests. The babies are weighed and measured by competent physicians who point out defects to the mothers and give them constructive suggestions for improving the child's general health. Free literature on infant care is frequently distributed. Baby "shows" of various sorts were held in connection with county fairs in a number of counties, including the lowland county of this survey, which has had one for three years. The mountain county would, no doubt, also find the mothers interested in the introduction of such a feature.

COMMUNITY SERVICE LEAGUES.

The activities of the State bureau of community service have been of especial significance to the rural districts of the State. Under the leadership of this bureau, a number of rural neighborhoods have been organized into "Community Service Leagues," with committees on education, farm progress, cooperative marketing, health organization and social life, and an executive committee which in consultation with the State bureau determines upon the line of work for each year and the special problems upon which attention is to be concentrated.

Two important acts of the 1917 session of the legislature gave a decided impetus to the movement for community organization. An article in the Community Center for September, 1917, comments on one of these acts as follows:

By this act [an "act to provide for the incorporation of rural communities," 1917, ch. 128], the people of each rural neighborhood—a common school district or uniting group of districts—* * * may secure the powers and advantages of incorporation usually reserved for cities and villages—the right to enact ordinances [through a legally-provided-for community assembly] and assure common contribution to pay for community improvements through the levying of taxes; they may nominate for the Governor's appointment a community judge or magistrate; and * * * may, through their duly chosen executive committee of "directors," take any and all necessary steps looking to a system of * * * cooperative community marketing.

A committee appointed by a conference which was called by Governor Bickett to prepare a statement concerning the purpose of this law concludes its report with these words:

"It will make the school and the schoolhouse the center and rallying point for all activities, agencies, and plans for the improvement of community life and the advancement of community progress and prosperity.

"It is applied democracy, and in accordance with the traditions and genius of our race. * * *

"In short, it makes progress legal and binding when favored by a majority of the community instead of its being probably only an ineffectual, effervescent mass-sentiment."

Through an "act to improve the social and educational conditions of rural communities"[1] it is the duty of the State superintendent of public instruction "to provide for a series of rural entertainments, varying in number and cost and consisting of moving pictures selected for their entertaining and educational value, which entertainments may be given in the rural schoolhouses of the State as herein provided."

HOME-COUNTY STUDY CLUBS OF UNIVERSITY OF NORTH CAROLINA.

An interesting organization of the State university—the North Carolina Club—is composed of university students and faculty members, "bent on accurate, intimate acquaintance with the Mother State." The society has entered upon its third year of study of economic and social problems in North Carolina, "her resources, advantages, opportunities, and achievements; the production and retention of wealth and the conversion of wealth into welfare and well-being; market and credits; organization and cooperative enterprise; schools and colleges, churches and Sunday schools; public health and sanitation; problems of urban and rural life; * * *."[2] Affiliated with the North Carolina Club are various county clubs of students, exploring the economic and social problems of their home counties. Nearly 70 "home-county" studies have been made by these clubs and prepared for publication in the home papers. In some instances the county officials are preparing to issue these county studies in pamphlet form for textbook use by students in the high schools, by teachers in the county institutes, and so forth. The subjects covered in the study of each county are as follows:

(1) The Historical Background, (2) Timber Resources, (3) Mineral Resources, (4) Water-Power Resources, (5) Industries and Opportunities, (6) Facts About the Folks, (7) Facts About Wealth and Taxation, (8) Facts About the Schools, (9) Facts About Farm Conditions, (10) Facts About Farm Practices, (11) Facts About Food and Feed Production, (12) The Local Market Problem, (13) Where the County Leads, (14) Where the County Lags, and (15) The Way Out.[2]

Such a searching study of the home State must prove of great value in the development of a trained and intelligent leadership which is one of the most essential factors in the progress of any State.

LAWS RELATING TO CHILD LABOR.[3]

Up to September 1, 1917, when the Federal child labor law went into effect, the employment of children was regulated only by the State law, which is meager and ineffective. The State labor law permits the employment of children 12 years of age or over in manu-

---

[1] Acts of 1917, ch. 186.

[2] University of North Carolina Record, No. 140, pp. 7, 8.

[3] The Federal child labor law was in effect at the time of the study, but it has since been declared unconstitutional by a decision of the Supreme Court of the United States (June 3, 1918).

facturing establishments, providing that no child between the ages of 12 and 13 shall be employed except in an apprenticeship capacity, and then only after having attended school 4 months in the preceding 12 months.[1] The State law also prohibits night work in any mill, factory, or manufacturing establishment—that is, between the hours of 9 p. m. and 6 a. m.—for children under 16 years of age.[2] By the passage of the Federal child labor act,[3] in effect September 1, 1917, the age at which children are permitted to work in manufacturing establishments, mills, factories, workshops, or canneries shipping in interstate or foreign commerce is fixed at 14 years, with the added provision that no child under 16 shall work more than 8 hours a day, 6 days a week, or between 7 p. m. and 6 a. m., in such establishments.

Prohibition of employment in agricultural pursuits is not specified in either the State or Federal law.

LAWS RELATING TO SCHOOL ATTENDANCE.

The school law of North Carolina makes definite provision for its enforcement; under the general supervision of the State superintendent of public instruction it charges the county board of education with the appointment of attendance officers, one to each township,[4] and provides that the county board, together with the county superintendent, may make rules governing school attendance.[5] Yet, as a matter of fact, in the counties of the survey at least, the law is very poorly enforced, due largely no doubt to a discouraging indifference on the part of the public, and to the lack of a system of special truancy officers. According to the census figures, North Carolina's rank in school attendance, as compared with the other States, is thirty-third.[6] In view of the fact that on account of the Federal child labor law[7] many children under 14 are released from the mills, a rigid enforcement of the compulsory-attendance law would seem particularly desirable.

CHILD-CARING INSTITUTIONS AND AGENCIES.

FACILITIES FOR DEALING WITH JUVENILE OFFENDERS.

The State juvenile court law[8] embodies the modern conception of the delinquent child as a ward of the State in need of guidance rather than as an offender to whom punishment should be meted. The

---

1 Pells Revisal of 1908, Supplement 1913, ch. 45 A, sec. 1081 b.
2 P. R., 1908, Supp. 1913, ch. 45 A, sec. 1981 ee (2).
3 39 U. S. Stat. L., p. 675 (act of Sept. 1, 1916).
4 P. R., 1908, Supp. 1913, secs. 4092a (5) to 4092a (6), as amended by 1917, ch. 208, sec. 2.
5 P. R., 1908, Supp. 1913, sec. 4092a (11), as amended by 1917, ch. 208, sec. 1.
6 Thirteenth Census of the United States, 1910. Vol. I, pp. 1118-1127.
7 The Federal child labor law was in effect at the time of the study, but it has since been declared unconstitutional by a decision of the Supreme Court of the United States (June 3, 1918).
8 Acts of 1915, ch. 222.

modern principle of probation is an important feature of the law—permitting the court to suspend sentence and place the child on probation for a specified period. The court has jurisdiction over adults contributing to the child's delinquency, juvenile offenders are tried before the county courts, and the law directs the court to hold separate trials for children as far as practicable. No child 14 years of age or under can be committed by the courts to any jail or prison inclosure where the child will be the companion of older and more hardened criminals, except where the charge is for a capital or other felony, or where the child is a known incorrigible or habitual offender; the child may be placed in a detention home or in the temporary custody of a responsible person pending the disposal of his case by the court.

Although most of the essentials of good juvenile court legislation are included in the law, it is lacking in certain respects: Separate sessions of the court for the trial of juvenile offenders are not obligatory; children 14 years or younger, if known as "incorrigible" or "habitual offenders," may be confined in jail or prison, where they are subject to the contaminating influences of adult offenders; and the probation system, except in a few of the larger cities which maintain paid probation officers, is dependent upon volunteer service.

The Stonewall Jackson Training School near Concord provides institutional restrictions and training for a limited number of delinquent boys—97 were enrolled at the time of this study—but, according to the annual report for 1916 of the board of public charities, it is handicapped by insufficient equipment and needs to be materially enlarged.

The 1917 legislature has provided for the issuing of bonds to erect an institution for delinquent girls,[1] which has been a most vital and urgent need. At the time of the study, throughout the State, no separate institution was available for this class of offenders. When the judge of a North Carolina court pronounces a girl, however young, guilty of a crime, he has no alternative but to place her in the State penitentiary. In 1916 alone there were received at the State prison, with no provisions at that time for a separation of young from older prisoners, 48 children under 20, 8 from 10 to 15, and 40 from 15 to 20 years of age.[2] Recent legislation[3] for the purpose of regulating the "treatment, handling, and work of prisoners" provides that "the races shall be kept separate, and youthful convicts from old and hardened criminals in sleeping quarters."

---

[1] Acts of 1917, chs. 255, 265.
[2] Annual Report of the Board of Public Charities of North Carolina, 1916, p. 30.
[3] Acts of 1917, ch. 286, sec. 24.

INSTITUTIONS FOR DEFECTIVE CHILDREN.[1]

A State school for the feeble-minded, the Caswell Training School at Kinston, affords facilities for institutional care and industrial training for 200 children, and had an enrollment of 181 on November 30, 1916.[2] Fifteen children, reported feeble-minded, were inmates of county almshouses [3]—obviously unsuitable institutions for their care, since they are unequipped for the special treatment and training necessary for the mentally defective. No suitable State provision has been made for feeble-minded negro children, who are committed to the county almshouses.

Seventeen children under 16—both boys and girls—were patients at the epileptic colony of the State hospital for the insane at Raleigh.[4]

The North Carolina school for the white deaf, located at Morganton, had a capacity of 300 and an enrollment of 281.[5] State schools for the blind—white and negro—at Raleigh had an enrollment of 286 white boys and girls and 69 negroes.[6] The negro school also has the care of 105 deaf negro children.

Along with a plea for an industrial school for delinquent girls and for an increase in the capacity of the Jackson Training School for Boys, the board of public charities in its report for 1916 mentions the need for a hospital for crippled children also—a hospital school where "the children are taught during the months when under treatment. * * * Many States have opened such institutions, and the wonderful cures have demonstrated that they are eminently worth while." [7] The first step toward an orthopedic hospital was taken by the legislature of 1917,[8] which appropriated $20,000 for this purpose, provided the amount can be duplicated from sources other than the State. A committee appointed by the governor has selected a site at Gastonia and is empowered to proceed when the necessary funds shall have been raised.

PROVISIONS FOR HOMELESS AND DEPENDENT CHILDREN.

The State orphanage for white children at Oxford has an enrollment of 375, and the orphanage for colored children, also at Oxford, 155.[9] Several private orphanges scattered throughout the State are caring for 1,690 children; also a children's home society at Greensboro, the only child-placing society in the State, has under its super-

---

[1] The figures given in this section are as of Nov. 30, 1916.
[2] Annual Report of the Board of Public Charities of North Carolina, 1916, p. 22.
[3] Ibid., p. 74.
[4] Ibid., p. 19.
[5] Ibid., p. 26.
[6] Ibid., pp. 24, 25.
[7] Ibid., p. 7.
[8] Acts of 1917, ch. 199.
[9] Annual Report of the Board of Public Charities of North Carolina, 1916, pp. 31, 33.

vision 442 children who have been placed in private homes.[1]   A number of dependent children, 37 in 1916, were cared for temporarily in the county homes or "almshouses"[2] designed for adults, totally unfitted, according to modern standards, for the special problems of child care. The board of public charities urges the county commissioners to provide otherwise for the children as soon as possible.

STATE BOARD OF CHARITIES AND PUBLIC WELFARE.

Since March, 1917, a new "State Board of Charities and Public Welfare," taking the place of the old "Board of Public Charities," has been given the duty to "study and promote the welfare of the dependent and delinquent child and to provide either directly or through a bureau of the board for the placing and supervision of dependent, delinquent, and defective children," and to "inspect and make report on private orphanages, institutions, and persons receiving or placing children."[3] This board hopes eventually to organize county boards of public welfare throughout the State, with a locally paid county commissioner of public welfare in every county.

---

[1] Annual Report of the Board of Public Charities of North Carolina, 1916, p. 38.
[2] Ibid., p. 74.
[3] Acts of 1917, ch. 170.

SCHEDULE USED IN VISITING FAMILIES DURING SURVEY.

[Page 1.]

U. S. DEPARTMENT OF LABOR.

CHILDREN'S BUREAU.

OUTLINE FOR STUDY OF CHILD WELFARE IN RURAL COMMUNITIES.

....

....

....

....

....

[Page 2.]

FATHER.　　　　MOTHER.　　　　BABY.　　　　ADDRESS.

S. No.　　B. C. No.　　D. C. No.　Township.　　COUNTY.　　STATE.

BABY—1. M. F.　2. L. I.　3. L. B., S. B.　4. At one year: Alive, Dead.　5. Date of birth ....　6. Date of death ....

23. Mother's occupations | Industries | Extent | Ages.

7. Feeding:

	1	2	3	4	5	6	7	8	9	10	11	12
(a) Breast only.......												
(b) Breast and other..												
(c) No breast........												

a. Specify (b) and (c)........................

FATHER—24. Occupation. | Industry. | E. O. W.

MOTHER—8. Marriage ages........duration........years.

9. Pregnancies.

25. Illness................

No.	Sex.	Mother's age.	Child's present age.	At'd't at birth.	Period.	Cause of death	Age at death
1							
2							
3							
4							
5							
6							

26. Physical history of children.

1
2
3
4
5
6

10. Before conf.: Saw phy'n, mwf., how often....Ur. exam., how often....
11. After: No. visits....　12. Drops in baby's eyes.........
13. Cord, how dressed.........
14. Instruction in inf. care.........
15. Nursing care in conf.: (a) Kind.........
　　(b) Duration........　16. How long in bed.........
17. Usual help with housework.........
18. Extra help in confinement.........

27. Home remedies.........

28. Distance from phy'n ....
29. From telephone ....
30. Distance from school ....
31. Education of living children .....

19. Usual duties.	Ceased.	Resumed.	Usual duties.	Ceased.	Resumed.
(a) Cooking ..			(f) Milking....		
(b) Cleaning .			(g) Churning..		
(c) Washing ..			(h) Chickens..		
(d) Ironing ...			(i) Garden....		
(e) Bulk family sewing.			(j) Farm......		

No.	Ages at school.	Total months' schooling.	Grade completed.	Can read and write	Reason for leaving.

20. Household conveniences.........

32.	Native white	Native black	Other	Can read	Read and write

21. Illness.........
22. Compl. of former pregnancies.........

	Native white	Native black	Other	Can read	Read and write
Mother.				Y.N.	Y.N.
Father.				Y.N.	Y.N.

[Page 3.]

	These columns are reserved for office use.

33.	Children's farm work—by seasons.	Hours.	Wages.		
......					......
......					......
......					......
......					......
......					......

34.	Children's other work.	Industry	Extent	Ages	Hours	Wages	
......							......
......							......
......							......

HOME—35. No. acres....No. improved....36. Rental $....per....Own, free (value $....
    per....) Worked on shares: Y. N. %........................
37. Mortgage $....Rate of int.... 38. Crops and stock........................
39. Equipment........................
40. Persons: Family....Others....Total....Specify others........................
41. No. rooms....No. used for sleeping.....Baby sleep alone: Y. N. with.....adults....
    children 42. House screened Y. N........................
43. Water: dg. w., dr. w., cist., sprg. Distance from house. Slope, up, down from house; up,
    down from privy. Casing........................
44. Toilet: none, privy, specify..... Slope, up, down from house. Condition........................
45. How often cleaned..... Disposal........................
46. Garbage: Burn, bury, fed stock..... 47. Rubbish........................
48. Manure.
49. General description of house and   Sketch of premises.
    premises:

0 25 50

Ft.

Symbols: D=dwelling. P=privy. W=well.
Sp=spring. St.=stable. Hp=hog pen.

[Page 4.]

50. Home economics: [Diet and clothing; income—(cash and other): indebtedness, other than mortgage:
    store credits and methods of purchasing; expenditures for stock and farm equipment; for hired help;
    method of crop disposal: distance from market, etc.]
....
....
....

51. Social life, recreation, use of leisure time, etc.:   Distance from nearest town.   R. F. D. Y. N.
    Publications taken.   Road.
[Give for each member of family: Membership in farm or civic association, club, lodge, grange, etc.: attendance at Farmers' Institutes; frequency of visits to town, participation in social events, etc.: also attitude toward farm life, desire to go to mill town or city, etc.]
....
....
....

Notes:
....
....
....

Informant.   Agent.   Date of visit.

MIDWIFE SCHEDULE.

U. S. DEPARTMENT OF LABOR,

CHILDREN'S BUREAU.

OUTLINE FOR INTERVIEW WITH MIDWIVES IN A RURAL DISTRICT.

1. Name and address .... 2. Col., white ....

3. No. births attended in 1915 ...... No. with M. D. ...... 4. Patients wh., col., both ....

SERVICES DURING CONFINEMENT: 5. How is patient prepared ....

6. How does midwife prepare herself ....

7. Antiseptics used ....

8. No. exams. usually made during labor .... 9. 2d and 3d stages of labor, how treated...................

10. Treatment of cord ....; of infected cord ....

11. No. cases infected cord ....; of umbilical hernia ....

12. Treatment of baby's eyes......................... 13. No. cases of infected eyes ....

14. Remains how long after birth .... No. calls after .... Patient discharged when ....

What exam. made previous to discharge ....

15. What advice given on infant care ....

16. What services performed other than obstetrical: Nursing, Y. N. Housework, Y. N.

ABNORMAL CASES: 17. No. treated in 1915 .... No. lacerations .... No. repaired by mwf. ....

Other abnormal cases: Specify...

18. Use of instruments ....; of anæsthetics ....

19. Bag: Equipment and condition ....

20. Under what circumstances does mwf. call phyn. ....

Names of phyns. called ....

21. No. stillbirths ...... No. infant deaths ...... Causes ....

22. Mothers' deaths: No. ...... Causes ....

No. cases of childbed fever ....

SERVICES DURING PREGNANCY: 23. Sees patient how often, and in what mos. ....

24. Does mwf. as a rule make phys. exam.: Y. N. Specify no. and kind ....

Urine exam.: Y. N. and in what mos. ....

25. Prenatal care: Advice given mothers ....

TRAINING OF MIDWIFE: 26. Where .... 27. Name school or phyn. .... 28. Diploma: Y. N.

29. Mos. attended ...... 30. Lectures per week ...... 31. No. births attended during training ....

32. Genl. education .... Can read and write: Y. N.

33. Yrs. practiced: Total ......; in township studied .... 34. Usual charge for conf. $...........

35. Does she register births: Y. N. How long after ....

36. License No. ....

37. Condition of house ....; of person ....

38. Approximate age ....

Enter notes and remarks ....

117

SCHOOL-SURVEY SCHEDULE.

U. S. DEPARTMENT OF LABOR,

CHILDREN'S BUREAU.

WASHINGTON.

SCHOOL SURVEY.

1. Name of school .... 2. White or negro........................ 3. Term ....
4. Graded or ungraded.................... 5. Highest class...
6. Teachers, number...................... 7. Salary...
8. Enrollment, total..................... Boys .... Girls ....

Attendance.	Total.	Boys.	Girls.
9. Average for year....................			
10. Average for November............			
11. Average for March.................			

School building:
12. Material .... 13. Finished, outside .... inside .... 14. No. rooms ......
15. Blinds or shutters at windows .... 16. Method of heating ....
17. Provison for coats, etc .... 18. General condition ....
19. Equipment ....
Sanitation:
20. Number of toilets, for boys .... girls .... 21. Distance apart ....
22. Drinking water, Dg. W., Dr. W., Sp .... 23. Drinking cup, individual, common ....
Surroundings:
24. Any attempt to beautify grounds with flowers, shrubbery, or trees ....
25. Playground, Yes, No.
School activities:
26. Library .... 27. School clubs (Audubon Soc., etc.) ....
28. Athletics ....
29. Industrial work ....
30. County commencement, No. attending .... 31. Exhibits and prizes ....
....
32. School entertainments ....
The school and the community:
33. Community gatherings held at the school, meetings of Community Club, Farmers' Institutes, etc.
....
34. Money raised privately or by school entertainments last year and how used.......................
....
35. No. of visits to parents .... 36. No. parents who visit school ....
Notes:
....
....
....
....
....
....

118

U. S. DEPARTMENT OF LABOR
CHILDREN'S BUREAU
JULIA C. LATHROP, Chief

MATERNITY AND INFANT CARE

IN TWO RURAL COUNTIES IN WISCONSIN

BY

FLORENCE BROWN SHERBON, M. D.

AND

ELIZABETH MOORE

❦

RURAL CHILD WELFARE SERIES No. 4

Bureau Publication No. 46

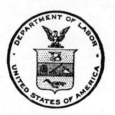

WASHINGTON
GOVERNMENT PRINTING OFFICE
1919

CONTENTS.

4 CONTENTS.

LETTER OF TRANSMITTAL.

U. S. Department of Labor,
Children's Bureau,
Washington, April 10, 1919.

Sir: Herewith I transmit the fourth report prepared by the Children's Bureau in its study of conditions affecting infants and mothers at childbirth in rural areas of the United States. A comparison of such vital statistics as are available for the United States with those of other countries shows 10 other countries with relatively fewer deaths among babies under 1 year of age and 13 other countries with relatively fewer deaths among women from conditions directly related to childbirth.

Considerably more than half the births in the United States occur in rural areas, and, although the mortality rate among babies under 1 year of age is apparently somewhat lower in the rural part of the birth-registration area than in the cities, the difference seems to affect only those babies who have survived the first month of life. For infant deaths during the first month—and these are more than two-fifths of all infant deaths—and for maternal deaths, there is no evidence of a lower average rate in rural than in urban areas. The need for clearer understanding of rural conditions and for constructive measures is plain.

The present unit in the rural inquiry followed the schedule and general plan prepared by Dr. Grace L. Meigs, as director of the bureau's division of child hygiene, and her assistant, Miss Viola I. Paradise. Valuable help in planning the details of the work in Wisconsin was rendered by the Wisconsin State Board of Health and by the extension division of the University of Wisconsin. The field work was done and the report was written by Dr. Florence Brown Sherbon and Miss Elizabeth Moore, of the Children's Bureau staff.

Respectfully submitted.

Julia C. Lathrop, *Chief.*

Hon. Wm. B. Wilson,
Secretary of Labor.

7

MATERNITY AND INFANT CARE IN TWO RURAL COUNTIES IN WISCONSIN.

INTRODUCTION.

OBJECT OF THE SURVEY.

This report is one of a series of studies undertaken by the Children's Bureau which deal with the conditions surrounding childbirth and infancy in typical rural communities. The subject of maternity care (including prenatal care) is emphasized in these studies because it is one of the main factors influencing a child's chance of being born alive, uninjured, and with sufficient vitality to carry him through the hazardous period of early infancy. How serious and important a problem this is, is indicated by the fact that two-fifths of the deaths of babies in the registration area of the United States—over 60,000 deaths in a year—are due to premature birth, injury at birth, congenital weakness, and malformations,[1] conditions which can be prevented to a great extent through and only through better care of the mother during pregnancy and at confinement. And even this large figure takes no account of the heavy losses—how heavy, no one knows—from stillbirths and miscarriages.

Furthermore, it is a well-recognized fact that even a baby sturdy at birth has a much better chance of life and health if he has a strong, well mother to nurse him and care for him. Yet it is estimated that in one year in the United States " at least 15,000 women * * * died from conditions caused by childbirth," [2] and the amount of sickness and even permanent invalidism among the mothers of the country caused by preventable complications of childbearing can not even be estimated.

Evidence coming to the bureau from many sources, especially through letters from country women themselves, indicates that the problem of securing adequate medical and nursing care at confinement is especially serious for country mothers; that in some districts and for many mothers such care is practically unattainable, either because of actual isolation or because of the expense resulting from

---

[1] Mortality Statistics, 1915, p. 645, U. S. Bureau of the Census. Washington, 1917.

[2] Meigs, Dr. Grace L.: Maternal Mortality from All Conditions Connected with Childbirth in the United States and Certain Other Countries, p. 7. U. S. Children's Bureau Publication No. 19, Miscellaneous Series No. 6. Washington, 1917.

distance from physicians and nurses. Indeed, this appears to be one
of the serious handicaps of country life as at present organized; and
studies looking toward means for relieving this situation were, therefore, considered urgent by the bureau. The first requisite in facing
this, as any, problem is knowledge of the facts.

Three studies of maternity and infant care in rural communities
were made in 1916, in representative districts of Kansas, North Carolina, and Wisconsin.

FIELD OF THE SURVEY.

As the field of the inquiry in Wisconsin, two counties were
chosen, one in the southern and one in the north-central part of the
State. These are referred to throughout the report as the northern and
the southern counties. Both are fertile agricultural country, in which
dairying is the prevailing type of farming. In both there is a considerable industrial population in some of the villages and in certain
places in the open country. Both have poor roads; hence travel in
the country is apt to be difficult, and many homes are almost isolated.
In other respects the two districts are widely dissimilar.

The northern county lies in what was originally lumber country
and is still largely in the transition stage from pioneer clearing of
" cut-over " land to more settled farming. While some farming communities are well-established and wealthy, the larger part of the
county still faces the necessity of ridding the soil of its brush, stumps,
and trees before crops can be raised. Consequently, like most pioneer
communities, these districts have little money to spend; and many
families live on isolated clearings or in remote settlements under
primitive conditions. The large majority of the settlers have been
German, with an important Polish contingent in addition; both these
nationalities cling to their foreign customs and habits of thought and
to a certain extent to their languages, making the district as a whole
distinctly foreign in its atmosphere. The northern county was
chosen in consultation with the State board of health because of the
large proportion—about one-sixth, according to preliminary figures—
of births attended by midwives. It was considered that a study in
such an area would throw light upon the problems of rural midwifery in general. In addition, the county is typical of conditions
prevalent over large parts of northern Wisconsin, Michigan, and
Minnesota, which were forest territory not much more than a generation ago.

In its general economic and sociological features the southern
county is typical of large farming areas on the prairies of southern
Wisconsin and Minnesota and northern Illinois. It is situated in the
older part of the State, where farming has been well-developed for

more than a generation and has changed little within that period; it is, therefore, a rich, well-established community. While about half its people are of foreign parentage, they are in the main thoroughly Americanized. This county was selected, on the advice of the extension division of the State university, because it is a prosperous but conservative community in which it was hoped that a survey by the Children's Bureau, and the children's health conference to be held in connection therewith, would increase the interest in public provision for the welfare of children. Furthermore, the State vital statistics, showing that this county had in 1914 an infant mortality rate of 115 per 1,000 births, one of the highest rural rates in the State, indicated that problems affecting the health of babies needed special attention.

Both counties were too large to make a survey of the whole area practicable; therefore a limited number of townships, with the villages therein, were covered. These townships were selected with a view to representing as fully as possible the variety and range of conditions in each county.

SCOPE AND METHOD.

The survey made in Wisconsin, like that in Kansas,[1] covers two main topics: The conditions affecting the health of the childbearing mother—the general living conditions of the family, the work done by the mother, and the care she received during pregnancy and at the time of confinement; and the care—especially the feeding—and survival of the babies. Throughout these rural surveys, the chief aim has been to give a picture of the district studied, rather than to indicate any connection between certain conditions and the infant mortality rate.

The information upon which the report is based was secured by the bureau's agents through personal interviews with mothers (or, in cases where for some reason the mothers could not be seen, with their near relatives) who had borne children within the two years preceding the survey, and who, when those children were born, were living in the territory covered. As the first step in finding families where there had been births, the names of the parents were copied from the birth certificates of this territory for the designated period. Secondly, a canvass was made in each district to find additional unregistered births. In nearly all cases the information was given by the mother herself. The mothers interviewed were appreciative of the object of the inquiry and answered the many personal questions with generous frankness.

---

[1] Moore, Elizabeth: Maternity and Infant Care in a Rural County in Kansas. U. S. Children's Bureau Publication No. 26, Rural Child Welfare Series No. 1. Washington, 1917.

Records were filled out for stillbirths as well as for live births within the given period, but not for miscarriages. No attempt was made to interview the mothers of illegitimate children, even in the few cases where such births were registered; in a study dealing with the provision for maternity and infancy in normal families it was considered that a few records of abnormal conditions would add nothing of value.

The records secured do not cover absolutely all the births which occurred, for some families had moved out of reach. The number thus lost was comparatively small, however, because the farming population in the areas studied is not migratory.

In the northern county the survey covered the births of the two years from July 1, 1914, to June 30, 1916; in the southern county the period was from May 1, 1914, to April 30, 1916. In each case this was the two-year period immediately preceding the beginning of the survey.

The report is based upon information concerning 614 families who lived in the selected districts—453 in the northern and 161 in the southern county. In 47 of these families, the mother had borne children twice during the two-year period of the survey and within the districts studied, so that the records cover the history of 661 confinements. Since nine pairs of twins and one set of triplets were born in this group, 672 births are included; 648 of these were live births and 24 still births.

SUMMARY OF FINDINGS.

The infant mortality rate in the northern county was low compared to the average for the United States birth-registration area; the stillbirth rate was somewhat higher than the rates found for six of the eight cities in which infant mortality studies have been made by the bureau. The death rate of mothers from causes connected with childbirth was high. Many births were attended by midwives in certain sections of this territory; a proportion as high as four-fifths was found in one of the Polish settlements. Moreover, it was not uncommon for mothers in inaccessible neighborhoods to go without any regular attendant at childbirth. Few women, even among those who had a physician at childbirth, secured any prenatal care; postnatal supervision was rare. Trained nurses were almost never employed for childbed nursing and practical nurses seldom. In many neighborhoods the midwives were the only nurses available who had had any obstetrical training. They gave some care during the lying-in period to about half their patients and also nursed a few mothers who had a doctor at confinement.

In this county the employment of midwives appears to be both a result of isolation in the Wisconsin forests and a survival of European custom. From the point of view of her patients the advantages of the midwife are: First, many foreign women prefer a woman rather than a man to help at childbirth; second, the neighborhood midwife is easier to secure than the doctor and more likely to be on time for the delivery; third, some midwives render nursing service during the lying-in period, which is highly appreciated; fourth, the midwife is much cheaper than the doctor; fifth, in the experience of most of these mothers the midwife whom they and their acquaintances have employed has seemed adequate to the situations which have arisen. On the other hand, some of them have had unfortunate experiences while under the care of physicians. Consequently they have come to believe that they get better service from the midwives.

The chief argument against the midwife is that, while an experienced midwife may be successful in conducting normal deliveries, she is a dangerously uncertain reliance if anything goes wrong; and there is always the possibility that something may go wrong. On an isolated farm it is even more unsafe than in the city to wait until complications have developed before sending for a doctor. A remark made by a Polish father aptly illustrates this point. His wife became sick during pregnancy and, though there was a physician 8 miles away, he sent to the county seat, 25 or 30 miles away, for a doctor whom he knew. He said: "When you get something for protection, like a doctor, you want the best there is. It was worth the money." Substitute the words "an attendant at birth" for "a doctor" in his phrase, and you have the crux of the midwife problem. This father employed a neighborhood midwife for his wife's confinement, two weeks later, because he and his wife regarded childbirth as a normal occurrence and did not realize that she then needed "something for protection—the best there is."

In the southern county the infant mortality rate was higher than in the northern county but the stillbirth rate was lower. Only one mother died at childbirth. Practically all the births were attended by physicians; there were no midwives in practice. The mothers, however, received much less prenatal and postnatal care from their doctors than their safety and the health of their babies required. Furthermore, the situation as to obstetrical nursing was far from satisfactory; trained nurses were difficult to secure and competent "practical nurses" or attendants were too few to fill the need for their services.

In neither district were the housewives on the farms obliged to provide for large crews of hired men at any special season, for dairy farming distributes the farm work more evenly through the year.

than does grain farming. But, on the other hand, it was common in both districts for the women to help with the milking and to have more or less dairy work added to their household duties. In the northern district half the farm mothers helped with the field work also, even in some cases with such heavy work as pitching hay and grain or clearing land; many of the Polish immigrant women did practically men's work in the fields in addition to their housework.

In both districts at the sixth month half the babies were exclusively breast fed; at 9 months of age only between one-fifth and one-fourth had been weaned. The record of these Wisconsin mothers for nursing their babies through the first nine months compares favorably with that of city mothers where the Children's Bureau has studied this subject, but is not so good as in the other country districts studied.

Birth registration proved to be defective in both districts, especially the northern.

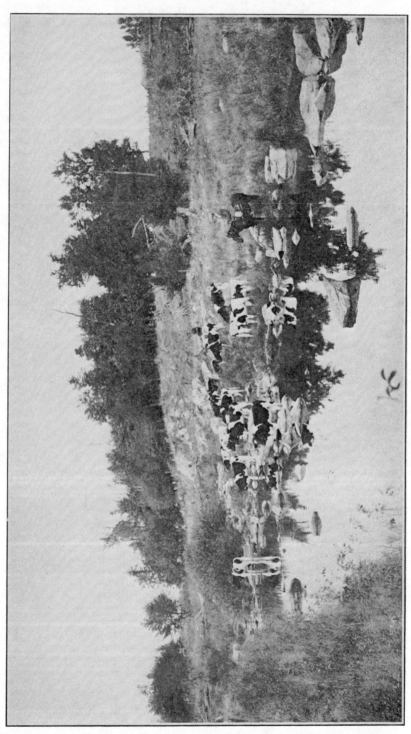

A TYPICAL NORTHERN COUNTY SCENE.

15–1

PART I. THE NORTHERN COUNTY.

ECONOMIC AND SOCIAL CONDITIONS IN THE COUNTY.

This county is located near the center of the northern half of Wisconsin, in the forest belt. It is one of the largest counties in the State, 30 miles wide and 55 miles long; it is nearly half as large again as the State of Rhode Island. The population in 1910 was a little over 55,000, an increase of 27 per cent in the preceding decade. Within the county at the time of the survey there were 12 incorporated villages, of which the largest had at the last census less than 1,000 population; and one city of approximately 17,000, which is the county seat.

Topography and soil.[1]

The Wisconsin River flows south nearly through the center of the county; its tributaries, some of which are important streams, drain the whole area. The sandy, alluvial soil which covers the river bottom, varying from less than a mile to 6 or 8 miles wide, is the poorest soil in the county; over much of its extent no attempt is made to raise crops of any kind.

Outside this valley, practically the whole of the county except the southeastern corner is a gently rolling country, rising to about 400 feet above the river. Nearly all of it is well drained. The uplands are broad and nearly level, while the numerous stream valleys, though deep, have gentle slopes. The soil of these uplands and valleys is clay or loamy clay, very fertile and giving good yields of all crops suitable to the northern climate. It is especially well adapted to hay and forage crops. At the time of the survey uncleared land of this type sold for about $25 an acre, while cleared land was valued as high as $100 an acre. In the belt of deeply weathered glacial clay, which extends over the western third and across the northern edge of the county, the older farming communities are exceedingly prosperous.

In the southeastern section the soil is much lighter, and in the valley of the Plover River decidedly sandy, though not so poor as that along the Wisconsin River. This soil is the result of much more recent glacial drift than that in the western part of the county and

---

[1] Data from Preliminary Report on the Soils and Agricultural Conditions of North Central Wisconsin, Bulletin No. XI, Wisconsin Geological and Natural History Survey, 1903.

is much cumbered with stones and even bowlders. In this district steep, stony ridges—glacial moraines—are a common feature of the landscape; and the intervening depressions are frequently so poorly drained that swamps result.

Climate.

As far north as this the winters, of course, are severe; but, while the temperature is low, this district does not suffer from the high winds or blizzards which are common farther west on the plains. Fuel is so plentiful throughout the county that the winter cold is not nearly so great a hardship as might be anticipated. The rainfall is usually ample—the year of the survey was an exception—for all crop needs and keeps the pastures luxuriant through the summer.

Agricultural development.

All this part of the State was originally forest country, covered with dense growths of hardwood, hemlock, and more scattered pine. The first settlers were lumbermen who came for the pine timber, most of which was removed years ago. Almost the only vestiges of those logging days are the great pine stumps still standing in many places among the lesser timber and brush; and an unpleasant reminder they are, for they are huge—sometimes as large as a small house—and extremely difficult to uproot. In more recent years the hardwood and hemlock have become valuable assets; many tracts of hardwood forest are still standing, but hemlock is now becoming somewhat scarce.

Farming began in certain parts of the county 40 or 50 years ago but did not become an important factor until within the past 25 years. The early agricultural settlements grew up around a number of distinct centers, often separated by miles of forest; this isolation of one part of the county from another still persists to a certain extent. At the present time all stages of development are represented, sometimes not many miles apart. In some of the older districts, on the rich clay soil, the farms are well improved, with ample buildings and wide stretches of cleared land. In such districts farm values are as high and people live as comfortably as in the southern part of the State. The present occupants are in many instances the children of those who cleared the land.

In other districts, pioneer conditions prevail to-day. Large areas of potential farms are still forest or what is called "cut-over land," covered with brush or small timber and full of stumps. Such tracts are largely in the hands of land companies—the successors of the earlier lumbering companies. It is still common for a young husband and wife to buy 80 acres, of which little or none is stumped, pay for it largely with a mortgage, build a rough two-room shack

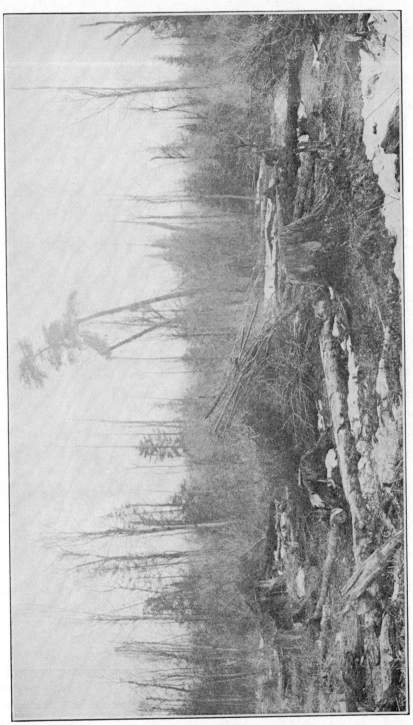

UNCLEARED CUT-OVER LAND.

16–1

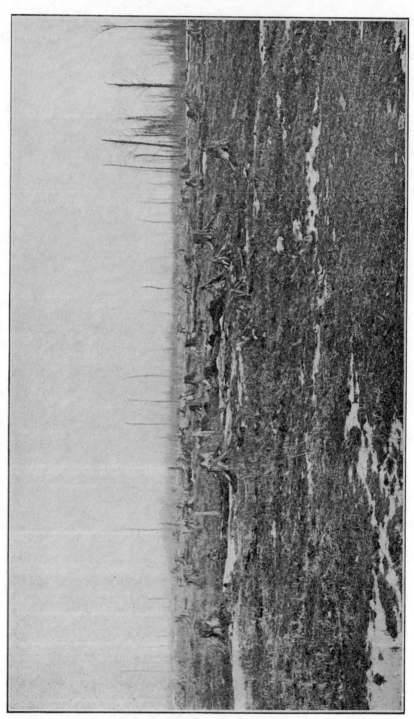

CUT-OVER LAND "BRUSHED" BUT NOT "STUMPED."

16–2

A CABIN IN A NEW CLEARING.

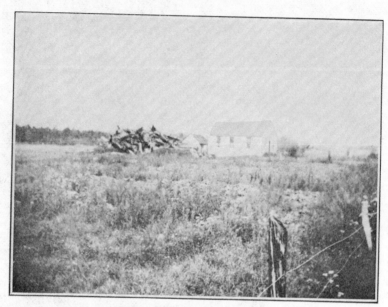

A SAMPLE OF UPROOTED STUMPS.

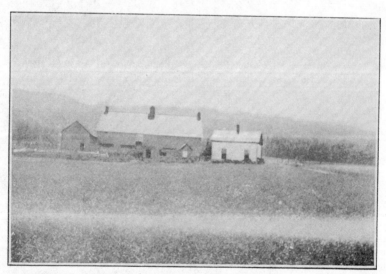

A NEW BARN ALONGSIDE THE OLD CABIN.

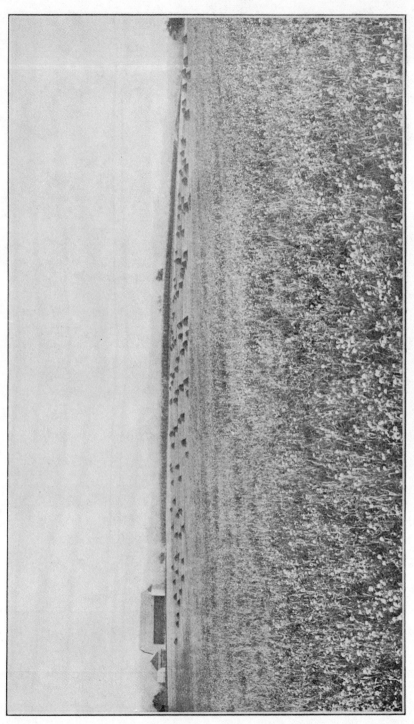

CLEARED LAND IN THE OLDER SECTIONS.

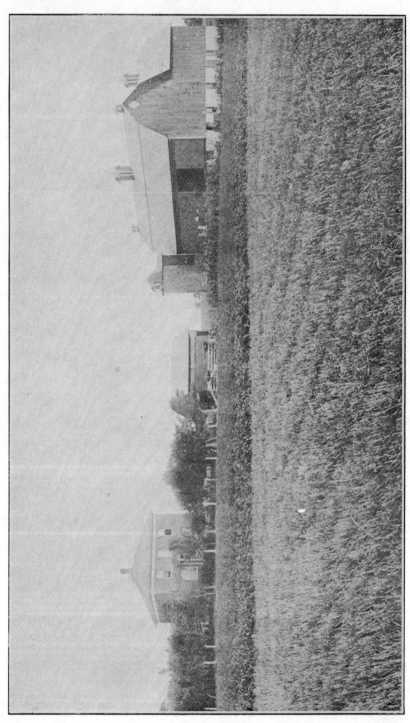

THE HOME ON A PROSPEROUS FARM.

of lumber from their own trees, and move onto the "farm." During the first few years, the husband often works out by the day during the summer and works on his land in the winter, felling trees and pulling stumps. Gradually, as they get pasture and hay land, they develop a herd of dairy cattle, building at first a rough barn shed for them. After a few years, perhaps 5 or 10, they build a large barn. And in a few years, usually not many after this, they build for themselves a substantial, well-finished, roomy house. But almost always the house comes after the barn, for it is a saying in this country that "the barn will build the house, but the house won't build the barn," a proverb which seems economically sound. And all this time the couple is rearing a family of children, not a small family, either, in most cases, but a healthy one. "Never had a doctor in the house except when the babies were born" is a common report. The last stage in the evolution of the farm is usually the payment of the mortgage.

Most of the land near the railroads where it is at all suitable for farming has been occupied for a good many years; the newly settled and unsettled districts are more remote. But accessibility was evidently not the only factor in determining which parts of the county were first chosen for farming, for two of the oldest-settled and richest townships have no railroad within 5 miles of their boundaries.

Although the State conservation commission in its 1909 report estimated that from 75 to 80 per cent of the land area of this county was suitable for cultivation, the 1910 census showed that only 54 per cent was included in farms, and only 35 per cent of this, or less than one-fifth of the total area, improved. Even with the large growth that has taken place since then there is still ample room for new settlers in this northern county.

Type of farming.

Over almost all the county, except on the comparatively small areas of sandy soil, dairying is the main source of the farmers' livelihood. The greater part of the farm land is in meadow or pasture, and the chief grain crops—oats, barley, and rye—are those used for feeding stock. Timothy, blue grass, and clover all thrive; clover does especially well, making good hay for milk production. Even on partly cleared land grass and clover will grow luxuriantly among the stumps; consequently such land can be utilized for pasture before it is stumped and ready for the plow. Milch cows are kept, and milk, cream, or butter is sold from almost every farm in these dairy districts. As throughout Wisconsin, cheese is the most important dairy product, and cheese factories are found in practically every countryside; but proportionately more butter is made here than in the southern county. In 1916 there were 118 cheese factories and 18 creameries (butter factories). Though few of the cheese factories are owned by the farmers, the milk producers are nevertheless commonly paid on the basis of the selling price of the cheese rather than at a flat rate.

In the sandy areas, notably in the Plover River Valley, potatoes are the chief crop. In fact, this is one of the main potato-raising districts of the State, and potato fields of 10 acres or more are common. Yields range from 90 to 150 bushels to the acre, sometimes running as high as 200 or 300 bushels in especially good years; but in the year when the survey was made (1916) the potato crop was an almost total failure. Farmers in the sandy districts also raise cucumbers on a large scale.

Roughly speaking, 80 acres is the standard size for a farm in this county; that is to say, it is the smallest farm on which it is considered that a family can live with reasonable comfort. This does not mean necessarily 80 acres under cultivation, for many dairy farmers manage remarkably well with as little as 20 to 40 acres cleared; but on a " forty " a farmer feels cramped as to his future as well as his present. On the other hand, the owner of more than an " eighty " is on the way to prosperity; farms larger than a quarter section (160 acres) are unusual.

Over one-third of the farms visited in the survey were from 80 to 120 acres in size; and the 1910 census reported the largest number— nearly one-half (43 per cent)—of the farms in the county in the group of from 50 to 100 acres. That the comparatively small size of the farms in this county does not indicate poverty is due both to the fertility of the soil and to the fact that practically all of it can be intensively cultivated as soon as it is cleared.

Farm ownership.

Tenantry is not a problem in this county, for tenants' farms were only 4 per cent of the total number at the last census. In this territory it is entirely possible for a prospective farmer with little capital to become a landowner. But the usual road to that goal is not through renting an already developed farm but through purchasing comparatively cheap, uncleared land under a mortgage and building up its value through the farmer's own labor. This means a hard struggle for both man and wife in the early years, with living reduced to the simplest basis; but such poverty as this is lightened by the hope and prospect of " winning out " to comfort and prosperity.

Rural density.

Outside the city and the incorporated villages, the population of the county in 1910 was 32,378. Since the unincorporated villages are all comparatively small, this is practically the open-country

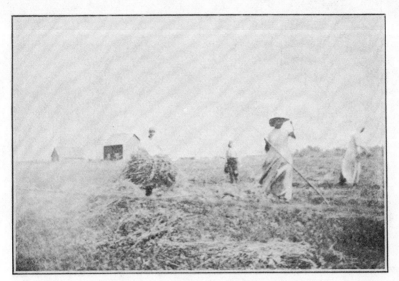

POLISH WOMEN IN THE HARVEST FIELD.

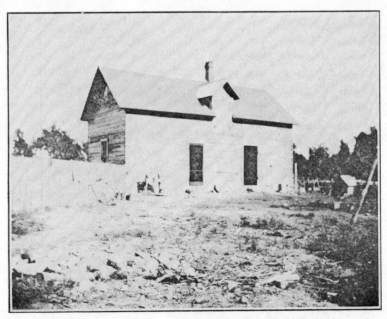

CABIN IN A POLISH SETTLEMENT, WITH COW STABLE, HAYLOFT, AND
DWELLING UNDER ONE ROOF.

18–1

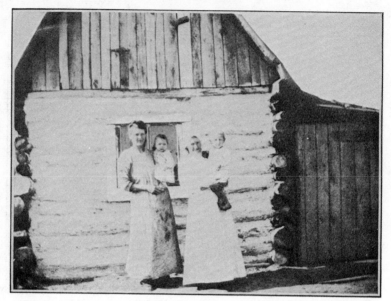

THREE GENERATIONS.

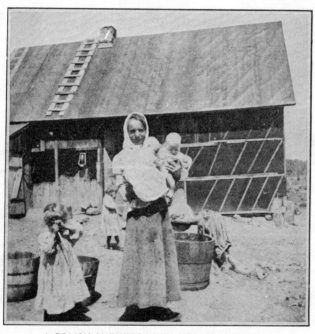

A POLISH MIDWIFE WITH HER OWN BABIES.

population and gives a rural density of approximately 20 persons per square mile. This average covers large variations in density between the thickly settled and the sparsely settled districts. Thirteen townships had 25 or more inhabitants per square mile; 1 of these is adjacent to the city and 2 contained unincorporated villages of some importance, while 9 lie in the northwestern section of the county in the region of the older German settlement and within the clay-soil area. On the other hand, 11 townships in different parts of the county had less than 15 inhabitants per square mile; some of these are situated where the land is poor, while others were merely undeveloped. Certain of these latter districts have had a large growth in population since the census year.

Nationality.

The great majority of both the early and the later settlers in this county were German; and over at least three-fourths of its area the county is strongly German in custom, language, and habit of mind up to the present day. There are a few Irish, Bohemian, Dutch, and Norwegian farmers in isolated groups; and in the southeastern quarter of the county there are two important Polish communities. The larger of these, in the Plover River Valley, originated a generation ago as an offshoot of a much larger Polish settlement farther down the river in the next county; this, therefore, is a well-established community. The other Polish settlement is the result of development during the past few years by a land company, which brought comparatively recent immigrants to rough, uncleared land.

According to the 1910 census, the population of the county (including the one city) was 26 per cent native white of native parentage, 52 per cent native of foreign or mixed parentage, and 22 per cent foreign born. For the whole county more than three-fourths (78 per cent) of the natives of foreign parentage had both parents born in Germany, and nearly three-fourths (72 per cent) of the foreign born hailed from Germany. Of course, these figures include the Poles of German origin.

The foreign element, as the census shows, is largely American born; but the Germans and Poles have been so numerous and have segregated themselves to such an extent that they have retained and handed down their foreign characteristics. So markedly foreign is the general atmosphere that the county agricultural extension teacher, upon being asked to name an American township, replied: " All are strongly foreign." Another indication of the persistence of foreign influences is the fact that not only half of all the foreign-born mothers visited in the county but also 16 American-born Polish mothers and 2 American-born German mothers were unable to speak English. In the older Polish settlement, though the majority of those born in the United States can speak English, it is not at all unusual to find those who can not; and Polish is still to such an extent the language of the family and the church that commonly children come to school lacking acquaintance with the English language.

Social organization.

The foreigners' among the farming population are mainly of peasant origin. Consequently, side by side with the advantages of peasant stock—strong physique, industry, and thrift—the community has the disadvantage of the peasant's strong attachment to his ancestral customs. While the rural illiteracy rate at the time of the last census was not excessive—2 per cent among the native born and 7 per cent among the foreign born—the farmers in the strongly foreign townships often do not realize the value for their children of any further education than the district or parochial schools can give. As might be expected, the mothers in these communities know nothing of modern principles of hygiene. Not only ancestral farming methods but also ancestral ways of feeding a baby or of caring for a woman at childbirth are considered fully satisfactory, while "newfangled notions" are viewed with suspicion if not hostility.

To be sure, certain districts are much more progressive than others; in general, the newer communities are the more open to new ideas. With one exception, all the larger villages have high schools.

Cooperative production, as exemplified by the cheese factories of the southern county, has not found favor in this county. In the western third of the county one of the national farmers' associations is well organized and has active locals. In this district cooperative buying and selling organizations are numerous and seem to be thriving; some of these ship and market cattle for their members, while others are engaged mainly in handling feed and flour. There are a few farmers' cooperative stores in other parts of the county, and a cooperative packing plant at the county seat.

This county, in its organized political capacity, has made certain provisions to meet public-health needs that are in advance of the average. To wit, there are a county tuberculosis sanitarium and a county hospital. The latter is located on the grounds of the county almshouse, but is under separate management. It was primarily intended for cases of sickness which would be county charges, but sometimes receives pay cases; it will care for obstetrical patients.

The county also has at the county seat an agricultural school, supported in part by the county and in part by the State. This is open to boys and girls who have completed the district-school course and gives instruction in agriculture, manual training, and domestic science. Although it has been in existence since 1902, it has never had a large patronage. One of the most important branches of the work of this school is its agricultural extension service—directed mainly toward the improvement of live-stock breedng, through the introduction of pure-bred stock and the formation of cow-testing associations. The extension officer working under the school practically takes the place of the ordinary county agent.

As a whole, it may fairly be said that none of the social-service agencies of the county, except perhaps the district schools, has come into helpful contact with the Polish settlements.

Means of communication.

The map of the county gives the appearance of ample transportation facilities, for the county is served by three main railroads and by two or three short branch roads. Nevertheless, 9 of the 40 townships in the county have no railroad within their borders, and parts of other townships are also remote from any railroad. Because of bad roads, intercourse with the outside world and with other parts of the county is seriously hindered and curtailed in those districts which lack railroad communications.

By reason of the location of the railroads, the county seat is accessible to the central and most of the eastern portions of the county and is the urban center for this area. But the western end, as well as sections along the northern and southern borders, are more accessible to cities in neighboring counties, and their interests gravitate in those directions.

Speaking generally, the roads of the county are poor. Only a few stretches—5 per cent of the total mileage [1]—have been surfaced with rock or gravel. Even what are considered the main roads, though fairly well graded, are for parts of the year almost impassable—those on clay soil in wet weather and those on sandy soil in dry weather. Some of the minor roads, which are the only means of approach to a large proportion of the farms, are so rough that the use of an automobile at any season is practically impossible, and even wagon hauling is difficult. One mother, who lived 7 miles from town at the very end of such a road, exclaimed, when told that the Government was working for the good of the children: "Well, tell them to fix a road through this section so that our children can go to school; it's only a little time of the year that they can possibly get through the swamp and forest."

Large areas were still without mail delivery at the time of the survey, notwithstanding the 31 rural routes then in operation. In the more inaccessible half of one of the townships included in the survey, about 40 families had no delivery service; some of these had to send as far as 12 miles for their mail.

---

[1] Public Road Mileage and Revenues of the Central, Mountain, and Pacific States, 1914. U. S. Dept. of Agriculture Bulletin No. 389.

Along the western border, telephone lines cover the settled districts reasonably well and most of the homes have telephones; but in the central and eastern sections, the lines do not, as a rule, reach any great distance back from the railroads and villages, or they serve only one important customer in a district—such as a creamery, saloon, or land office—leaving many farms miles away from any telephone. Only 20 of 280 country families visited in these districts reported a telephone in the house; while 120 were 2 miles or more from a telephone; and 40, 5 miles or more. In one township, a third of the families had to send at least 5 miles to reach a telephone, and in another the situation was nearly as bad.

This lack of telephone facilities is keenly felt by many families in these isolated neighborhoods; but, for some reason, the farmers and the company have not been able to come to any agreement as to the terms on which lines should be built and telephones installed.

Industries.

Aside from farming, the chief industries of this district are still those dependent upon the supply of wood. There are still some logging camps in the county, though most of the timber now marketed is brought in by the farmers from their own land. Sawmills providing lumber for local use are fairly common; and in the city there are large saw and planing mills and woodworking factories of various kinds. Away from the city, along the Wisconsin River, are three large paper mills, each with its mill village or settlement; these consume such quantities of pulp wood that they must send outside the county for much of their raw material. A tannery provides a market for hemlock bark.

In the north-central part of the county, on both sides of the river, there are quarries which are said to produce an unusually good quality of granite. But they are a comparatively unimportant factor in the life of the countryside, for they employ only a small number of men.

SELECTED TOWNSHIPS.

In the northern county, the survey covered 7 townships and the 6 villages lying therein. These were selected primarily with a view to representing both the districts where midwives are employed and those where they are not. Preliminary information, furnished by the State board of health or obtained from local sources, indicated certain townships in which at least half the births were attended by others than physicians. From this list 4 townships were chosen in which both the number of births and the proportion of midwife cases were large, and in which other conditions were varied. These townships happened to lie in the central part of the county. Therefore, the

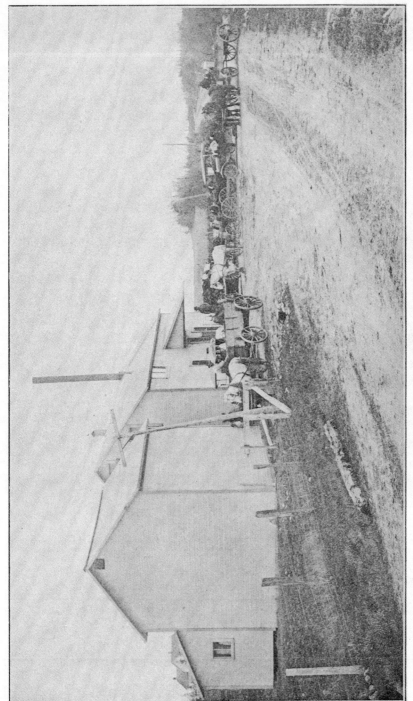

WHERE THE MILK GOES—A COUNTRY CHEESE FACTORY.

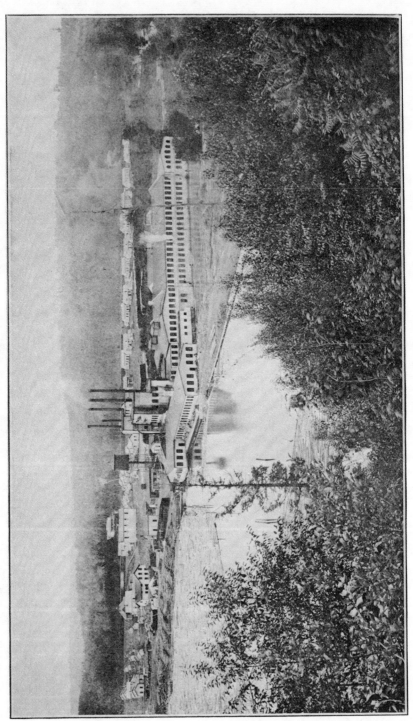

A PAPER-MILL VILLAGE.

3 other townships, in which practically all the births were attended by physicians, were selected, 2 from the western border and 1 from the eastern border, in order to cover as far as possible the different sections of the county.

Four of the selected townships are strongly German; one is almost exclusively Polish; one about half German and half Polish; and one of mixed nationalities—Norwegian, German, Polish, and American. One of the important Polish settlements and half the other were included; thus the Polish element was represented out of proportion to its importance in the county as a whole.

Two of the German townships belong in the older and comparatively well-developed districts, though in each there are sections where conditions are still primitive. One of these is counted among the most progressive communities in the county, the other among the most conservative. The other two are in the main more recently settled, with large areas of wild land.

The villages comprised five which are rural community centers, and one paper-mill town which had practically no organic relation to the countryside. In this latter village were found a number of Polish mill hands, though the township in which it lies is German. A second paper mill is located within one of the townships covered, and many of its operatives live near by; but there is nothing which could be called a village. Two of the villages lie on both sides of the county line; consequently, only part of each was covered in the survey.

FAMILIES INCLUDED IN THE SURVEY.

The large majority of the 453 families visited in the northern county lived in the open country; less than one-fifth (87) were villagers.

Nationality.

In the northern county live large groups of persons of German and Polish nationality, who, even when born in the United States, are practically unassimilated. They have retained to such an extent the customs and language of the German and Pole, respectively, that it was thought best, in order to give a true picture of the life and customs of this community, to group them according to their nationality rather than according to their country of birth.[1] The parents in the families visited have been classified in four nationality groups:

1. The native-born fathers and mothers of native parentage on both sides, who for the sake of brevity are referred to as the American group.

---

[1] The term " nationality " is thus used to designate a racial group inheriting common customs and a common language—its meaning in discussions of problems of immigration. In this sense it has no implications in regard to allegiance or citizenship.

2. The German group, comprising those of German "nationality" born abroad together with those born in the United States whose fathers were foreign-born Germans (the mothers of this group are sometimes referred to as the German mothers).

3. The Polish group, consisting similarly of foreign-born Poles and of those born in the United States whose fathers were foreign-born Poles (the mothers of this group are sometimes referred to as the Polish mothers).

4. The "miscellaneous and other foreign" group, consisting of all others of foreign birth or of foreign or mixed parentage. The last three groups are combined into—

5. The "foreign" group.[1] Where it is necessary to differentiate those born in Germany or Poland or abroad from those included in the "nationality" or "foreign" groups, the former are specifically designated as born in Germany, born in Poland, or foreign born.

Among the 898 parents whose nationality was reported, 162 (18 per cent) were natives of native parentage on both sides (the American group); 359 (40 per cent) were of German birth or parentage (the German group), of whom only 72 were of foreign birth; 273 (30 per cent) were of Polish birth or parentage (the Polish group), of whom 167 were foreign born; the miscellaneous group consisted of 104 persons, of whom 29 were of foreign birth. The foreign born of all nationalities, therefore, formed a little less than one-third (30 per cent) of the whole group, while the native parents of foreign or mixed parentage made up over half the total (52 per cent).

As the figures show, the German was the largest group; it was in the majority in three townships and one village and formed the largest nationality group in another township and village. Even these proportions understate the importance of the German element in the county as a whole, because while both the main Polish settlements were included in the survey, it was impossible to cover more than a sample of the German districts. Four-fifths of the German parents visited were born in the United States.

The Polish group formed the majority in the two townships in which lie the two large Polish settlements; in one of these practically all the Polish parents were foreign born, while in the other most of them had been born in the United States. In this latter community, where all but 3 out of 53 families visited were Polish, 17 native Polish mothers were encountered who were unable to speak

---

[1] On the schedule the nationality of each of the grandfathers of the baby was recorded. Since in nearly all families both grandparents on either side were of the same nationality, the nationality of the grandfather given on this record was usually that of the grandmother; even when the grandfather was foreign born and the grandmother native she was practically always of the same nationality as her husband. On the other hand, when the grandfather was native but the grandmother foreign born, the specific foreign nationality was not recorded; such cases have been included of necessity in the miscellaneous group. They embraced only 2 fathers and 9 mothers out of the 906 parents included in this study.

English. The husband of one of these women, himself foreign born but with a good command of English, told the agents that he would like to move away from that district in order that his wife might learn English. Nearly all—52 out of 58—the foreign-born women in this county who were unable to speak English were Poles.

Among the mothers visited in the northern county the illiteracy rate was much higher than in the census figures—5.4 per cent for the native born instead of 1.6 per cent and 26.7 per cent among the foreign born instead of 6.8 per cent. These high rates are largely chargeable to the Polish women, for while only 1 per cent of the mothers of native parentage were illiterate, and only 4 per cent of the German mothers, 28 (36 per cent) of the 78 foreign-born Polish mothers and 12 (21 per cent) of 58 born in the United States were unable to read and write in any language.

Father's occupation.

As was to be expected, nine-tenths of the fathers living in the country were engaged in farming. Nearly all these were farmers on their own account; only 7 farm laborers and 2 farm managers were included. Eighteen of the nonfarmers were paper-mill men, most of whom lived in a group in the country near a large paper mill; 5 fathers were cheese makers; 3 worked in the quarries, 4 in the building trades, and 2 at lumbering.

In this county, a large proportion—between one-fourth and one-third—of the farmers found it necessary to eke out their incomes by some kind of supplementary work, as loggers or woodcutters, masons or carpenters, saw-mill or paper-mill hands, or farm laborers. This was especially true of the Poles in the new settlement; since most of them had for the basis of their farming operations only 20, 30, or 40 acres of practically uncleared land, inevitably almost everyone resorted to day labor of some kind. A number of them walked daily 6 miles or more to the nearest paper mill.

The fathers living in the villages represented a greater diversity of occupations—masons, carpenters and builders, blacksmiths and other mechanics, storekeepers, saloon keepers, bankers, laborers, teamsters, etc. The largest group (27) was made up of the paper-mill hands. A few farmers and farm laborers lived in the villages.

Land tenure.

Ten per cent of the fathers included in the survey were tenants. This is much larger than the proportion of farms operated by tenants given in the census reports; to wit, 3.5 per cent. There is no reason, however, to believe that the proportion of tenants was actually greater in the selected townships than in the county at large.

To some extent the apparent difference between the two figures may be due to an actual increase in tenantry since the census date;

but it seems more probable that the chief explanation lies in the fact that the older farmers, who are more apt than the younger men to be landowners, are as a rule not in the count when the fathers of young babies are enumerated.

More than half the landowning fathers were carrying mortgages on their farms and many were newcomers, struggling through the early stages of land clearing. Therefore it is entirely natural that in many of these families as well as in the tenant families expenditures were carefully pruned down to what was regarded as absolutely necessary.

MATERNITY CARE.

Childbearing is an experience which comes often to these country mothers. Thirty-three of those interviewed had borne children twice within the two-year period of the survey; nearly two-thirds (65 per cent) of those who had been married at least two years had borne a child or had had a miscarriage more than once on the average in every two years of their married lives. For 42 of them, this meant 10 or more pregnancies. This condition is reflected in the high birth rate of the rural districts of the county—30 per 1,000 population in 1914 and 1915.[1] For such mothers, injuries from overwork or neglected complications are all the more menacing, because their effects become cumulative.

Availability of physicians.

The American Medical Association directory for 1916 lists 48 physicians in this county, the majority of them located at the county seat. This means one doctor to about every 1,300 inhabitants, which is nearly twice as large a number of persons per physician as the average for the United States (691[2]).

Most of the villages had resident physicians at the time of the survey; but five, including one place of between 400 and 500 inhabitants, had none. This latter was included in the survey; a doctor from the city held office hours there twice a week; but whenever he was needed in an emergency he ordinarily had to come 7 miles by road. There are large areas where a country family may be from 10 to 15 miles from a doctor. It is in exactly these sections that the roads are roughest and most apt to be in bad condition, and that often there is no direct road to the nearest doctor. Some of these neighborhoods which are practically isolated from medical service were included in the territory covered by the survey. Sixty-six of the 395 confinement cases in the open country occurred in families living 10 miles or more from a doctor; for only 8 of these

---

[1] Twenty-sixth Report of the State Board of Health of Wisconsin, 1916, pp. 316 and 318.
[2] American Medical Association Bulletin, Jan. 15, 1917, p. 99.

cases was a doctor secured. And in this county, outside the villages where there was a resident doctor, only two-fifths of the families were living within 5 miles of a physician's headquarters.

How serious may be the delay in getting a doctor when an emergency arises was shown by a tragic experience of one of those country families, that lived 12 miles from a doctor and 6 miles from a telephone in an isolated district of rough roads. One evening in the winter, when the snow was deep, the 6-year-old child had a nose-bleed which could not be stopped. At midnight the doctor was sent for, but he lost his way in the night, had to go back to town, and did not reach the home until 3 o'clock the next day. The bleeding had continued all the while, with the result that the child died just after the doctor arrived. This family—which had seven other children— " never had a doctor in the house " except this one time.

Attendant at birth.

Before the survey was begun it was known that a large proportion of the births in the county were attended by midwives. The investigation showed that the true proportion was even larger than the official figures indicated, because many births attended by midwives were either not registered or registered under the father's name as informant. As has been explained, four of the seven townships, with the three villages therein, included in the study were chosen because maternity care was largely in the hands of midwives. In these townships and villages 50 per cent of the 335 confinements for which records were secured were attended by midwives, while 8 per cent had no professional attendant. In one Polish township, only 5 out of 59 confinements were attended by physicians. In the other districts, where midwives were practically unknown, of 151 confinements 139 were physicians' cases; 3 had no regular attendant; and only 9 were attended by midwives (8 of these in one township). The proportions for all districts together were: Physicians, 58 per cent; midwife, 36 per cent; other attendant or none, 6 per cent.

Of the 28 mothers who had no professional attendant at confinement during the survey period (2 of them twice during the 2 years), 22 belonged to the Polish group, 2 were foreign-born German, and 1 was Indian. Twenty of these confinements were attended by a neighbor, four by the father, three by the grandmother, one by an aunt; and two mothers—one of whom was herself a midwife—delivered themselves, as they had done at six and seven previous confinements. None of this group of mothers was giving birth to her first baby and half had managed with similar informal assistance at previous births. Among the other half who had had either a physician or a midwife at each previous confinement, not a single one had had a physician each time. Five mothers, including the Indian, had never had either a doctor or a midwife present at confinement; one of these had borne 11 children, one 8, one 7, one 6, and one 3.

Such a situation comes about sometimes without any particular choice on the part of the parents, as shown in the case of one Polish family living at the end of an almost impassable road. The father stated that there was never time to go for help because his wife was usually in labor less than an hour; consequently he always tied the cord and cared for the mother. Several mothers in the group reported labor of less than an hour's duration; as one expressed it, the baby " came alone," or as the Polish women say, " it was born in two pains," with the consequence that " there was no one on hand but a neighbor," and sometimes even the neighbor was late. With the majority, however, there was doubtless an element of deliberate intent in the situation, even if unacknowledged. Among the Poles especially the opinion is not uncommon that a mother should be able practically to deliver herself, and that a physician is not only superfluous but even undesirable. One father stated vehemently: " I would not let a doctor come near my wife." His wife, who had borne eight children, said that she always delivered herself, cut the cord, and washed the baby before going to bed, calling only upon a neighbor or her husband to hand her supplies. That such a practice can not be counted upon for safety even when everything has repeatedly gone well is exemplified by the experience of this same mother. At her ninth confinement, which followed almost immediately after the agent's visit, spontaneous delivery was impossible because of a face presentation; after she had been in labor three days, the doctor had to be summoned to turn the child.

One of these women, who had lived all her married life within 2 miles of a doctor, had tried all kinds of obstetrical care in the course of her 20 years' experience. She had had 3 miscarriages and had borne 15 children. Two of the children were stillborn; both these births—instrumental deliveries following protracted labor—were attended by physicians. Two other children had died before they were a day old, and a third at 8 days; all these were delivered by physicians, in one case after 2 days' labor. Of the 10 living children, 4 were delivered by a doctor, 2 by a midwife, 1 by a neighbor, and 3 by the father. Two of the babies (including the last), who were ushered into the world by their father, were born after very brief labors.

In the cases of 23 mothers who are counted as physicians' patients, the doctor did not arrive until after the birth had occurred, sometimes only a few minutes late but occasionally as much as two hours. In the majority of cases these doctors had to come 5 miles or more, sometimes over bad roads; only one of these births (a protracted labor which suddenly terminated while the doctor was away) occurred in the doctor's home town. Most often, some neighbor or relative who was present tied the cord and attended to the baby; but in a few instances this was left for the doctor. One mother reported that her baby "just laid till the doctor came" and apparently suffered no harm by the two hours' wait. Usually the doctor examined the mother and baby after he arrived; thus the mother was to that extent protected from complications. Occasionally, however, a story was told of a doctor who came late and neither looked at the baby nor examined the mother.

In some instances the attendant midwife also failed to reach her patient on time. Naturally this happens less often in a midwife's practice, both because she is apt to be closer at hand than the doctor and also because she seldom has other patients to delay her.

Hospital confinements.

In the northern county there are two general hospitals at the county seat, one of 60 and one of 24 beds. These and the county hospital are available for obstetrical work; a large hospital just outside the county line is easily accessible to the people along the western border. At the worst, in order to reach one of these hospitals, a railroad journey of several hours might be necessary for the people near the eastern border, since the connections are poor; and in the isolated districts it might take two hours or more if the roads were bad, to reach the railroad.

In spite of facilities near at hand, the only mother included in the survey who was confined in a hospital went to Milwaukee—not as an emergency measure but as an insurance against possible difficulties. However, hers was a notable exception to the general attitude on this subject. By most families in the county the idea of going to a hospital for confinement would undoubtedly be regarded as preposterous; certainly it is almost never done.

Obstetrical service by physicians.

The use of obstetrical forceps was much more frequent in this county than it was found to be in the Kansas survey. In 10 per cent (48 cases) of all the deliveries included in the survey instruments were used, instead of in less than 5 per cent as in Kansas; this was 17 per cent of the confinements attended by physicians in the selected districts. Twenty-one of these forty-eight cases were first births, seven were stillbirths, and one child died within the first few hours. No physician used the forceps in any large number of cases; but if the doctors who had the most cases in the area of the survey (at least 10 cases each) are grouped according to their use of instruments, it develops that out of 86 births attended by one group only 5 were instrumental, while among 49 attended by another group, 13 (over one-fourth) were forceps cases.

One of the great difficulties in rural obstetrical practice is the matter of waiting for normal dilatation. A physician in general practice may have other patients critically ill or may have other impending obstetrical cases; and it is very difficult for him to go miles into the country, many times entirely away from a telephone, and to wait 10 or 15 hours or more for nature to take her course. The saving of time effected by the use of instruments is a great temptation.

The large majority of the lacerations recognized by the mothers had been repaired, though in a couple of cases the operation had been unsuccessful. But four mothers reported what they considered severe lacerations which had been neglected by the attending physician. A few other mothers felt strongly that they had suffered from the doctor's carelessness at the time of confinement.

Nearly half the country mothers attended at confinement by a physician were never revisited after the baby was born, and only one-fifth received more than one subsequent visit. This is practically the same situation as that found in the lowland county in North Carolina, but somewhat worse than in western Kansas or in the southern part of Wisconsin (see p. 63). Evidently the vital importance of postnatal supervision is not recognized in any of these country districts. Since postnatal visits far out in the country are difficult for a busy doctor to make, as well as expensive for the family, there is every incentive to take for granted the safe progress of mother and baby; but this is doubly dangerous in districts where even telephone messages are hard for the family to send. That the lack of " after care " is not due wholly to inaccessibility is indicated by the fact that out of 35 mothers attended by physicians in villages where there was a resident doctor, 7 (one-fifth) received no postnatal visits and 10 received only 1.

Midwives.

The midwife is a factor definitely to be reckoned with in a study of maternity care in this county. As has been mentioned, a large proportion of births in certain communities were attended by midwives; in all, records were secured for 175 midwives' confinement cases. Because of the importance of the problem, it was decided to secure directly from these women certain additional facts about their training and methods.

In classifying the attendant at birth, any woman who was considered by the neighborhood competent to take the responsibility for delivering a child and was engaged for that purpose was counted as a midwife. Twenty-four women were so classified; some of these attended only one or two of the births included in the survey, but all had had considerable experience and were looked upon as part of the neighborhood's resources in providing for childbirth. Of the 24 midwives included in the list, 6 had each delivered 10 or more children for whom schedules were secured, while 2 —1 German and 1 Polish—delivered each more than 30. A number had a much larger clientele than the schedules indicated, even during the survey period, because they practiced outside the territory covered by the survey.

As thus used the term "midwife" does not necessarily imply training or legal status. Of 14 midwives concerning whom the information was obtained, only 2 had attended a training school of any kind, though several had been taught by physicians and worked under their supervision; and only 2 out of the whole list of 24 held an official certificate entitling them to practice.

The Wisconsin law provides that no midwife may practice for pay without a certificate of registration, issued by the State board of medical examiners; the requisites for such certificates are (1) presenting a diploma from a reputable accredited school of midwifery, together with evidence of good character, and (2) passing an examination given by the board.[1] In Wisconsin there is no school of midwifery known to the authorities; consequently only women trained outside the State can qualify for the examination.

Only two of the women who were found to be acting as midwives were reported by the State board of medical examiners as registered. These were both professional midwives living in the city and taking occasional cases in the country; the two attended only 3 out of the 175 widwife cases included in the survey. It is only to be expected that women living in isolated neighborhoods and attending perhaps only two or three confinements a year, should not trouble to secure certificates. But that midwives with large practices should fail to do so is a more serious matter. From the midwife's point of view, there are several reasons for this. One woman, with a large practice and good training, was ignorant of the necessity of a State certificate, considering her diploma all sufficient. Others knew that they were debarred because they had no diplomas to present, having never attended a school. Yet others feared the expense and trouble of going to Milwaukee or Madison for the examination; to poor, illiterate Polish women who could not speak English such a prospect naturally seemed appalling. And though most of these women were aware that a "license" was required—and were therefore chary of admitting that they received pay for their services—they had practiced unmolested for so long that they felt under no necessity to comply with the law. Certain of these unregistered midwives had filled out birth certificates in their own names for years.

In part, the employment of midwives seems to have been a natural—almost an inevitable—result of the isolation of many of the early settlements and of many neighborhoods at the present day,

---

[1] Statutes 1917, secs. 1435b, 1436f–12, and 1436f–13.

making it expensive and often practically impossible to secure a doctor. Under such circumstances it frequently happens that one of the neighbor women who are called upon to help in emergencies develops special skill in such work and soon finds herself more and more drafted into service. In these communities the women are often in labor only a short time—a few hours at most—and deliveries usually proceed without difficulty. If thrifty pioneers have once had the experience of paying the bill of a physician who arrived too late to be of any service—at least so it appears to them— they are apt to choose a neighboring midwife for the next occasion. When to such conditions come settlers like the Germans and Poles, who have been accustomed to the services of midwives in "the old country" and prefer them to physicians, midwifery is likely to become an established institution.

A few of the midwives encountered in the course of the survey made their living by the practice of midwifery, but the majority "went out" mainly as an accommodation to their neighbors. They were farmers' wives, living in sparsely settled districts where there would not be enough obstetrical cases to support a professional midwife. Some who had previously been in active practice would have preferred to give up such strenuous work as they grew older; only, as one elderly Polish woman said, "If I go not, what becomes of the women?"

Half the midwives were Polish women practicing in Polish settlements; nearly all the rest were German. Midwives attended 31 per cent of the confinements of German mothers and 61 per cent of those of Polish mothers, while only 16 per cent of the births to American mothers of native parentage were in the hands of midwives. Polish immigration is so recent as compared with the German, and the Polish people have mingled with other nationalities so much less even than the Germans, that it is not surprising that the Polish women have clung more tenaciously than the German to the old-world custom of employing midwives. From all accounts it seems probable that the midwife was as commonly employed in the German settlements a generation ago as she is to-day in the Polish settlements. The really surprising fact is that Polish mothers born in America employed midwives much more and physicians much less than did the immigrants, though they were less likely to go without any attendant. Why this should be is not clear. Inaccessibility of physicians could not have been the chief cause of this difference, for they were about equally inaccessible to the two chief settlements. Several of the foreign-born Polish women who employed a physician had to have a version or an instrumental delivery performed; others had had difficulties at previous confinements which made them anticipate the necessity for a doctor.

As a general proposition there is no question that the difficulty of securing a doctor is one of the important factors leading to the employment of midwives in the country districts. In most of the communities studied the midwife was a neighbor of her patrons and was employed in preference to doctors who were a long distance away. Taking all the selected districts together, three-quarters of the midwives' patients were 5 miles or more from a doctor, while three-fifths of the doctors' cases lived within 5 miles. Where there was no doctor within 10 miles, a midwife was employed in three-fourths of the confinements and in another one-ninth there was no regular attendant. But in the country where there was a physician within 5 miles, a midwife was employed for only one-eighth of the confinements.

The greater convenience of securing a midwife in isolated neighborhoods does not explain the whole situation in the county, however, for a midwife was employed in over one-third of the village cases where there was a doctor in the same village. One of the German midwives living in the city told the agents that she had sometimes driven as far as 30 or 40 miles out into the country to care for women at childbirth. And in one of the German districts included in the survey the midwife, who depends upon her work for her livelihood, lived in the village where there were three doctors and was called upon both in the village and in all the surrounding townships in preference to these doctors. She had practiced in that neighborhood for 20 years. In the village she attended two-thirds of the births scheduled and in one of the adjacent townships nearly half; the majority of her patients were German, but a number were American of native parentage. One of the village physicians, when asked how it happened that the doctors did so little of the obstetrical work, replied: " Well, to tell the truth, it is largely our own fault. We don't like that kind of work and have always more or less turned it over to Mrs. M."

Mrs. M. was a well-educated woman, with a diploma from a school of midwifery; she gave the impression of being both cleanly and capable and had that reputation with the local doctors also. She said that she used carbolic-acid solution in cleansing her hands and in preparing the mother. She sometimes made several examinations during labor, but " sometimes there is not time to make any." She gave douches of " plain water," but boiled the apparatus each time. She carried a bag with cotton, gauze, umbilical tape, two syringes, and a supply of carbolic acid.

Among her patients she was highly esteemed; some of them she had attended at every childbirth—six, seven, or eight times—as long as they had lived in her territory. One of her regular patrons explained the attendance of a physician at one birth by saying that she "wanted Mrs. M. that time but could not get her." More than one mother "tried a doctor once" and had the midwife every time afterwards. Mrs. M. frequently acted as nurse when a physician was in charge of the case. One or two mothers had her as nurse until the last confinement, when, because the doctor could not be secured, the midwife took charge. She was apparently careful to call a doctor when anything seemed to her to be going wrong, and almost never failed to do so in case of a miscarriage.

Mrs. M.'s ordinary charge was $5. She expected her country patrons to furnish transportation and did not ordinarily revisit unless they sent for her; in the village where she lived, however, she customarily made two daily visits for 9 or 10 days. Naturally her village patients were enthusiastic over the service secured; one of these mothers said that she liked the midwife much better than a doctor, "she does lots more for you." She gave no prenatal supervision to her country patients, but occasionally "dropped in" to advise those living in the village.

Typical of the German neighborhood midwife was Mrs. R., whose family homesteaded 40 years ago in an isolated neighborhood 9 or 10 miles from town, where they still live. Her first three children were born in Germany, under a midwife's care. On the Wisconsin clearing eight more were born; she never had a doctor in the house for any cause during all those 40 years; and at childbirth sometimes had not even a neighbor's assistance. She brought with her from Germany a textbook on midwifery, and soon became the neighborhood's mainstay for care at childbirth. At one time she held a State certificate but allowed it to lapse. She did not like to discuss her practice or methods—she speaks no English—but said that in all her experience in that neighborhood she had known of only one stillbirth and no maternal deaths at childbirth.

Records were secured of 16 births which she had attended during the two years of the survey, of which 5 were her own grandchildren. She was then 65 years old, and said that she did not want to "go out" but the neighbors would not let her alone. No one would admit that she made any charge, but "we just gave her something," usually about $2 or $3. She rarely saw her patients in her professional capacity either before or after confinement, even when the baby was her own grandchild.

Of a different type was a much younger woman who had a large practice in one of the paper-mill villages, 7 miles from a resident doctor. She began her work casually, through being summoned in an emergency to help the doctor from the city. He thought her so capable that he called upon her frequently after that, and before long recommended her as able to do as well for these women as he could. For several years before her death the large majority of the births in the village were in her hands. She studied assiduously and even went to a hospital in Chicago for a few weeks. Of all the midwives, she gave the most attention to her patients—advice during pregnancy as well as care during the puerperium—and seems to have been really devoted to the work and to her patients. She insisted that her patients stay in bed 10 days; during that time she made two visits daily, bathing mother and baby and doing everything possible to make them comfortable. Sometimes she even took home and washed the soiled linen "so as to have something clean to put on them the next day." For all this service she charged $12 to $15.

The Polish midwives, as a class, gave the impression of being much less cleanly than the German ones. But some of them seem to have developed skill in their work and to be remarkably successful. A neighboring doctor with a large practice among the Poles begged the agents to try to get one of these midwives to "wash her hands occasionally"; but almost in the same breath he acknowledged that he had never known a Polish woman to get a puerperal infection.

One Polish midwife, herself an immigrant, delivered more than half the babies born in the recent Polish settlement; most of her neighbors regarded her as indispensable to their safety. She was seldom called until labor began; many were the tales of her running 2 or 3 miles to "be on time for the baby," since neither she nor her patient had a horse. She practically supported her family through her own work in the fields and among the neighbors, for her husband had been disabled by an accident in the mill. When her patients were within walking distance she usually made one or two visits a day during the lying-in period and sometimes did the absolutely necessary housework. Her statement as to compensation was: "Sometimes 50 cents, sometimes $2, sometimes $5, sometimes they forget to pay anything." She had no schooling and no formal training, but had picked up some traditional midwives' lore from her grandmother and had worked under a physician's supervision in another State before coming to Wisconsin. She said that she used carbolic acid in the water with which she washed her hands.

In the older Polish settlement the obstetrical practice was divided among a number of neighborhood midwives, most of them old women and illiterate. Four of them were interviewed. All were crude and primitive in their methods, without any training for their work; according to their statements they carried no equipment; and, with the exception of one who had a bottle of bichloride tablets given her by a doctor, they made no pretense of using antiseptics. Before making an examination they all " washed their hands and greased them with lard or any grease they had." All claimed that they called a doctor whenever complications appeared but that the necessity seldom arose. However, a patient of one of these women—her own daughter-in-law, from whom a schedule was secured—was allowed to be in labor three days with what was probably a breech presentation before a doctor was called. Only one made a practice of revisiting her patients. One charged $2, the others took " what they give." These four women together probably cared for about 40 cases a year.

Seldom was the midwife consulted during pregnancy; in only one-seventh of the midwives' cases did the mother see her attendant until labor began. Only one midwife gave her patients any considerable prenatal supervision. On the other hand, nearly two-thirds (65 per cent) of the midwives' patients were visited after confinement, in contrast to a little over half (54 per cent) the physicians' patients; half the midwives' patients (89) received at least two postnatal visits. The case is, of course, not exactly parallel with a doctor's practice, because the midwives who made more than one visit to their patients after confinement were really acting in the capacity of obstetrical nurses; moreover, the midwives usually lived closer to their patients and seldom revisited unless they did live near.

No one of the midwives interviewed used instruments or anæsthetics, or repaired lacerations. They seldom interfered with the expulsion of the afterbirth; without exception they reported that it was their custom to wait for it to " come " naturally. As a rule, they used common twine to tie the cord. All stated that they called a physician immediately if they recognized an abnormal condition. However, it seems fairly certain that at least some of them were willing to perform versions.

Among the 178 births attended by midwives for which records were secured, there were 4 stillbirths and 6 deaths under 2 weeks of age. There was 1 maternal death, due to sepsis developing about a week after confinement.

Nursing care.

In none of the districts studied was there a resident trained nurse; but families in the central part of the county could secure trained nurses from the county seat. One of the hospitals gives a nurses' training course, and there are said to be about 18 trained nurses located in the city. Two country mothers—in addition to one who went to the city for confinement and the one mentioned who went away to a hospital—had trained nurses at the time of childbirth; one of these nurses was the mother's sister; thus only one was employed.

In this county the practical nurse was replaced in the midwife districts by the midwife as a semiskilled childbed nurse. Of 486 confinements, 24—practically all in communities where there were no midwives—were nursed by practical nurses and 93 by midwives, giving together a proportion of about one-fourth who had semitrained nursing care. In 86 out of these 93 cases the midwife was the attendant at birth as well as the nurse. As has been said, these women seldom remained in the home or did the housework, but rather made visits once or twice a day.

The remaining three-fourths of the mothers did as most country women do at childbirth—depended upon relatives or neighbors for their nursing care. It is difficult to see how the great majority of country mothers would manage if they could not call upon their mothers and sisters for help in such emergencies. There are not nearly enough nurses of any grade to do all the childbed nursing in any of these country districts in Wisconsin; and, aside from the difficulty of securing hired girls, those who can be secured could hardly be trusted to give as conscientious care as the mother's own " folks." Of course hardships sometimes occur, as in the case of one mother who was left to care for herself and her baby for two days, with only a daily visit from a neighbor. On the third day she became seriously ill; then her mother-in-law and the neighbor " stayed a day and a night, and worked over her all day "; but after the fever subsided she had to care for herself again.

Prenatal care.

Less than one-fifth (19 per cent) of the mothers attended at birth by physicians had any medical care or supervision during pregnancy; only a very few (9) who were attended by midwives came under a doctor's care during pregnancy. In the districts covered, in only one-eighth of the recorded pregnancies did the mother have any medical prenatal care. In the villages nearly one-third of the mothers who had a doctor at childbirth had some care from him during pregnancy; but in the country only 1 in 6. As was to be expected, the mothers of the foreign group sought medical care during pregnancy much less than mothers of the American group; one-fourth of the native mothers of native parentage had prenatal care, but only one-eighth of the German mothers, and only 1 in 50 of the Polish mothers. Taking the three foreign groups together only 1 in 32 of the foreign-born mothers and approximately 1 in 10 of the native women of foreign parentage had any prenatal care.

Where a mother gets to town only once or twice a year, or where the town in which the family does its business has no resident physician, it is hardly to be expected that she will secure medical supervision during pregnancy; certainly not so long as she regards such care as a superfluous luxury. This is emphatically the case in the foreign groups, who consider a physician, even at confinement, an unnecessary expense. Over a large part of the northern county, a campaign of education of the general public will probably be necessary before the mothers as a rule will be willing to seek or accept prenatal care.

For the purpose of classifying the care received by mothers during pregnancy, the following outline of requirements for *adequate* medical prenatal care was drawn up after consultation with Dr. J. Whitridge Williams, professor of obstetrics in Johns Hopkins University:

1. A general physical examination, including an examination of heart, lungs, and abdomen.

2. Measurement of the pelvis in a first pregnancy to determine whether there is any deformity which is likely to interfere with birth.

3. Continued supervision by the physician, at least through the last five months of pregnancy.

4. Monthly examinations of the urine, at least during the last five months.

Though this standard is no higher than is necessary to insure the early detection of abnormal symptoms and conditions, it is not a standard which is generally attained in private or public practice, either in cities or in rural districts.

Patients whose supervision fell short of these requirements but included at least one personal interview with the physician, with a physical examination and with measurement of the pelvis if a first pregnancy, and one urinalysis are classified as having had *fair* care.

As the facts were reported by the mothers, only 2 of the 63 mothers who came under a doctor's supervision during pregnancy had adequate care according to this standard; neither of these was carrying her first child. Nine had fair care—only 1 of these was a first pregnancy and in this case the pelvis was measured; 7 out of the 9, moreover, saw the physician only once and had no subsequent urinalysis. Two others received care which would have been fair if they had not been primiparæ. Of the 52 who had inadequate care, 5 did not see the physician; 29 who saw the doctor received no physical examination; and 40, or three-fourths, had no urinalysis. Evidently the importance of testing the urine for albumin—the only sure way of detecting the beginning of toxemia or " kidney trouble "—needs especial emphasis in this community.

MATERNAL MORTALITY.

Three maternal deaths connected with childbirth occurred in the selected districts during the survey period. The causes of death were reported as "toxemia, uremic eclampsia, pregnancy," "puerperal embolism of the heart," and "septicemia." Two of the three were doctors' patients. The one who died of septicemia was attended at confinement by a midwife; the mother became ill after having been up and around the house at the end of a week, and then called in a physician. She died six weeks later, after two operations. Her baby lived and thrived. The full record could not be secured for the mother who was reported to have died of toxemia, because the family had moved away; she bore stillborn twins at that time. The third mother "felt fine" during her first pregnancy, but had a difficult forceps delivery, followed by constant hemorrhage, which her husband believes was the cause of her death. Her baby was stillborn.

The county death certificates show 17 deaths outside the city from causes connected with childbirth in the period of the survey. There were 2,540 registered births during this period, which gives 7 maternal deaths per 1,000 births.[1] In 1915, when the estimated population of this rural area was approximately 42,500, there were 8 maternal deaths connected with childbirth, or a maternal mortality rate of 19 per 100,000.[2] These rates are only slightly higher than the rates for the birth-registration area and the death-registration area of the United States. But the rates for the registration areas are, in their turn, considerably above the rates in certain foreign countries.[3]

MOTHER'S WORK.

Rest before and after confinement.

One-fourth of the mothers visited remained in bed for the customary period of 10 days; more than half, however, were in bed less than that time; and only one-fifth longer than the 10 days. In fact, 104 mothers (over one-fifth of the total) were up from bed in less than a week—45 of them in less than four days. This state of affairs

---

[1] The rate is usually stated on the number of maternal deaths per 1,000 live births, but since the number of live births could not be accurately determined, the rate is stated as the deaths per 1,000 registered live births and still births. Owing to the probable omission of many births from registration, the number of registered live and still births probably falls somewhat short of the total live births in the district for the period of the survey.

[2] In 1915, in the death registration area of the United States, the death rate from puerperal fever was 6 per 100,000 population, and from other puerperal affections 9, giving a total rate for causes connected with childbearing of 15 per 100,000. Mortality Statistics, 1915, p. 59, U. S. Bureau of the Census.

In 1915 in the birth-registration area the death rate for all causes connected with childbearing was 6.1 per 1,000 live births. Computed from Birth Statistics, 1915, and Mortality Statistics, 1915, published by the U. S. Bureau of the Census.

[3] Meigs, Dr. Grace L.: Maternal Mortality, Table XII, p. 56. U. S. Children's Bureau Publication No. 19.

shows an alarming disregard 'for the mother's safety, either on her own part or on the part of other members of the family. Even while they were in bed some of these hard-working women were not free from household cares. One mother was found by a neighbor propped up in bed the day after confinement " with her dough board in front of her, trying to make biscuits "; this same mother had bathed her baby that morning.

Nearly twice as large a proportion of country as of village mothers secured less than 10 days' rest after confinement. An equally great difference was found between the customs of the American and the foreign group in this respect. In this county even the American mothers had inadequate opportunity for recuperation after child-birth, for one-third of them got up in less than 10 days; but half the German mothers and over two-thirds of the Polish group ran the same risk of injury. The Polish mothers took least care of them-selves; in fact the records indicate that 7 days in bed instead of 10 was their standard. Nearly half the 88 foreign-born Polish mothers stayed in bed less than a week. One did not go to bed at all after her baby was born but got supper and milked the cow the same even-ing; another was in bed less than a day; and two more, only one day.

The difference between the mothers of the American and the for-eign groups in this respect is, of course, largely a matter of physique and racial custom, but also is influenced by economic conditions. The American and German families as a whole are in better circum-stances than the Poles and are therefore better able to arrange for the relief of the women from the pressure of work. This is only a general rule, however; there are American mothers hard pushed by their work even in the first weeks after childbirth, and on the other hand Polish mothers on prosperous farms who could have help if they saw the need.

Getting up from bed too soon does not always mean " pitching into " the housework immediately, but for many mothers it does. Thirty mothers began to do their cooking or cleaning within a week after the baby was born, and three even did the washing the first week. Though a fortnight was the generally recognized standard for rest from housework, about one-third of the mothers took up the lighter work within the first two weeks. After that time the majority began to do the heavy work as well; only about two-fifths waited as long as a month before doing any washing or ironing.

As was the case with the mothers in other communities studied, the large majority of those interviewed in this county kept up their lighter housework until the time of confinement, some from necessity or custom and some because they had found that they felt better if they kept active. Fifty-one reported that they did no housework for at least the last two weeks before confinement; most of these mothers reported poor health during those last weeks, and one-half of them had a hired girl during that time. Almost twice as many—one-fifth of the total—did not do their washing and ironing in the last two weeks, but only a small proportion discontinued even this heavy work through the last three months of pregnancy.

In addition to the few mothers who kept a hired girl regularly, in 179 cases the mother had hired help with the housework during the lying-in period; this is not quite two-fifths of the total.

Usual housework.

In many farm homes the indoor work is simplified to the last degree. The floors are bare or covered with linoleum; the articles of furniture are few and plain; there are few curtains or ornaments. The family dining table is covered with oilcloth and stands in the kitchen conveniently near the cookstove. Even in the matter of dishes and utensils there is economy. The everyday clothing is apt to be of a character which requires the minimum amount of washing and ironing. In some country families the amount of washing, sewing, and cleaning actually done is small. These facts must be kept in mind in estimating the burden which farm women are called upon to bear. The woman who tries to maintain a more elaborate housekeeping standard and also meets the farm's demands upon her strength often breaks down under the strain.

Only three country mothers and seven village mothers among those visited kept a hired girl for the greater part of the time.

Nearly half the mothers visited had had five or more children. At the time of the survey nearly half had households of more than 5 persons in addition to the baby; about one-seventh had more than 8 in the house; and families of 12 or more were sometimes found. Many of the larger households, of course, contained other adults; but the typical family consisted of the parents and three or four small children. A family of this kind, where none of the children is old enough to be a real help, makes as much work for the housewife as a larger one with older children.

Large families were more common in the country than in the villages. Often where the families were largest the houses were smallest, for a farmer who is engaged in clearing cut-over forest land ordinarily can not build a commodious house until long after the family has outgrown the original cabin. The resulting overcrowding is strikingly shown in the figures. Two or more persons— not counting the baby—to every room in the house may surely be considered overcrowding; and while few village families—less than 1 in 20—showed this condition, 1 in 4 of the country families was living with 2 or more persons to a room. Such a state of affairs makes efficient housekeeping almost an impossibility, especially through the long winters when the children must spend so much time in the house and " underfoot." On the other hand, only about one-third of the country families were living with less than one person per room.

Water supply.

Almost invariably wells furnish the water for drinking and for household use. The water situation as a whole was far from satisfactory. In the first place, a large proportion of the wells in some of the recently settled districts were so shallow as to be most insanitary. In the new Polish settlement the condition was atrocious in this respect; around many of the homes the ground was almost solid rock, and there would be either no water at all or an open hole in the ground—perhaps not more than from 8 to 12 feet deep and filled with water so roily that even an uninformed family recognized its unfitness. Secondly, though the well water is hard, few families had a rain-water supply. Thirdly, water in the house was almost unknown. Less than 1 in 10 (31) of all the country families visited in this county were provided with this elementary convenience; only 2 of these had running water; while none had a bathroom or water-closet. In the four townships in the central part of the county, only 7 families out of 249—in one township not a single family—had inside water. Eight families had an engine to run the house pump, while 13 barn pumps were equipped with engines.

Just half the families who had to carry water had their source of supply within 25 feet, and about one-tenth had to go 100 feet or more. In this county it was the usual thing for the mother to have to carry the household water herself. The hardest feature of the situation is that in most instances every bit of water must be carried up several steps, often of the roughest construction. Moreover, all household waste must be carried down these same steps.

None of the villages included in the survey had a public water supply available for family use; consequently each family had to provide its own water just as though living in the country. About one-sixth (14) of the village families had water inside the house. In most cases this was the usual hand pump; only three families had running water, bathroom, and water-closet. In the paper-mill village, a strictly " company " town, there were only 11 wells for 81 dwellings.

Other household conveniences.

Sinks for the disposal of waste water add almost as much to the housewife's convenience as does water in the house, and in most cases they are probably less costly; 30 country and 7 village families had sinks.

Aside from sewing machines, which were common in both farm and village homes, the one mechanical labor saver possessed by a large number of· rural families is the washing machine. In this county, however, only about one-fourth of the mothers in the country and one-fifth of those in the villages had a washer. Twelve country mothers, and two in the villages had their washing machines run by engines.

A little intelligent care in planning homes would make work much easier for the housewife. Houses are commonly built upon high, damp-proof and frost-proof foundations. It almost never occurs to the builder to locate the pump on a porch or platform level with the kitchen floor. Fuel also is stored in a heap some distance from the house, or in a separate woodhouse if it is sheltered. The cellars often have no inside door, hence every trip to the cellar involves going outdoors.

Boarding hired men.

Dairy farming has no such " rush season " as have other types of farming whose main output is some one crop such as cotton, corn, or wheat. The dairy farm has, it is true, a busy time when its chief homegrown feed crop—hay or corn or whatever it may be—is harvested; but the bulk of the work, the care and feeding and milking of the herd, goes forward steadily day by day throughout the year. One result of this is that the labor force must be kept nearly uniform through the year; if hired men are needed, they are apt to be kept on hand all the time; and it is often possible for the family ‚to manage the work without outside help.

The small farms of the north country seldom require hired labor. Consequently only 95 mothers out of 327 whose husbands were farmers or farm managers boarded hired men during the time covered by the records, while 40 had hired men as usual members of their households. In a number of cases these men were carpenters and masons rather than farm hands, for house and barn building was often in process. Having a regular hired man ordinarily involved doing his washing as well as providing his bed and board, but this would not usually be the case with builders or temporary help.

Work for the dairy.

Dairy farming, however, has disadvantages for the housewife as well as the advantage of relieving her of harvesting crews. In the first place, it almost invariably—at least on these Wisconsin farms—burdens her with the care of the dairy implements, pails, cans, and separator. The milk pails are always on hand to be washed and scalded. The sale of cream is probably the method of disposing of dairy products which is usually easiest for the housewife, since cleaning the separator, though troublesome, is not heavy work. On the other hand, if she is called upon to operate the separator as one of her chores she does hard work, requiring much muscular effort. Next in order comes the sale of whole milk, which removes the separator but substitutes numerous 10-gallon milk cans—heavy, awkward objects to lift and clean. This is the form in which milk is most commonly sold. A mother who washes cans for a 10-cow dairy farm up to the time of confinement and begins again two or three weeks afterwards, as did many mothers in the northern county, runs a decided risk of injuring herself. Last, and most arduous for the housewife, comes the sale of butter. This involves a separator to clean and perhaps to run, the care of the cream and its storage vessels, usually the churning, and almost always the butter to "make up," even if someone else runs the churn. Many mothers in this county made butter for sale. About one-third of the farm women (103) stated that they churned and made butter either for the family's use or for sale. The usual type of churn was the rotary or barrel churn, but a considerable number still used a dasher churn.

Milking.

The women commonly helped with the milking; among the German and Polish families, if the herd was small, the milking was apt to be left entirely to them. Three-fourths (256) of the farm mothers milked; and most of those who milked during pregnancy kept it up until the time of confinement. One Polish mother got up to milk her cow on the fifth day after her baby was born and then went back to bed again for two days.

Other chores.

The care of the garden and of the chickens was the commonest form of outdoor work done by the mothers. More than three-fourths of all the mothers, both in the country and villages, worked in the garden. The care of chickens was an almost universal duty but did not usually mean a great deal of work, because most families raised only chickens enough for their own use.

Many mothers cared for the pigs and calves, and a few for other stock, but this was not an important part of their work. In the newer districts some of them had to chop or saw the household supply of firewood in addition to a multitude of other tasks. Nine did this up to the day the baby was born and one started in again a week afterwards.

Field work.

In half (168) the farming families the mother reported having done more or less field work during her last pregnancy or the year following. Such work ran the whole gamut from "raking a little hay" or "driving team for the unloader" or "picking potatoes" to "planting, hoeing, and digging potatoes, cultivating and picking cucumbers, cutting corn and oats, carrying oat sheaves into the barn, and sawing stove wood," or "raking and loading hay, hoeing and digging potatoes, cutting and grubbing brush, pitching rocks, and cutting stove wood and pulp wood for sale"—in addition, of course, to milking, gardening, caring for chickens, and all the housework.

In the main the women who did field work belonged to the German and Polish groups. Furthermore, though many German women helped in the fields, few of them did anything like the amount and variety of field work which was the common lot of the Polish women. On the small farms of the recent Polish immigrants it was a usual arrangement for the women to do the bulk of the farm work as well as much of the land clearing while the men worked away from home for wages. It was a common sight in harvest time to see a group of these women helping one another in the field, often cutting oats among the stumps with hand sickles. A few of these Polish mothers even cut cordwood, at $1.50 a cord, to provide the necessary groceries for the family, while the husband's wages went to meet the mortgage or the doctor's bill.

Undeniably a moderate amount of outdoor exercise is good for most women; and probably many women can do strenuous outdoor as well as indoor work without injury if they have been accustomed to it, as most of these northern farm women had been from girlhood. But it must be borne in mind that the records under discussion deal with a special group of women, each of whom had borne a child during the period which the record covers. For such women the possibility of injury from heavy work is closely connected with the question of how near it came to the time of childbirth. When a mother rakes hay on the day her baby is born and again eight days afterwards. the question of risk of injury assumes a different aspect from that which it would have at another time.

Field work has the additional disadvantage of depriving the baby of his mother's care. These hard-working country mothers almost always managed to nurse their babies, either taking them along to the fields, or more commonly returning to the house when necessary; but in the intervals a young baby was often left in the hands of children hardly old enough to meet such a responsibility. One baby was said to have been fatally injured by being dropped by an older child who was acting as nurse. Another Polish baby was burned to death while his mother was out helping her husband in the woods; the other children ran out from the burning house, but left the baby in his cradle.

Inevitably most of the field work done by these mothers, such as planting, haying, harvesting, gathering potatoes, had to to be done when the crop called for attention, without regard to the convenience of the worker. As one overworked mother remarked, " the work has to be done." It would not be surprising, therefore, to find that mothers whose babies were born in the summer had helped with the rush work close to the time of childbirth. As a matter of fact 36, the majority of whom were Polish, reported having worked in the fields within four weeks of confinement; considering the urgent need for the women's help on many farms, this is not a large proportion, but from the point of view of the safety of mother and baby the matter is seen in a different light. Nineteen of these mothers worked up to the day of confinement; five were in the fields in a week or less afterwards.

On the whole, the urgent work like haying and harvesting grain was responsible for less of the work done near the time of childbirth than was work like tending the potato crop or clearing land, which is less pressing at any particular time. The probable explanation of this fact is that the latter class of work was common only among the Polish women, who do not plan to spare themselves during pregnancy, while the women of other nationalities, who often help with the rush work, would not usually do this close to the expected time of confinement or soon afterwards.

Haying time is the season of greatest work pressure on the dairy farms of this section of the country. It ordinarily comes in July and lasts from two to four weeks; immediately thereafter comes the grain harvest (oats, rye, barley), making with the haying a busy season of about two months. But the farms of this county produce so much more hay than grain that haying brings much more work than harvest. And in this northern country the mother would often go into the hayfield herself if help were needed. On many a small farm the farmer and his wife and children managed the haying together, with no outside help.

Three-fourths of the mothers who did any field work helped with the haying. Mostly they raked or shocked, or drove the wagon or the unloader team, or stood on top of the load to pack the hay as it was thrown up; some women, however, did all work at haying, including loading and unloading, pitching hay on and off the wagon. With the mothers of the German group haying was the most common field task, and half the 62 who reported working in the fields did no other field work. In spite of the fact that haying is usually a " rush job," involving a serious loss if the crop is not attended to promptly, only 10 mothers worked in the hayfield within a month before or after confinement; four of these worked up to the last day before the birth.

Haying and harvest work are commonly regarded as one continuous task; thus a mother would report in one phrase that she " drove team for haying and harvest " or " pitched hay and grain " or "helped with all work at haying and harvest." Nevertheless, only about half as many mothers (56) worked in the harvest as at haying; over half these harvesters were of the Polish group. They took part in all the necessary occupations—cutting, raking, binding, shocking, loading, and unloading, and especially "driving team." Only two mothers helped with harvesting up to the day of confinement.

Next to haying, work with the potatoes was the commonest field task. Mothers reported tending the potato crop through all its stages, from planting, through hoeing, spraying, and "bugging," to digging and picking. Planting and digging are the heaviest work, and were reported by 75 mothers. Since the Poles are the chief potato raisers of the county, it is natural that the majority of Polish mothers who did any field work worked "in the potatoes." For only a few of them, however, was this the only task; the usual report included haying and harvesting and clearing land as well. Eight mothers worked with the potato crop up to the day of confinement, and five began again in a week or less afterwards.

In the pioneer districts many mothers also helped clear the land—cutting brush, grubbing roots, picking and pitching rocks, and even pulling stumps. All this is heavy work but not especially rush work. Of similar character are the various lumbering tasks reported by a few mothers, who even cut and skidded logs, or cut and piled pulp wood and cordwood for sale; in the Polish settlement cutting and bringing in the stove wood was commonly a woman's job. Preparing the fields—plowing, driving drag, handling manure—was work which the women were seldom called upon to perform.

Of the other miscellaneous tasks reported, one of the most arduous, because of the constant stooping, was picking cucumbers—a common crop in the sandy areas. The mothers who cared for the ginseng bed, who pitched pea vines, or who made maple sirup for four weeks in the spring, represented unusual phases of farming for this district.

How all this work may affect the life of the individual mother is illustrated by the following stories:

A Polish family of mother, father, and two children lived on a clearing of 7 or 8 acres back in the woods 8 miles from town. The mother did her housework and cared for her chickens and pigs up to the day the baby was born, in September, and dug potatoes a week before, in spite of frequent fainting spells and a "bad" leg; during the preceding summer she cut brush, stove wood, and pulp wood, picked stones, hoed potatoes and garden, and raked and loaded hay. She said that the farm work, which she never had done until she came to the country three years before, was easy for her except when she was pregnant; but then it was hard. Her husband nursed her and the baby—except that she bathed the baby—and did the housework for a week; after that she got up and cooked the meals, one week after a difficult instrumental delivery. At the end of two weeks she was doing her chores, including milking the cow; two months afterwards, in the heart of winter, she was again cutting brush and wood in the forest, leaving the baby and a 2-year-old child in the care of their 8-year-old sister.

A Polish family with two small children came to a stony 40-acre tract, of which only 5 acres were cleared, and struggled to pay for the land with the father's wages as a day laborer. A baby was born in October of the first year; the mother was in good health and worked up to the last day, milking, caring for chickens, pigs, cow, and calf, picking stones, sawing and piling stove wood. In the summer she had made hay and earlier in the autumn had hoed and dug potatoes. After the baby came the father did the housework three days and the midwife did one washing; by the end of one week everything—including chores and sawing wood—fell upon the mother's shoulders again. Another baby was born in April of the second year. The mother had a fall a month before confinement which kept her in bed the whole month; but up to that time she had done everything as usual. Her husband did the housework for a week after the confinement on this occasion, and she stayed in bed a whole week, with daily visits from the midwife; afterwards she was more careful about her chores also—did nothing out of doors for two weeks. But after the fortnight she milked two cows; churned; made the garden; tended chickens, pigs, and cattle; hauled manure; chopped, sawed, and piled wood; and after three weeks she began to plant the potato crop. When the baby was 2 months old the father went away to Milwaukee to work, leaving all the farm work to the mother. At that time the oldest of the four small children was not yet 5. This mother was used to heavy work, for as a girl in Germany she had worked as a farm hand, "hauling manure, pitching grain—everything."

A Polish father and mother—living on a 40-acre farm, of which they had brushed 10 acres and stumped one and a quarter since they bought it, about three years previously—said that they did all the farm work together, "half and half." This included clearing land and cutting cordwood, as well as raising crops. There were three small children, the oldest $2\frac{1}{2}$ years of age. Throughout every pregnancy the mother was afflicted with persistent vomiting; two of her babies had been delivered with instruments, after protracted labor. The second baby was born in the dead of winter; the mother ran the separator and milked up to the last day, and cared for the stock until a week before confinement, when her husband came home from the paper mill; but she did no field work after the potatoes were dug. The father did the housework and took care of her for two days; on the third day she got up, cooked, and did the milking. She did the washing and ran the separator a week after the baby was born and was out cutting wood six weeks afterwards. In the summer she picked stones, made garden, looked after the cattle, and worked in the hay and harvest fields; in the autumn she dug potatoes again. The third baby was born the following spring. The father worked in the paper mills all winter until about three months before the baby was born; but, even after his return, the mother did her share of the work; she picked stones up to the last week, milked, ran the separator, worked in the garden, and cut cordwood and brush until the last day. Again she stayed in bed only three days, with her husband as nurse, and immediately thereafter began to cook, care for the house, and milk. Four days after confinement she worked in her garden and planted potatoes in the field; a week after, she did the washing and ran the separator; six weeks afterwards she was working in the hay field. She had done farm work practically all her life in Poland, beginning at 14 to do heavy work like spading, reaping, binding, and loading grain. She said that her work had never injured her in any way.

A German mother, living on a 20-acre clearing near the end of a rough " blind-end " road 13 miles from town, drove team at haying and harvest, shocked hay, and bound oats every summer. Her fourth baby was born early in September, two weeks after she ceased her work in the fields—and she complained of being " weak in the back " that summer. The next baby was born in April of the second year and was 3 months old before his mother went out to work " in the hay." She stayed in bed only three days each time, though she had a hired girl for a week. After the last confinement she began to get the meals as soon as she got up; she washed, milked, churned, and made butter after two weeks, with the help only of her 7-year-old daughter. The time before, she did all the housework after one week but no outside work, except tending the chickens, until spring.

A German mother, living on an 80-acre dairy farm 16 miles from town, had four small boys, the oldest 10. She said that she always helped with all the work on the farm—it had to be done. All through her last pregnancy, which terminated just in haying time, she was badly nauseated and miserable generally; yet up to the last day she milked five cows, made butter for sale, cared for her garden and chickens, and made hay. She had some fever after confinement but got up the fourth day, when her mother left, and did her housework; the next day she milked; a week after confinement she washed, churned, and began to look after her garden and chickens. When the baby was three weeks old she was again doing " all work " on the farm; haying was then over, but harvesting was in full swing.

A German mother with two small children lived on a 40-acre farm, of which about one-third was cleared, in the sandy country. Before the third confinement (in September) she was troubled with headaches, varicose veins, and swollen hands and feet; but she kept up all her housework and chores—milking and feeding two cows and tending chickens—and cut corn the last day. Two weeks before, she had hoed potatoes and a week before that picked cucumbers. She had a neighborhood midwife at confinement, who washed the baby the first time; the father did the housework for one day. On the second day after confinement the mother got up, washed the baby, and cooked the meals; one week afterwards she was churning, milking, and looking after the stock; but she had the washing done twice. When the baby was 5 weeks old she went to the field to dig potatoes. This woman had never done any farm work until the family came here six years ago to uncleared land, and she said that it was too hard for her. At the time of the interview she was " nearly used up " from picking cucumbers in the sun.

A German mother with six small children did all the housework with the help of the two older children—girls of 8 and 10. Her next baby was born in the winter, at the season when there were two hired men on hand to help with the logging. During the winter the mother felt miserable and did no outdoor work except to care for the chickens. But in the summer and autumn, both the year before and the year after confinement, she planted, sprayed, and dug potatoes; in the summer when she was pregnant she also pitched and unloaded both hay and grain. She said that she had been accustomed to this kind of work from the time she was about 13 years old. The summer following the birth of the last baby she did not make hay nor harvest, but instead she boarded masons and carpenters for three months while a new barn was being built.

INFANT WELFARE.

Infant mortality.

The term "infant mortality rate" means the number of deaths under 1 year of age per 1,000 live births. In ordinary statistical usage, such a rate is computed by dividing the registered deaths in a given area by the registered live births in the same period. Its value is dependent upon the completeness of both birth and death registration, and it has the further disadvantage that the infants who die are not necessarily the same ones who were born in the period and district under consideration. In its studies the Children's Bureau computes the infant mortality rate by following up each child born alive, to determine whether or not it was alive at the first birthday, the number of deaths in the group per 1,000 live births giving the rate. A rate of this kind, if based on a thorough canvass, can be obtained even where birth registration is incomplete, and gives a reliable index of the chances of death or survival in the group. In computing such a rate it is necessary to exclude all children born within a year of the time the study was carried on, since it can not be assumed that all those who were alive at the time of the agent's visit would live to the first birthday.

For the rural portion of the northern county—i. e., the whole county exclusive of the one city—the rate, based on birth and death certificates, for 1914 and 1915, together, is 73 per 1,000.[1] With complete birth registration the actual county rate would probably have been lower than this; but even as it stands, it is lower than the average for the rural parts of the urban counties (counties containing cities of at least 10,000 population) of the State, which was 83 in 1914 and 78 in 1915.[2] The birth and death certificates for the townships chosen showed that taken altogether these districts were fairly representative of the county in respect to infant mortality.

---

[1] Twenty-sixth Report of the State Board of Health of Wisconsin, 1916, pp. 316–318.
[2] Ibid., p. 310.

The infant mortality rate, based on the death or survival of the babies for whom schedules were secured, turned out to be considerably lower than the preliminary figures based on the certificates. Namely, out of 237 babies born alive a year or more before the investigation, 14 died before they were 1 year old, giving an infant mortality rate of 59 per 1,000. Fourteen of the 238 babies born alive within the year had died before the visit was made, and a few more deaths in the first year of life might be expected in this group (giving a rate probably somewhat in excess of 59 per 1,000). Therefore, the babies in this county have a considerably better chance of survival than the average. Even the rate given by the survey, however (59 per 1,000), should not be accepted as satisfactory. It should always be remembered that any deaths among babies means something wrong somewhere, and every community should set as its aim the preservation of all its children.

Premature birth and congenital debility were responsible for a greater number of deaths, 9 out of 28, than any other group of causes. Of similar significance is the fact that 7 of the 28 deaths occurred within the first day, and 15 (more than half) before the child was 2 weeks old, in contrast with a proportion of 38 per cent of deaths under 2 weeks in the death-registration area in 1915.[1] The main line of attack in efforts to reduce infant mortality must clearly be directed toward improved maternity care. That this condition is general throughout the State was one of the conclusions reached in a State-wide study made by Dr. Mendenhall,[2] who says:

In Wisconsin the infant death rate is falling and is in general not excessively high; but there is no decline in the deaths the first few weeks of life. The work done to save the babies has not as yet affected those who die at birth, who are too injured, too diseased, or too weak to live. The health of the mother and the care she receives in pregnancy, in confinement, and in the lying-in period must be studied if we wish to save the children who die at birth.

Excluding children born within the year preceding the investigation, the mothers interviewed had borne during their entire childbearing history, 1,821 live-born children and had lost 162 of them before they were a year old—an infant mortality rate of 89 per 1,000.

In this county (see Table II, p. 91) the mothers of the American group had lost a somewhat larger proportion—97 per 1,000—of their babies than the German mothers—71 per 1,000. Among the babies of the Polish mothers, however, the infant mortality rate had been much higher—114 per 1,000. The Polish mothers of both foreign and American birth had lost more than 1 in 10 of their babies; the American-born Polish mothers had the worst record of any group—an infant mortality rate of 134 per 1,000. Within the survey period,

---

[1] Mortality Statistics, 1915, p. 645.   U. S. Bureau of the Census.   Washington, 1917.
[2] Mendenhall, Dr. Dorothy Reed: "Prenatal and natal conditions in Wisconsin," in Wisconsin Medical Journal, Vol. XV, No. 10 (March, 1917), p. 353.

also, the deaths among the babies of the Polish mothers were excessive. This is not surprising, in view of the unhygienic standards of living and of feeding and caring for the children prevalent in the Polish communities. The German mothers born in the United States succeeded in bringing through the first year a larger proportion of their babies than the American mothers; but the foreign-born Germans did not do so well.

Stillbirths and miscarriages.

Another problem dependent for its solution upon better prenatal and obstetrical care is that of the loss of potential child life through stillbirths and miscarriages. This is evidently an important problem in this county, for both the stillbirth and miscarriage rates were high.

Within the two years of the survey the mothers interviewed in the northern county had 19 stillborn children—38 per 1,000 births. This is somewhat higher than the average stillbirth rate—34 per 1,000— in the seven cities where this problem has been studied by the Children's Bureau; apparently, therefore, rural conditions as exemplified in this district have not operated to cut down the stillbirth rate. That it might be much lower is indicated by the fact that the stillbirth rate in the Kansas study was only 11 per 1,000 births.

For the two-year period studied, the German mothers had proportionately more than twice as many stillbirths as the mothers of the American group, and also a higher proportion of stillbirths than the Polish mothers (see Table III, p. 91). When all the pregnancies of these mothers throughout their childbearing history are taken into account (see Table IV, p. 92), the stillbirth rate, 2 per cent, is lower in the total and in each group than when only the last two years' history is included; but the relations between the different nationality groups are the same. The mothers of the miscellaneous foreign group had the highest percentage of stillbirths—6 per cent; next came the German mothers, with a rate of 3 per cent; then the Polish, 2 per cent; and the American mothers had the low rate of 0.9 per cent. Without question the Polish mothers had the least adequate care at childbirth, but nevertheless they show the lowest stillbirth rate of any foreign group.

The mothers interviewed reported two or three times as many miscarriages as stillbirths—6 per cent of their total issues. This is the highest rate found in any of the Children's Bureau rural studies and nearly one-fifth higher than the average rate for all the cities studied (5 per cent). Again we find the German, and especially the "other foreign," mothers having more miscarriages than the Polish mothers; there was little difference between the American and the German groups in this respect.

Feeding customs.

Breast feeding was general. Only a few (13) babies were artificially fed from birth; 26 (6 per cent) were weaned before the middle of the first month. Only a small proportion, less than one-fourth, had any other food than breast milk before the middle of the third month. Nearly half the babies were still exclusively breast fed in the sixth month; but the proportion fell in the seventh month almost to one-fourth because of the custom of beginning other food besides milk at about 6 months of age. Only one-sixth of the 6-months-old babies had been weaned and not quite one-fourth (23 per cent) of those 9 months old. Breast feeding was continued well into the second year; at 12 months, half (55 per cent) the babies were still nursing; at 15 months over one-third; and at 18 months one-sixth; a few had not been weaned even by the second birthday. This custom, common in country districts, of nursing babies beyond the first year is disapproved by most medical authorities.

It is usually believed that foreign-born mothers resort to artificial feeding less than do native mothers. In this county such did not prove to be the case with the younger babies. In the early months, as indicated by the percentages in the first and third months, the American mothers of native parentage had a better record both for exclusive breast feeding and for not weaning their babies than the mothers of the German or the Polish group, or the whole group of foreign-born mothers. For the later months, however, as shown by the percentages for the sixth and ninth months, a larger proportion of the babies of foreign-born mothers were breast fed, indicating that these mothers continue nursing longer than do the American mothers. The Polish mothers continued exclusive breast feeding in these months to a greater extent than either the German or the American mothers. In the sixth month the percentage of babies weaned was lowest in the Polish group; but for the ninth month it was the German mothers who had the smallest proportion of their babies artificially fed (see Table V, p. 92). The foreign-born mothers postponed weaning somewhat longer than the native mothers, especially those of native parentage.

The proportion of infants weaned was smaller in the villages than in the country districts throughout the first year of life.

Birth registration.

In the northern county 110 children whose births had not been registered were found by the canvass. This was 24 per cent, nearly one-fourth, of the live births in the area. More than one-half (61) of these unregistered births occurred in one township; in the rest of the selected districts, the percentage of nonregistered births was only 14. The township where registration was so poor—61 failures out of 109 live births—contained the recent Polish settlement, in which only 6 out of 48 live births were reported. Elsewhere in this township, however, the registration was worse than the average; and the township clerk had made no effort to enforce registration in the Polish settlement, although he was aware that the Polish midwife was reporting none of the births she attended. In the older Polish settlement, where practically all the births were attended by midwives, scarcely any went unregistered; this was due primarily to the activity of the clerk, who saw to it that births were reported to him even if only by word of mouth.

Of the 110 unregistered births discovered in this county 42 were attended by physicians and 44 by midwives. Outside the one Polish settlement where registration went so largely by default, only 15 unregistered births were attended by midwives; as a whole, therefore, the midwives may be said to attend to the registration of their cases at least as well as do the doctors. In one township the midwives had adopted the practice of having their cases reported by the father under his name as informant, with the result that the records showed practically no births attended by midwives.

In the northern county much will have to be done in the way of education of physicians and local registrars, as well as of parents and midwives, as to the importance and obligation of registering births before satisfactory registration is secured.

No unreported deaths of live-born children were discovered, but there were no death certificates for 6 of the 19 stillbirths, and no birth certificates for 5.

On the whole, the impression left after the visits with the mothers in this northern county was that they had met the demands of their strenuous pioneer life with notable success. In spite of the serious deficiency of adequate medical and nursing service and notwithstanding the heavy work done by these child-bearing women, most of them had experienced remarkably little difficulty in bearing and rearing their children. This, of course, does not remove the obligation of the families to lighten the mothers' work as far as possible, nor of the community to see that adequate care is provided. No mothers nor children should be subjected to avoidable risks; even though serious trouble may be infrequent, it is none the less calamitous when it does occur.

PART II. THE SOUTHERN COUNTY.

ECONOMIC AND SOCIAL CONDITIONS IN THE COUNTY.

This county lies in the southwestern quarter of the State, to the south of the Wisconsin River. It is approximately 25 by 30 miles in extent. The population in 1910 was between 22,000 and 23,000; it had remained practically stationary since the census of 1870, tending, however, to decrease. The decrease in the last decade was general throughout the county except in a few villages; in all probability it has continued during the years since 1910 except in the mining district. Within the county are 10 villages ranging from about 200 to 1,100 population; and two cities, of about 1,800 and 2,900. The smaller of these two cities, located near the center of the county, is the county seat. The larger is a center of an important zinc mining district.

Topography and soil.[1]

This part of the State is a beautiful rolling or hilly country, with many fine trees, ample farm buildings, fertile fields, and pastures full of cattle. The watershed between the Wisconsin and Pecatonica Rivers crosses from east to west through the middle of the county, forming a broad, level ridge nearly 500 feet above the Wisconsin bottom. This ridge and the valleys of the streams leading down from it in both directions are the important features of the local topography.

The streams flowing northward toward the Wisconsin River have cut deep narrow valleys, with the result that the whole northern half of the county is rugged and hilly, with precipitous ravines and cliffs in many places. In this area the soil both on the hills and in the valleys is silt loam of good quality, the valleys being considered exceptionally fertile where they are not subject to floods. But along the sides of the valleys are many steep, rocky bluffs which are useless to the farmer; and the hillsides, even where the soil is good, wash out in gullies if they are cultivated, and consequently can be utilized best as pastures. In the rougher parts of this section, the oak woods which originally covered all the hills are still standing, giving a wooded appearance to the whole landscape as seen from the ridge.

Along the ridge and in belts extending southward lies a rich rolling prairie which toward the west widens out into a nearly level

---

[1] Data from a soil survey made by the Wisconsin Geological and Natural History Survey.

plain. This prairie soil is fertile, and practically all of it can be cultivated; corn and small grains thrive, and the pastures of grass and clover are almost incredibly luxuriant.

The stream valleys leading southeasterly from the prairie reproduce in a general way the soil and topography of those to the north, except that the hillsides are not so steep nor so rocky.

Type of agriculture.

In the early days—from about 1829, when the agricultural development of the prairie uplands began, until about 1870—wheat was the chief crop of this county; this was followed for a time by flax. The soil depletion resulting from the continued cultivation of these crops was one of the causes of the change to dairying and stock raising which took place about 35 years ago.

At present dairying is the predominant branch of farming throughout almost the entire county; the chief exception is the western end of the prairie, where corn grows unusually well and many farmers make a specialty of raising or fattening market cattle and hogs. Elsewhere almost every farm produces milk for sale. Dairy farming is particularly well adapted to the hilly districts, comprising fully two-thirds of the county, because it provides an advantageous use for the hillside pastures; farms in these areas almost always include some bottom or hilltop land upon which the necessary grain and forage crops for winter feeding can be raised.

Nearly all the milk produced is sold to local cheese factories. In 1916 there were 131 of these factories; they are to be seen every few miles through the countryside, while there were only 7 creameries. A large number, probably more than half, of the cheese factories are owned by cooperative associations of farmers in the neighborhood. Where the farmers own the whole plant, they usually pay the cheese maker a fixed salary; where the cheese maker owns the machinery and furnishes the materials, he is allowed to charge a certain rate per pound for making the cheese and to take what profit he can out of that, while the rest of the proceeds goes to the farmers. There is keen competition between the managers of cooperative plants and the owners of factories in the same neighborhood, who pay a flat rate for milk, as to which shall yield the milk producers the larger return.

Since dairy farming was introduced—i. e., since about 1880—there has been little change in the agriculture of the county. The amount of land included in farms increased only 8 per cent during this period, and the acreage of improved land only 11 per cent; in the later years, along with the decrease in population, the number of farms has been growing smaller, and their size somewhat larger.

The proportion of land improved (59 per cent at the last census) is not far below the figure of 65 to 70 per cent, the proportion of the total area of the county which the State conservation commission estimated to be fit for cultivation.[1] In brief, this county is, and has been for a generation, a well-settled district with a stationary or diminishing population and a stable type of agriculture well suited to its physical characteristics.

The ordinary farm at the present day runs well over 100 acres in size. According to the last census, the largest group of farms— one-third of the total—was that containing from 100 to 175 acres, and over half of all the farms were between 100 and 260 acres. Nearly half the farms visited in the course of the survey contained at least 200 acres.

Rural density.

Excluding the cities and villages, the rural population of the county in 1910 was approximately 13,400, which gives a density for the open country of between 17 and 18 persons per square mile.

Economic conditions.

This county has the reputation of being one of the notably prosperous counties of the State. Certainly in so far as fertility and land values go it bears out its reputation; prairie land and arable tracts along the creeks have a market value of from $100 to $150 an acre. As a rule, the farms, especially on the prairie, present a prosperous appearance. Houses, barns, silos, and other buildings are ample in size and as a rule well built and well kept, though often without modern improvements. Both meadows and grainfields ordinarily yield good crops; nearly every farm is well provided with live stock, while valuable herds of cattle are not uncommon.

In spite of its prosperity this county has employed no agricultural agent and has allowed its county fair to lapse. There are no cooperative undertakings except the cheese factories.

In this community farming has been long enough established to develop the tendency of well-to-do farmers to retire and rent their farms to tenants. The point was reached long ago where a prospective farmer could not find new land out of which to make a farm but must acquire one ready-made from a previous owner; and land is valued so high that a farm means a large investment. Naturally, therefore, a certain amount of tenancy results. In 1910,[2] one-fifth of the farms in the county were operated by tenants, a slight increase over the 1900 figure; this is not an excessive proportion, though it is considerably larger than the percentage (14) for the State as a whole.

---

[1] First report of the Conservation Commission of the State of Wisconsin, 1909, p. 42.

[2] Thirteenth Census of the United States, 1910, Vol. VII, Agriculture, pp. 902, 922.

It so happens that in this district the tenant in most instances occupies a dwelling which the owner built for himself before retiring; thus he is comfortably housed and has good farm buildings. It takes considerable capital for cattle and other equipment before a man can farm even as a tenant in this district; consequently the really poor renter is seldom found, except as an occasional immigrant (usually Swiss) undertakes the seemingly impossible.

After an enterprising farmer has rented a farm for a time he usually attempts to buy his land, and with prices as high as they are this almost inevitably means a burdensome mortgage. A farmer in this case is apt to have a worse time financially than a tenant. On the other hand, farm owners who have their land paid for, or who have inherited a farm, are as a rule in very comfortable circumstances.

Nationality.

This county is predominantly native American; at the last census only 14 per cent, or less than one-seventh, of the population was foreign born. The American born were about equally divided between those whose parents were native and those whose parents were immigrants. English, German, and Norwegian were the chief foreign nationalities represented, both among the foreign born and those born in the United States. In the main, these nationalities are well assimilated into the community, and the atmosphere is nowhere strongly foreign. The more recent immigration, of smaller volume, falls into two distinct classes—farmers, chiefly German Swiss, many of whom came into the county as farm hands and subsequently took farms in the rougher districts which the native farmer considered hopeless; and mine laborers of various Slavic nationalities who are found in small groups in the mining settlements.

Literacy and education.

As might be expected of a well-established, prosperous, native farming district, there is little illiteracy. Outside the larger city (the only one of over 2,500 population), the illiteracy rate among the native born was only 0.6 per cent, while among the foreign born it was only 7 per cent.[1] All the American-born mothers visited in this county and all but two of the foreign born were able to read and write.

The country schools are all one-teacher schools, and the salaries paid are low, $320 a year being the most common stipend. The villages do better in this respect, for they have graded schools and the teachers receive a slightly higher salary, most commonly $450. Nine-tenths of the country schools had an eight-months' term; 9 of the 10 villages in the county, as well as the two cities, maintain high

---

[1] Thirteenth Census of the United States, 1910, Vol. III, Population, pp. 1087, 1099.

schools. Consequently secondary education is fairly accessible to country children in most parts of the county and would be within the reach of nearly all if the roads in winter were better.

Means of communication.

Two main railroads and three branch lines cross the county; most of its area is sufficiently equipped with railroad facilities, though there are isolated neighborhoods. However, the railroads are so located that intercommunication is difficult. The lower half of the Wisconsin River drainage slope has practically no railroad communication and consequently almost no intercourse with the rest of the county; its urban center is a large city in the adjoining county. The two cities in the county, though they are only about 12 miles apart, have no direct railroad connection with each other, and none with large sections of the county. This situation is an obstacle to the county's uniting on any common plans or undertakings, for habitual travel and lines of interest follow the railroads almost exclusively.

One reason why this community is so dependent upon its railroad facilities is that its highroads are often difficult to travel. In 1914[1] there were only 20 miles of sand-clay roads, 5 miles of macadam, and no gravel roads—only 2 per cent of the total mileage surfaced. In some townships the dirt roads are well kept and even dragged regularly; but in spite of good care they are bound to be heavy in wet weather—which means several months of the year. In the hilly country it is so difficult to get about during the winter and spring that some families away from the main roads reported that they had been practically marooned for long periods. Many of the hill roads are hardly more than ungraded tracks, painfully steep and rocky. But the worst roads of all are in the mining district, where the heavy hauling from the mines will ruin even a macadam road within a short time.

A peculiarity of this part of the State is that many homes are located so far back from the highroads that it is necessary to cross two or three fields, opening gates along the way, or to drive a long distance across the hills over a rough farm road in order to reach the dwelling. This condition is said to have arisen from the fact that the houses were built before the roads were located; but whatever the explanation, it certainly aggravates the isolation of many a family. One mother, whose home was reached only by climbing one of these rough, hilly private roads, told the agent that she was able to go to town only once a year and had no neighbors within walking distance.

The county is well supplied over most of its area both with rural mail delivery and with telephone lines. Among the families visited,

[1] Public Road Mileage and Revenues in the Central Mountain and Pacific States, 1914. U. S. Department of Agriculture, Bulletin No. 389.

only five had to go as far as half a mile and only one as far as a mile to reach a telephone, while the large majority had their own telephones.

SELECTED TOWNSHIPS.

The study covered 3 of the 14 townships in the southern county. These were selected to represent different localities. One is just south of the Wisconsin River, embracing some bottom land but lying largely in the rough, hilly country; this township includes one village of between 300 and 400 inhabitants. The other two are on the southern border of the county; both include some prairie and some more hilly land along the streams. One of the two latter townships is purely agricultural and contains no village but only a couple of small hamlets. The other lies partly in the mining belt and includes two villages, in both of which mining is an important factor.

FAMILIES INCLUDED IN THE SURVEY.

In the southern county less than one-fourth (38) of the 161 families visited were village people; the others lived in the open country.

Nationality.

Half (51 per cent) the parents in these families were native born of native parentage. In this county, as distinguished from the northern, the generation of parents who were the children of immigrants had largely lost their foreign characteristics and did not stand out as a distinct factor in the community. This group formed a little over one-third (35 per cent) of the total; about one-fifth were of German (paternal) parentage, and the rest of various other nationalities. Only about one-seventh (14 per cent) of all the parents were foreign born; of these one-third were German. These German immigrants nearly all came from Switzerland. In the mining districts five Serbian mothers and two Polish mothers had babies who were included in the survey. Of 20 foreign-born mothers, all but 7—4 German Swiss and 3 Serbian—could speak English; in no instance had a native mother of foreign parentage so far escaped amalgamation as to be unable to speak the language of the country where she was born and reared.

Father's occupation.

In this county 87 per cent of the fathers in the country families visited were engaged in farming; 3 farm managers and 10 farm laborers were included in this group of 107. Eleven zinc-mine employees formed the largest group of nonfarmers. Three cheese makers, 1 storekeeper, and 1 " odd-job " laborer completed the list.

In the villages, the zinc miners were in the majority; the others were scattered among the usual village occupations.

Land tenure.

The proportion of farmers included in the survey who were tenants (44 per cent) was twice as high as the census figure of 20 per cent for the entire county. Forty-four per cent is a high proportion of tenancy and indicates that the fathers, who were financially responsible for the care of the mothers and babies with whom this survey is concerned, were not as well able to meet this responsibility as census data for the county would imply.

MATERNITY CARE.

Of the 161 mothers visited in this county, 14 had borne children twice within the two-year period of the survey; half (52 per cent) those who had been married at least two years had borne children or had a miscarriage on the average more than once for every two years of their married life.

Availability of physicians.

The American Medical Association Directory of 1916 lists 22 physicians in the county; this gives approximately 1,000 persons per physician, which is somewhat less than in the other county but still higher than the average for the United States. All but one of the villages had resident physicians at the time of the survey; nevertheless there are a few places where a country family may be 10 miles or more from a doctor. The central part of the Wisconsin River slope is the most isolated district, and it is there in the hills that the roads are worst. A distance of 10 miles may be a serious barrier here when travel is difficult because of mud or snow. Only 2 out of the 135 confinements in the selected country districts occurred where there was no doctor within 10 miles, while half (49 per cent) these families had a doctor within 5 miles. But at 12 confinements the attending physician was summoned from 10 miles or more away.

The one village without a doctor in the southern county was included in the survey. This place is 4 miles from a railroad and, though there was a physician at the nearest railroad point and two others 6 miles away, the doctors had to use roads cut up by the hauling of ore from the mines—a state of affairs not conducive to a rapid response to a call.

Attendant at birth.

No midwife was practicing in any of the districts where the investigation was carried on nor, so far as could be learned, anywhere in the county. All the confinements in the villages were attended by physicians; and nearly all—130 out of 135—of those in the county. At the remaining five births there was no attendant except the father or grandmother or a neighbor. One of these cases was a sudden triple birth, in the middle of the night, at which the astounded father was compelled to assist after a fruitless attempt to summon help over a disabled telephone. Fortunately he had had previous experience in such emergencies, and nothing went wrong. It was not the family's intention to do without a doctor, but three out of five times they had been unable to have one on hand at the birth. In another of these families the doctor had been summoned but failed to arrive in time to be of any service. The other three families deliberately dispensed with the doctor's services; in one instance, because of poverty; in one, because the grandmother did not approve of having a doctor at childbirth; and in the third, because the father had called a doctor on two previous occasions but the physician had not arrived on time; so he decided that "we were just as well off without."

Among the mothers who are counted as physicians' patients were 13 whose doctor did not arrive until after the birth had occurred, sometimes only a few minutes late but in two cases as much as an hour. Most of these doctors had to come 5 miles or more.

Hospital confinements.

There is a general hospital of 30 beds at the county seat, a private hospital in the same city, and two small private hospitals in the other city. Certain districts are more accessible to hospitals outside the county; in no case would it be necessary to travel more than two or at most three hours by rail to reach a hospital somewhere. Of course for a good many families it is more difficult to get to the railroad than to make the train trip; yet patients do manage to reach a hospital when it seems imperative, though the delay in an emergency may be serious. The general hospital at the county seat reported caring for 18 obstetrical patients in 1916, 10 of whom came from outside the city. However, only three mothers from the townships studied went to hospitals for confinement during the period covered; all these went outside the county. These mothers had no especial reason to anticipate complications at confinement—and none arose except an instrumental delivery in one case—but chose the hospital as the most convenient method of providing the necessary care.

Obstetrical service.

The use of obstetrical forceps proved to be even more common here than in the northern county. Whereas less than 5 per cent of the deliveries in the county studied in Kansas were effected with instruments and 10 per cent in the other Wisconsin county, the proportion here was 14 per cent, or 25 cases. Eleven of these instrumental deliveries were first births. One resulted in a stillbirth and two in deaths within two days. The use of forceps was largely concentrated in the practice of one physician, who performed 15 instrumental deliveries among 35 confinements attended within the survey period; if his cases are deducted, only 7 per cent of the remaining deliveries were instrumental. The physician who had the largest obstetrical practice in the selected districts of that county delivered only 1 out of 46 children with forceps.

It is, of course, difficult, as has been said, for a country doctor with a large area to cover to visit his patients as regularly as is possible in city practice. Furthermore, the charge which a physician must make for additional visits miles away from his headquarters seems to many country families an expense which they are unwilling to incur unless the necessity is forced upon them. Nevertheless a mother is exposed to unjustifiable risks when, as happened to nearly one-third of the country mothers in the survey, her doctor never sees her after the day the baby is born. Only about one-fourth of the country mothers attended by physicians had more than one visit from the doctor subsequent to the delivery. In the villages the doctors revisited the majority of their obstetrical patients at least twice, ·but two mothers in villages where there was a resident physician were never seen by the doctor after the delivery of the baby. It should be noted that the mothers in this county received considerably more postnatal care than those in the north.

Nursing care.

In none of the districts studied was there a resident trained nurse; during part of the time none could be secured anywhere in the county. Consequently, aside from the expense of her salary, having a trained nurse for confinement or any other sickness involved both the trouble and the expense of bringing her from outside the county; moreover, many country families, even when they can afford a trained nurse, do not appreciate the importance of adequate nursing care. Only two country mothers, and none in the villages, employed a trained nurse at confinement; another secured a trained nurse two weeks afterwards after blood poisoning had developed; another had her sister, who was a trained nurse, to help the practical nurse in charge of the case.

In each of the country districts and in two of the villages studied there were practical nurses, women who had had considerable experience in obstetrical nursing—they were sometimes called baby nurses. These were the main reliance of the families who made a point of getting the best available care; many of them were held in high esteem, and in a number of cases the family sent away to a neighboring village or city to secure such a nurse who stood in good repute. However, the history of one young mother showed the danger of untrained and possibly ignorant nurses. In her inexperience she intrusted her first baby to a so-called practical nurse who had taken a correspondence course and "thought she would start out nursing." She fed the baby cows' milk and sweetened water the first three days. Then after nursing one day, he was sick and would not take the breast. The nurse tried various kinds of food, consulting the doctor only by telephone; she also "kept the baby asleep with dope nearly all the time." Finally, on the tenth day, he died in convulsions.

More than one-fourth (49) of the mothers visited were nursed during the puerperium by these practical nurses, but in only a few cases (10) did they do the housework. The remaining three-fourths of the mothers, with few exceptions, had to depend upon neighbors or relatives for nursing care.

Prenatal care.

The superiority of postnatal supervision in the southern county is accompanied by a much greater amount of prenatal supervision than was found in the northern county. Twice as large a proportion of mothers attended at birth by physicians had some prenatal care in the southern county (38 per cent) as in the northern (19 per cent). The difference between the counties is not great for village mothers but is very marked in the open country, a fact that is undoubtedly related to the greater isolation of the country districts studied in the northern county. In neither county can the situation be regarded as satisfactory; but any community where, as in the southern county, more than one-third of the mothers consult their physicians during pregnancy, has evidently begun to realize that prenatal care is worth while, both for the alleviation of present discomfort and for the prevention of later complications. Nevertheless, much ignorance on this point survives. For instance, one mother, living in comfortable circumstances on a large farm, stated that she vomited throughout pregnancy and was much troubled with headaches, swollen feet, and swollen eyes (symptoms suggestive of toxemia), but did not see the doctor at all—"just worried along." Her baby was stillborn at eight months.

The standards used in the study for classifying the medical prenatal care reported by the mothers are described on page 38.

According to these standards, none of the mothers in the southern county had adequate care; 13 had fair care, of whom only one was a primipara (carrying her first child); 9 other primiparæ had care which would have been fair except for the failure of the physician to measure the pelvis. Merely sending for medicine or advice, without a personal interview, was counted as no care. Of the 65 patients who had some care, 11 never saw the doctor, but merely sent the urine for examination; 19 others received no physical examination; 21 had no analysis of the urine made; 23 saw the physician only once.

MATERNAL MORTALITY.

In the selected districts in the southern county only one mother died at childbirth in the two years of the survey. The cause stated on her death certificate was pernicious anemia, with parturition and nephritis contributory. The account given by her family agrees with this diagnosis; the mother had suffered from pernicious anemia for three years, and during her last pregnancy she was in very poor health, the doctor under whose care she was having found albumin in her urine. The child was born prematurely and lived only a few hours; the mother died five days later.

The county records show during the survey period only one other death from causes connected with the puerperal state. This makes 2 maternal deaths out of 887 registered births (live and still born).[1]

MOTHER'S WORK.

Rest before and after confinement.

More than one-third of the mothers visited (38 per cent) remained in bed for the customary period of 10 days; one-fourth, or less than half as large a proportion as in the other county, stayed in bed less than this time. Only 9 (1 in 19) were in bed less than a week; and, on the other hand, more than one-third stayed in bed longer than 10 days.

A considerably larger proportion of mothers in the country than in the villages secured less than 10 days' rest after confinement. In this county, as well as in the other, there was a notable difference between the mothers of native parentage and those of foreign birth or parentage in this respect; 17 per cent of the former and 34 per cent of the latter stayed in bed less than 10 days.

With these mothers, getting up from bed too soon commonly meant " pitching into " the housework immediately. In nine cases the mother was out of bed in less than a week, and five of these mothers were doing their cooking or cleaning within that first week, while four even did the washing before a week was up. As a rule, however, the mothers in the southern county did no cooking nor cleaning during the first two weeks after childbirth; and, while many undertook the laundry work at two or three weeks, half of them obtained a respite of at least a month from this heavy work.

As often occurs, the large majority of the mothers kept up their lighter housework until the time of confinement. Twenty did no housework for the last two weeks or more; in most instances these were mothers who had a hired girl during that time. It was recog-

---

[1] See note 1, p. 39.

nized by many of the women that washing and ironing is too heavy work for a pregnant woman toward the end of her pregnancy; consequently one-third of the mothers did not do their washing in the last two weeks. But even this part of the housework was discontinued throughout the last three months by only a small proportion.

In addition to the few mothers who kept a hired girl regularly, in 87 instances the mother had hired household help for the lying-in period. This is the same proportion—one-half—that had " help " in the Kansas rural survey. Apparently village mothers found it no easier to get help at such times than did those living in the open country.

Usual housework.

Even on the prosperous farms of the southern county, practically all the housewives were obliged to do without hired help; even those who could afford to pay fair wages frequently could not secure a hired girl; many families who could afford to pay good wages for temporary help in time of sickness often, of course, could not meet such an expense regularly. Only three country mothers among those visited kept a hired girl for the greater part of the time; six village mothers had regular hired help, though a village housewife usually needs help less than does one in the country.

There were not nearly so many large families here as in the north; only one-third (instead of half) of the mothers visited had households of more than five persons in addition to the baby. The most usual family consisted of the parents and two or three small children; very large families, such as some of those in the north, consisting of 12 or more persons, were practically unknown.

In this county, there was little of the house crowding which was found to be common in the newer communities, not only in northern Wisconsin but also in western Kansas. Only 1 in 15 of the country families in southern Wisconsin was living with more than two persons to a room; on the other hand, more than three-fifths had more than one room per person (not counting the baby). This is one advantage of the commodious farmhouses seen throughout the southern part of the State. Half the village homes where a baby had been born also had at least one room per person.

Water supply and other household conveniences.

Well water is almost universally used for drinking. In this county, the well water is so hard that most families have a supply of rain water also for general household use; and available soft water makes an appreciable difference in the housework. Since the cistern or tank is naturally built near or under the house, it is comparatively easy to connect a hand pump in the kitchen with the cistern and thus give an inside water supply. Of 123 country families in this county, 25 reported water in the house; 21 of these had only rain water and had to bring their well water from outside. Of course, this arrangement is a great improvement over having to carry all the household cleaning and wash water from outside, for the purposes for which well water is required—drinking and cooking—take a much smaller quantity than do the cleaning and washing.

Even when the cistern pump or the rain-water barrel is outside, it is apt to be much nearer the house than is the well, for the barn has often a powerful attraction for the well. Partly as a result of that fact, the majority (52 per cent) of the families who had to bring in the household water had to carry it less than 25 feet and few (about 1 in 11) had to carry it as far as 100 feet.

Only two homes had running water piped into the house; one of these had a bathroom and water-closet. It is not uncommon in these districts to find the barn well, but not the house well, equipped with a windmill or engine to do the pumping; 16 families had an engine connected with the barn pump; and 14, one connected with the house pump. On the other hand, it was common for mothers in this county to tell the agents that they never had to carry the water, the men always carried it in for them; others reported that the men carried the water through the winter or carried the wash water. As in the other county, the water usually had to be carried up steps to the kitchen.

Both Wisconsin counties compare favorably with the one in Kansas as to nearness of the water supply to the house, and the southern county—but not the northern—as to the proportion of homes having inside water.

In this county, also, none of the villages included in the survey had a public water supply. About one-fourth of the village families had water inside the houses, but only one of these had running water with bathroom and water-closet.

Thirty-one country and 12 village families in the southern county had a sink for the disposal of waste water; this is just a few more than had inside water. Half the mothers in both country and villages had a washing machine; however, only one in the villages had a power washer, while 15 in the country were so provided. One ran her churn, and another the separator, by engine power.

Boarding hired men.

The large farms of the southern county naturally needed hired men more often than the smaller ones in the northern county. Consequently, in the southern county 54 mothers (out of 98 whose husbands were farmers or farm managers) reported that they had had to board "hands"—usually only one—during the period covered by the survey.

Work for the dairy.

In the southern county it was almost the rule that the dairy farms sold their milk to the cheese factories; on many farms the whole supply was hauled off immediately after the morning milking, leaving almost no milk even for the family's use. This relieves the house-wife of the tasks connected with butter making or the sale of cream, but usually burdens her with many heavy milk cans to clean. In one southern township the cheese-factory manager said that the men were beginning to wash the cans, and he " couldn't see but that they did it about as well as the women "; but it is usually considered a woman's job. Only one-fifth of the mothers living on the farms of the townships included in the survey reported that they did churn-ing; many of these made butter for their own families only. A good many others made butter but had some one else run the churn.

Milking and other chores.

As a rule the women of the southern county do little work outside the house, but half those on farms milked.

The care of the garden and of the chickens was the commonest of the outdoor chores done by the mothers here as elsewhere. About two-fifths of the mothers, both in the country and villages, worked in the garden. The care of chickens was a common duty, but in this county also the flocks were seldom large.

Field work.

Practically none of the mothers in the southern county did any work in the fields; field work for women goes absolutely against the local standards. One mother said indignantly, when asked about her work: " Mothers who work outside just don't care for their babies right." Three of the five who reported any field work were German; two of these helped with the haying, one husked corn two or three hours at a time, one picked corn and potatoes. One of the others picked apples and potatoes; one drove the plow and cultivator. The German mother who said she pitched hay two months before con-finement was the only one who did any really heavy work; none of the five worked in the fields within a month of confinement.

INFANT WELFARE.

Infant mortality.[1]

Among the 90 live-born babies for whom records were secured in the southern county who were born at least a year before the survey began, 7 died before they were a year old; this is equivalent to an infant mortality rate of 78 per 1,000, or 1 death to 13 live births. Of the 83 babies born during the year just preceding the survey, 9 had died before the agent's visit, or 1 in 10 (108 per 1,000). It is evident

---

[1] For definition of the term, see p. 50.

that this figure, though considerably higher than that for the preceding year, is probably less than the true infant mortality rate for this year; for some deaths in this group may have occurred after the agent's visit but prior to the first birthday, since most of these babies at the time of the agent's visit were not yet one year old. In other words, at least 16 out of 173 babies in this county—approximately 1 in 11—died before they reached their first birthday. The probability is that the true proportion was somewhat higher than this.

In this county, according to the official figures, the infant mortality rate was 115 per 1,000 in 1914; in 1915 the rate fell to 88.[1] The combined rate for the two years was 102, or just a little over 1 in 10. It appears, therefore, after allowing for the differences between the two methods of computing the rates, that the agreement is reasonably close.

One death in 10 is the average rate for the United States birth-registration area, which in 1915 was 100 per 1,000. But it was slightly higher than the rate of 94 in the rural part of the birth-registration area, and is certainly higher than should exist in a prosperous rural community. The average for all the rural counties in Wisconsin was 76 per 1,000 in 1914 and 73 in 1915;[2] and several counties are credited with rates lower than 50 per 1,000.

In the southern county, and in the two counties together, the proportion of deaths was less among the babies of the country districts than among the village babies. Of the 260 country babies in the two counties, 14 died—an infant mortality rate of 54 per 1,000. This is still somewhat higher than the corresponding rate of 40 per 1,000 which was found among the babies of the open country in Kansas.[3]

Premature birth was responsible for half the 16 deaths in the southern county, in contrast with one-fifth of the deaths under 1 year of age in the registration area.[4] An excessive proportion—10 out of 16 deaths—occurred before the baby was 2 weeks old; 6 of these were deaths within the first few hours. Evidently, therefore, the effort to reduce infant mortality, in this county as in the other, must be directed primarily toward better maternity and prenatal care.

Excluding children born within the year preceding the investigation, the mothers interviewed in the southern county had borne during their whole child-bearing history 415 live-born children and had lost 34 of them before they were a year old—an infant mortality rate of 82 per 1,000. For both counties there had been a much higher pro-

---

[1] Twenty-sixth Report of the State Board of Health of Wisconsin, pp. 315 and 317, Madison, 1917.

[2] Twenty-sixth Report of the State Board of Health of Wisconsin, p. 310. Madison, Wis., 1917.

[3] Maternity and Infant Care in a Rural County in Kansas, p. 40. U. S. Children's Bureau Publication No. 26.

[4] Mortality Statistics, 1915, p. 645. U. S. Bureau of the Census. Washington, 1917.

portion of deaths than had occurred in the country families of the Kansas survey (55 per 1,000) or in the white families of the lowland county in North Carolina (48 per 1,000) ; the Wisconsin rates are about the same, however, as that in the mountain county in North Carolina (80 per 1,000).

In the southern county, the mothers of foreign birth or parentage had lost a somewhat larger proportion of their babies than the mothers of native parentage. (See Table II, p. 91.)

Stillbirths and miscarriages.

Within the two years of the survey the mothers interviewed in the southern county had 5 stillbirths, 28 per 1,000 births. This is somewhat lower than the stillbirth rate (34 per 1,000) for the seven cities where this problem had been studied by the Children's Bureau. That it might be still lower is indicated by the fact that the stillbirth rate in the Kansas study was only 11 per 1,000 births.

The mothers of this county had had a smaller proportion of stillbirths (2 per cent) among all their issues than among the births of the past two years. Both in the survey period and during their whole history the mothers of native parentage had borne more stillborn children than the mothers of the foreign group; but they had lost a smaller proportion through miscarriage. (See Tables III and IV, pp. 91, 92.)

Feeding customs.

As in the other county, only a few babies were artificially fed from birth. Over four-fifths of the 3-months-old babies were exclusively breast fed—a proportion even larger than in the northern county. In the sixth month, the proportion was still over half; in the seventh, it fell to only one-third. A large percentage of the babies not exclusively breast fed received some breast milk throughout the first nine months. Only one-sixth of the 6-months-old babies had been weaned; the proportion weaned had increased by the ninth month to only one-fifth (20 per cent). Breast feeding was continued in the second year for a large number, three-fifths of the 12-months-old babies received some breast milk, and at 15 months one-third were still nursing. Practically all were weaned, however, before they were 18 months old.

When the customs of the different rural counties where these surveys have been carried on are compared (see Table VI, p. 92), the mothers of the two Wisconsin counties are found to have given their babies breast milk without any other food to a less extent than those in the western Kansas county, but to a much greater extent throughout the first eight months than the mothers of the mountain county in North Carolina. And the proportion artificially fed was throughout the first nine months higher in these two Wisconsin counties than in any of the other rural districts studied.

In all the rural counties the proportion weaned was lower throughout the first nine months than in any of the four cities—two middle western and two eastern—included in Table VI (see p. 92). Up to the fourth or fifth months a larger proportion of the Wisconsin babies were exclusively breast fed than in any of these cities; but in the later months the percentages of exclusive breast feeding are higher for the cities.

Birth registration.

In the southern county, 17 live-born children, born in the area studied, were discovered by the canvass to have been omitted from the register of births. This was 10 per cent of the total live births included in the survey; 15 of these 17 births were attended by physicians.

So far as indicated, therefore, by the selected districts, no great improvement would be necessary to bring birth registration in the southern county up to the minimum census standard of 90 per cent completeness. In both counties all the unregistered births discovered by the canvass were reported to the State board of health and investigated by it.

In the southern county it was found that three infant deaths (out of 16) had not been recorded. Failure to register deaths indicates an even more serious violation of the law than does the deficiency of birth registration, because the need for death registration is more widely recognized, and in general the registration of deaths is much more widely enacted and observed than is birth registration. Through the requirement of a burial permit before interment, the registration of deaths can also be enforced more easily than that of births. Furthermore, if many deaths are omitted the apparent infant mortality rate is an understatement of the true mortality rate, and a community when it becomes sufficiently interested to look up the figures may fail to appreciate the actual conditions.

The southern county is of interest mainly as an example of one of the most prosperous agricultural sections of the United States— the prairie lands of the northern Middle West. The conditions revealed by this survey are undoubtedly typical of the lives of a larger proportion of the farm women of the country than are those, in many respects more striking, found in isolated districts in the South and West. Moreover, there need be no financial difficulty in the community's providing adequately for the health of its mothers and children, even though some of its families would be unable to do this individually.

PART III. ACTIVITIES IN WISCONSIN ON BEHALF OF THE HEALTH OF MOTHERS AND BABIES.

This section of the report deals with work undertaken up to the close of the year 1917, for the protection of the health of childbearing mothers and of young babies in the rural districts of Wisconsin. Some of these activities are State wide in their scope, and it is believed that the account of these is complete. Others are local; and of these the report covers in full only the two counties in which the survey of maternity care was made.

No account of conditions in Wisconsin would be complete without mention of the active spirit of cooperation among the various public-health agencies. Often several different organizations are found working together on a common enterprise, with the result that the credit for accomplishment belongs not to any one but to the whole group.

WORK OF THE STATE BOARD OF HEALTH.

Birth registration.

Wisconsin is one of the States recognized by the census as having an adequate birth-registration law. Each township or incorporated village is a separate registration district for vital statistics, the township or village clerk acting as local registrar. The clerk is required by law to send the original birth and death certificates to the State office, and a copy of each to the county registrar of deeds; village clerks must also keep a local record, but in the township such a local register is not provided for. The county files of copies are also notoriously incomplete; hence it is necessary in most instances to send to the State office to find out whether a birth has been registered.

Within recent years the State board of health has been progressively increasing its efforts toward the strict enforcement of the birth-registration law. In 1917, it adopted the policy of prosecuting all failures to register which came to its attention, unless the offender presented an adequate excuse and gave his written promise to observe the law in the future. Knowledge of unregistered births is secured (1) from reports by local registrars, (2) from inquiries by parents, and (3) from checking hospital records of births. During 1917 the board also requested each county medical society to devote a meeting to birth registration, and where a society complied with this request the deputy State health officers were frequently sent to talk on the subject.

Since 1914 the board has sent to parents a card certifying to the receipt of the birth certificate for their child. This practice is undoubtedly a stimulus to the parents' interest in birth registration. During the course of the survey many mothers spoke of having these "papers" or wondered why they had not received them. The State board is said to receive about 200 inquiries a month from parents who failed to receive their cards.

In the latter part of 1917 the United States Bureau of the Census made a State-wide birth-registration test in Wisconsin, covering the births of two months. These tests were based not upon a canvass but upon live births reported to the census agents by postmasters, mail carriers, etc., throughout the State. In the outcome, 95 per cent of the births thus reported in each of the two counties studied in the Children's Bureau survey were found to have been registered.

Educational literature.

The State board of health publishes a bulletin on the care of babies, which is sent out to any citizen of the State making a request for it. The revised edition of this pamphlet, printed in 1917, contains a section on prenatal care—the mother's personal hygiene and the complications which must be guarded against. On the birth-registration certificate card is printed a notice that anyone may secure this bulletin free of charge, and many requests result from this notice. The pamphlet on the feeding of children published by the agricultural extension division of the State university (see p. 78) is also distributed by the State board of health.

Prevention of blindness.

The law [1] in Wisconsin requires that every obstetrical attendant must use a 1 per cent silver nitrate solution in the eyes of each newborn infant as a preventive measure against ophthalmia neonatorum or "babies' sore eyes," and provides for the gratuitous distribution of the proper solution. In accordance with these provisions, the State board of health sends out once a year to each physician, registered midwife, and health officer in the State a case containing six dozen ampules of silver nitrate solution, each designed for the treatment of one case. Additional supplies are sent as requested; about 2,000 requests are received in the course of a year.

It is the opinion of the executive officers that this prophylactic is very generally used. The law also requires that cases of inflammation of infants' eyes must be reported to the State board of health. Only about 10 such cases a year are reported.

Campaign against venereal disease.

Because of the direct causative connection of venereal disease with infant mortality, the efforts of the State board of health for the

---

[1] Laws of 1915, sec. 1409a–1.

prevention and cure of these diseases should be mentioned. Diagnostic service is provided by the various laboratories under the control of the board and by the State psychiatric institute; diagnoses are made free of charge for any licensed physician. The board of health publishes a pamphlet on the dangers of venereal diseases and the necessity of treatment by a physician; it also posts placards in suitable places giving the same information.

LOCAL PUBLIC-HEALTH ADMINISTRATION.

In Wisconsin the townships and villages are important organs of local government. Among other functions, they are the units for local public-health administration. There are township, village, and city health officials, but none representing the county; next above the local unit stands the deputy State health officer, who is a full-time employee of the State board of health and has under his jurisdiction one of the five sanitary districts into which the State is divided. Each township or (incorporated) village board either acts itself as the local board of health or appoints such a board; this board then appoints the health officer, who may or may not be a physician. In townships and villages the clerk acts as registrar of vital statistics.

At the time of the survey the State registrar stated that somewhat less than half the local health officers in the State were physicians. In the 10 townships where the survey was made, 5 of the health officers were physicians and 5 were farmers; of the 5 incorporated villages, 4 had medical health officers—the fifth had apparently neglected to provide itself with any.

The local board also fixes the compensation of the health officer. Judging from the survey, $10 a year is the usual rural salary; in some cases the annual salary is supplemented, and in others replaced, by payments " by the visit," but the largest sum paid to any of these officers for the year preceding the survey was $18.25. Several had no compensation during that period because they " had put in no time "; one had been paid only $5 in five years, for posting quarantine twice.

As a rule, almost the sole duty of these local rural officers is conceived to be the posting and removal of quarantine notices and fumigation for the severe contagious diseases—scarlet fever, diphtheria, and smallpox. Only a few of the rural health officers interviewed made any serious attempt to placard measles or whooping cough or to disinfect after tuberculosis. If the officer is not a physician, he ordinarily depends upon instructions from the attending physician as to when and how long to quarantine, and in such cases the physician is often paid by the township to do the fumigating. It is only in very rare instances that a sanitary complaint is brought to the health officer's attention, while it is practically never conceived to be his duty to seek out insanitary conditions.

The general laxness found in the rural districts in enforcing or observing isolation of measles and whooping cough should be combated in the interest of the babies as well as that of the older children. A small, but not a negligible, proportion of infant deaths is always found to be due to these diseases. Whooping cough is especially apt to be fatal to young babies. In Wisconsin in 1915, 124 babies under a year old died of whooping cough, almost eight times as many as died from diphtheria.[1] In the families visited in the course of the Wisconsin survey, eight babies had died of whooping cough before they were a year old, in contrast with only two deaths from diphtheria. One township clerk, in discusssing measures needed for the protection of children's health, complained especially of the habit of some parents of carelessly exposing other people's children to the diseases which their children had, and urged that persons doing this be made liable for the results of their indifference. In that particular neighborhood such carelessness had extended even to scarlet fever.

WORK OF THE STATE BOARD OF MEDICAL EXAMINERS.

The law charges the State board of medical examiners with the duty of enforcing the medical practice act, including the examination and registration of midwives. Obviously a law drafted for the purpose of protecting the mothers of the State from untrained midwives does no good if not enforced. And that it is not enforced in the rural districts the survey furnishes ample proof.

The secretary of the board writes that a couple of years ago the midwives on a list made up from the birth-registration records " * * * were notified that they must become registered by examination or cease to practice. Beyond this notification the State board of medical examiners have been able to do nothing. We found after this investigation that the greatest majority of midwives were women along in the fifties and sixties, of foreign birth, who were unable to comply with the law, due to the fact that they must pass a written examination in the English language. The law provides for gratuitous service and service in the case of emergency, and their attention was called to the fact that such service was the only kind which they could render under the law. I think most of them understand the situation, but of course we have no way of knowing how they are complying with these requirements."

The attorney for the board stated that in the course of his connection with the board, extending back to its organization in 1897,

---

[1] Mortality Statistics, 1915, p. 549. U. S. Bureau of the Census. Washington, 1917.

he remembered only one or two prosecutions of midwives for practicing without registration. (Prosecutions for malpractice have
been more frequent.) He stated that the law permits anyone to give
either gratuitous or emergency service, and that in case a physician
or registered midwife could not be secured in time for a delivery
it might be lawful for an unregistered midwife to charge for her
services, the law being ambiguous on that point.

It is obvious from the foregoing, as well as from the findings of
the survey, that there is absolutely no supervision of the midwives
who are in practice. The medical practice act makes no provision
for any such supervision.

WORK OF THE STATE UNIVERSITY.

The State university reaches the rural mothers and fathers of the
State in various ways through its extension service. There are two
separate extension departments, one known as the university extension division, and the other as the extension service of the college of
agriculture or more briefly as the agricultural extension division.

University extension division.

The university extension division gives several correspondence
courses in health subjects. Three of these bear directly on the health
of mothers and babies and were planned and are conducted by a
woman physician. They are entitled "The Prospective Mother,"
dealing with the care of the mother during pregnancy, confinement,
and the puerperium, and also with the care of the newborn baby;
"The Child in Health," dealing especially with infant feeding and
general hygiene; and "The Child in Disease," dealing with the prevention of the ordinary sicknesses of childhood as well as with
home nursing. While the enrollment in these courses has not been
large, the students have been widely scattered over the Northwestern
States.

Another phase of the educational work of the extension division
is the series of weekly health articles which it furnishes to the press
of the State. These articles are so widely published that it is estimated they reach at least 300,000 readers a week. In this series, there
have been a considerable number of articles dealing with various
phases of infant hygiene, and also a few dealing with maternity
care.

The community institutes conducted by the university extension division (sometimes in cooperation with the agricultural extension
service), in nearly all cases have made a feature of popular instruction in hygiene and the prevention of disease; frequently they have
included talks by physicians on the care of mothers and babies. The
programs are planned and advertised with the object of attracting

country people as well as townfolk, and the majority of the institutes have been held in places of less than 2,500 population—a third in villages smaller than 1,000 population. Consequently, these institutes are to be counted among the forces working for the improvement of rural health conditions.

Agricultural extension division.

During the three years 1915, 1916, and 1917, the agricultural extension service has made health talks one of the main features of its agricultural schools, which are held for a few days at a time in small towns and villages. These health talks and conferences have been given by the woman physician who wrote the correspondence courses. At each place the series usually includes a general meeting on community health problems and two or three informal meetings or conferences especially for women, at one of which maternity care is the main topic, and at the others child hygiene and infectious diseases. This service has reached each year the women of 15 to 20 rural communities. The interest of the women in these topics, especially in maternity problems, has been marked; and the meetings are often followed by letters of inquiry from perplexed mothers. The care of the childbearing mother as a community problem is sometimes discussed at the general evening meetings also.

As has been mentioned, the agricultural extension division has also published a bulletin on the feeding of children; this gives detailed instructions for feeding through the third year.

WORK OF THE WISCONSIN ANTITUBERCULOSIS ASSOCIATION.

The Wisconsin Antituberculosis Association is, in the scope of its work, really a general public-health organization, because its managers believe that all health problems are intimately linked together; and that the influences which build up the individual's strength are a main reliance in combating all forms of disease alike—that, for example, a sturdy, healthy baby is not only more apt than a weakling to survive the perils of infancy but also less apt to develop tuberculosis in after life. Consequently this association has been one of the instigators and promoters of most forms of infant-welfare work undertaken in the State. It has joined in the campaign for the education of mothers in the care of themselves and their babies and has added its quota to the instructive literature on this subject in the form of circulars and printed charts giving directions for infant feeding.

The greatest contribution of the association, however, has been the promoting and supervising of public-health nursing. The status of this work in rural communities is discussed on pages 79 to 81. The Wisconsin Antituberculosis Association employs four field nurses, two supervising nurses who spend part of their time in visiting the nurses throughout the State, and two demonstrating nurses who are available for short-time demonstrations of community nursing. The association also holds periodical conferences of the public-health nurses of the State, keeps in touch with them through correspondence, and furnishes them with educational literature and with blank forms needed in their work. It acts as an employment agency for communities wishing nurses, and for the past two years it has maintained training courses in order to help fill the dearth of adequately trained public-health workers.

Another valuable contribution is the research work by which the association has directed attention to health conditions in rural communities. Its tuberculosis survey of Dunn County in 1911 was a pioneer rural study, a forerunner of subsequent studies in many States dealing with health conditions among country school children and with infant mortality in rural districts. The research work of the association was influential in securing the passage of the State law authorizing the employment of county public-health nurses by county boards of supervisors, and of other enactments for the promotion of the public health.

RURAL PUBLIC-HEALTH NURSING.

At the close of 1917, 140 public-health nurses were at work in Wisconsin. A large proportion of these were in the city of Milwaukee, the majority were in smaller cities, and only 5 were doing strictly rural work. These 5 were all county nurses; 2 of them were employed by county boards of supervisors, 2 by the trustees of the Milwaukee County institutions, and 1 was supported by the sale of Red Cross seals. The last 3 concentrate their efforts chiefly upon tuberculosis work.

The legislature passed an act in 1913 authorizing county boards to employ nurses.[1] None did so, however, for two or three years afterwards. In 1916 a nurse was employed by Chippewa County; Waupaca County was added to the list in January, 1917; Lincoln in August; and Eau Claire voted the appropriation in the autumn. All these counties are in the north-central part of the State, in the same general section as the northern county of the survey. At the close of 1917 the nurses' positions were vacant in two of these four counties because no one could be found to fill the places;[2] consequently the nurses then in the service of county boards numbered only two, as has been stated. In both these counties the nursing work which was started as an experiment for a year only was made permanent at the next annual meeting.

---

[1] St. 1917, sec. 679–10m (constituting Laws 1913, ch. 93).
[2] These positions were filled early in 1918.

In each of these two counties—Lincoln and Waupaca—the nurse made school visiting and the inspection of school children the main feature of her work for the first year; one of the nurses expected to be able to make the round of her schools in about a year, the other in a year and a half. Both have been called upon to aid in checking school epidemics of contagious diseases. Both nurses established women's rest tents at their county fairs, where a simple health exhibit was displayed, literature was distributed, and the nurse was on hand to talk with mothers who wanted information or advice.

In Waupaca County the nurse helped with the Baby Week celebration in the largest village in the county. She also tries to hold a mothers' meeting whenever she visits a school; at these meetings she explains her work, and the mothers ask questions. Interest centers largely upon the inspection of the school children and the meaning and cure of the various defects found.

In Lincoln County the nurse took up her work in the summer with the belief that tuberculosis should be the first point of attack, but upon consulting the county records she found that the deaths from tuberculosis (22) were far overshadowed by the stillbirths (33) and deaths under 1 week of age (14) which, as she said, "are practically the same thing as stillbirths." In other words, she found that her biggest problem in life-saving would be that of prenatal and natal care. She has not been able to start any organized work along that line because of the pressure of school work beginning with the opening of the school term. But she says that she has spoken about prenatal and maternity care whenever she has had a chance to address an audience of women, and that she has found them much interested in the subject. Some women's organizations, at her suggestion, have undertaken to provide maternity outfits for mothers in need. The nurse has made an attempt also to get in touch with prospective mothers and has found it possible to establish such relations with a few pregnant women that she could give them advice on prenatal care. She has met with no midwives in her territory, though it is largely German.

In spite of the fact that neither of these two counties is excessively large—only about half the size of the northern county of the survey—each of the nurses felt strongly that her territory was much too large for one nurse. One had thought of dividing her county into four or five districts; then she believed that the work could be adequately handled.

The 1917 legislature made it legally possible to employ nurses in smaller units than counties.[1] By the terms of the act "the local board of health, health commissioner or health officer of any town [-ship], village or city may employ public health nurses"; "towns,

---

[1] St. 1917, sec. 1411g, as amended by Laws of 1917, ch. 123.

villages, and cities may * * * employ public health nurses jointly," on the same principle of sharing the cost according to population as joint-district high schools are now supported in many places. So far no action has been taken under these provisions, but such an arrangement seems to be the logical next step in the development of rural nursing.

In the southern county of the survey, there has been no public-health nursing in the rural districts. The county seat employed a school nurse on part time for the year following the survey (see p. 83).

In the northern county, the county seat has had a full-time school nurse for several years. In the city also is a small children's infirmary, in charge of a trained nurse who devotes part of her time to visiting nursing. She occasionally makes calls in the country, mainly for the purpose of getting sick children into the hospital. The county is so large, however, and so many districts are almost inaccessible that only exceptional cases come to her notice. This same infirmary nurse keeps a register of nurses, both trained and practical; she fills calls for trained nurses outside the city as well as in, and sometimes even outside the county, but says that she has never sent a practical nurse outside the city.

In the year following the survey one of the largest paper mills, located in one of the townships included in the survey, employed a visiting nurse primarily to care for the mill employees and their families. So far as her time allows, she also accepts other cases on call from the attending physician and examines the children in neighboring village and rural schools. It is of interest in connection with the subject of maternity care that for the first seven months of her service she reported having made 24 prenatal calls and 329 obstetrical nursing calls upon 33 patients.

LOCAL EDUCATIONAL CAMPAIGNS.

Baby Week.

Baby Week was widely celebrated in Wisconsin in both 1916 and 1917. The State-wide direction of the movement was primarily in the hands of the State federation of women's clubs; much assistance in providing speakers, literature, and exhibits and in suggesting programs was given by the Wisconsin Antituberculosis Association and especially by the university extension division. There is no way of telling to what extent the celebration reached the rural districts. However, the list of places published by the university extension division as observing Baby Week in 1916 contains a large proportion (over one-third) under 2,500 population, showing that the interest in Baby Week was by no means confined to the cities.

In 1916, a Baby Week celebration was held in each of the counties included in the survey; in the southern county this took place in the mining town (the larger of the two cities) and in the northern county in the county seat. In the latter, an elaborate program of lectures, demonstrations, and exhibits was presented; the main feature, however, was a Baby Health Contest, which lasted through four days. In this county, an effort was made to include the rural districts in the campaign. Extension meetings were held in seven villages; demonstrations were given by members of the State agricultural extension faculty, and speakers gathered for the city meetings brought to the smaller places the message of better care of mothers and babies. Twenty-five or thirty country babies were brought to the Baby Contest in the city, and these were included in the follow-up work during which a nurse employed by the central committee was sent out to visit the mothers of all babies registered in the contest.

In the following summer (1917) the committee which had charge of this "Better Baby Campaign" in the northern county employed a trained nurse—the demonstrator from the Wisconsin Antituberculosis Association—for three months' intensive work in the city. Infant-welfare stations were opened in four public schools, at each of which a weekly conference was held, with a doctor and the nurse in attendance; babies were examined by the doctor, talks on the care of babies were given by the doctor and the nurse, and literature was distributed. The nurse called once a week at the home of each of the 97 babies enrolled at the stations; she also supervised a few prenatal cases, making regular visits and examining the urine. No rural work was undertaken this year.

Children's health conference.

In 1916, in connection with the Children's Bureau survey, a children's health conference was held in the county seat of the southern county. This was undertaken, cooperatively, by the Children's Bureau, which furnished the physician and an assistant for the examination of the children; by the university extension division, which provided the exhibit, demonstrators, and speakers; by the State board of health, which sent a speaker; by the Wisconsin Antituberculosis Association, which furnished speakers and an organizer; and by a local committee of women who arranged places of meeting, provided supplies, and advertised the conference.

The central feature of this campaign was the physical examination of children by the Children's Bureau physician. This differed from a baby contest in that children were not scored nor prizes given. Its object was to teach mothers how to observe their own children and how to promote their health by suitable care and feeding, as well as to point out to the mothers defects which needed to be remedied either by better hygiene or by a physician's care. In spite of cold weather and heavy rains which practically cut off the attendance of country families, 77 children were brought to the conference for examination.

As a result of the interest in children's health aroused by the conference, the local committee undertook to persuade the school district meeting to employ a school nurse. They were successful in this attempt, and a part-time nurse was employed in 1916–17; but, in the following year, "the authorities did not feel disposed to retain the nurse."

CONCLUSIONS.

The southern county in Wisconsin is an example, such as might be found anywhere throughout large sections of the Middle West, of a prosperous farming community on fertile soil, where the land is cleared, crops are abundant, and the necessary farm improvements—houses, barns, fences—as well as live stock have been provided. Therefore there should be no difficulty in financing any cooperative undertakings for the common good upon which the community may decide.

The northern county represents a different range of conditions. As a community engaged in converting "logged-out" land into farms and homes, it illustrates conditions common in the forest belt of Michigan, Wisconsin, and Minnesota. Its foreign settlements, also, are a feature common in those States and others as well, and it has certain characteristics common to most communities in the pioneer stage. As a whole it is still engaged in building up its farming capital—land values, buildings and dwellings, and live stock— out of meager beginnings. Many a farmer finds it beyond his means to provide adequate shelter and sometimes even adequate food for his family, while conveniences and comforts are for the present entirely beyond his contemplation. Even in those neighborhoods and families which have passed beyond that stage, the memory of pioneer hardships is still vivid and the habit of pioneer economy still strong. Consequently it is difficult, and probably seems more difficult than it really need be, to secure money for anything beyond the most primitive needs of the community. However, it should not be impossible to persuade the farmers in even the newest settlements that the protection of the health of their own wives and children is a matter of vital concern to them. Fortunately the influence of the county seat and of certain of the smaller centers could probably be counted upon to support a progressive public-health campaign.

Without question, the most urgent of the common needs in both counties, from the point of view of general utility as well as from that of providing for the safety of mothers and babies, is for good permanent roads which will remain usable throughout the year. None of the other needs can be adequately met until such roads cover the county so thoroughly that no home, even on the remote hill farms or forest clearings, shall be a mile and a half—or even half a mile—from a passable road.

The provision of a county public-health nurse would probably be the most useful " next step " which the county authorities could take in the interest of the mothers and babies on the farms and small industrial settlements. As we have seen, four counties in Wisconsin have already decided to provide such a nurse; there seems no good reason why the children of other counties in the State should not have the advantages provided for these children.

Such a nurse could be of service to country and village mothers in many ways, some of which can be foreseen from the experience of other communities and some of which would appear only as her work developed to fit the local needs. In many counties rural public-health nursing has begun with school nursing, including both the inspection of school sanitation and the examination of the pupils; but some counties might find it a good plan to begin with infant-welfare work. The nurse might establish a series of periodical mothers' meetings in different local community centers, usually in the villages but sometimes in a township hall or an accessible country school, where she could weigh babies, give simple demonstrations in infant care and home nursing, and talk with mothers who wish her advice. How to keep a baby well through the summer; what to do before the doctor comes, in an emergency such as croup or convulsions; how to nurse a sick child or a mother and newborn baby at home—these are all questions about which women are anxious to learn all they can. It is often a good plan to combine meetings of this kind with the establishment of a women's rest room in the village, where mothers coming to town for shopping and trading may find toilet facilities and a clean, quiet place in which to care for their children. A local committee should be organized to supervise the rest room and to help the nurse in her work. Such a rest room may in time be developed into a local health center, with exhibits and literature for distribution. Similar exhibits and mothers' conferences held in connection with a rest tent at the county fair have proved popular in other counties where they have been established by the nurse.

As these meetings became well established, the program might be widened to include such an examination of children by physicians as constitutes the main feature of a children's health conference and of many Baby Week celebrations. The experience of other communities, as well as the popularity of the examination held at the county seat in each of these counties in the year of the survey, shows that mothers are usually eager to take advantage of such an opportunity to secure expert advice about the health of their children when it is brought within their reach and fully explained to them.

The nurse's meetings with the mothers would usually in the beginning concern themselves with the health of babies and the younger children but would naturally develop to include advice as to the mother's care of her own health, especially during pregnancy. The experience of the Lincoln County nurse shows that Wisconsin mothers are keenly interested in this subject also. A nurse who has had special training and experience in prenatal work can be of great help to the prospective mothers in the country, and to their physicians. She will so advise the mothers about daily details of their care of themselves that they will be able to avoid much discomfort and disability; she will urge them to see their physicians early for a thorough preliminary examination and later when necessary; she will urge them to send samples of urine regularly to be examined; or, if asked to do so, she may make these tests and report the results to the physicians.

In a territory so large and so difficult to get about in as are both these counties—especially the northern one—it would be impossible for any one county nurse to do any home nursing; in the northern county it would probably be impossible for her even to make the round of the rural schools more than once in two years. Therefore an effort might be made to arrange, possibly through private contributions or through the interest of an industrial plant in the health of its employees (as in the northern county), for a demonstration in some limited neighborhood of the advantages of a community nurse, who would be available to help the mothers in time of sickness, to nurse them at confinement, and to show them how to apply the principles of hygiene in their own homes. On the basis of such a demonstration, the county could in time be divided into nursing districts, each consisting probably of from two to five or six townships, with a trained nurse employed in each district. The last legislature made it legally possible to provide community nurses for such districts from public funds, on the same principle that joint-district high schools are now in many places supported by a village and two or more townships. At least three such districts would be needed in the southern county and at least six in the northern, in order to bring the district nurse into intimate contact with the people who need her help.

Each nursing district would normally center around some village which is a natural community center; each would have as a nucleus of interest the school inspection, the mothers' conference, and other lines of work previously established by the county nurse. The county nurse would, of course, take the lead in organizing the nursing service in the districts and should supervise the work in order to unify it and keep it up to the highest possible standard of usefulness.

The need which is felt by the largest number of country mothers in connection with their confinement care is the need for better nursing and household help. Therefore, they would undoubtedly

welcome the establishment of a service of supervised trained attendants—competent women who have had some training and experience
in home care of the sick and who will do the housework as well as
the nursing. In several communities it has already been proved
that women can be found willing and anxious to do this work. The
register of " practical nurses " now kept by the infirmary nurse at
the county seat in the northern county might serve as a nucleus for a
county-wide register. With a combination of county and district
public-health nursing, it should prove feasible in these counties to
conduct a county training course for attendants under the direction
of the county nurse and to keep a register in each district from
which mothers could obtain help in case of sickness. The attendants
should always do their nursing under the supervision of the district
nurse; this supervision by a trained nurse is essential to the success
of the plan.

Even in the foreign districts of the northern county, where the
midwife is now the main reliance for childbed nursing as well as
for delivery, it should be practicable in time to make the supervised
trained attendant popular, for the more competent midwives are in
the main old women and none so trusted seem to be rising up to take
their places. In view of this fact, it seems probable that even in
the Polish settlements mothers will gradually come more and more
to engage physicians for confinement and to need some one to take
the midwife's place as nurse. A trained attendant would necessarily
cost more than families of this nationality have been used to paying
the midwife, but she would also give them more service, because she
would remain in the home instead of making visits.

In both sections of the State there are hospitals to which mothers
who need hospital care at confinement can be taken. Many isolated
neighborhoods are at present almost out of reach of any of these
hospitals so far as emergency service is concerned, but improvement
of the roads would relieve this difficulty. A campaign of education
in which the public-health nurses would naturally be the main
agents is evidently needed to induce mothers (and physicians) to
make use of the hospital facilities now available.

The State board of health has as yet no special division or officer
charged with the duty of promoting the health of the children, the
work which it does along this line being handled by the general ad-
ministrative officers. It is the hope of the board that the next legislature may see fit to provide means for the establishment of such a
bureau. A bureau of child hygiene would be of great service to
mothers and children throughout the State and especially to those
in rural districts who are out of reach of the various infant-welfare
activities of the cities. It would serve to correlate many of the
lines of work now carried on in the State, and could also undertake

new activities. All kinds of work for the prevention of infant mortality and of children's diseases would naturally fall within its scope. Like the Kansas Division of Child Hygiene, it might also find means to carry on an extensive campaign of education and advice as to the best standards of prenatal and maternity care. As the survey has indicated, this is one of the urgent needs in rural Wisconsin and therefore promises to be one of the most fruitful lines of activity opening before a child-hygiene bureau.

APPENDIX.

TABLE I.—*Per cent of physicians' obstetrical cases receiving postnatal visits.*

Districts.	Number of confinements attended by physicians.	Per cent receiving specified number of postnatal visits.			
		None.	One.	More than one.	Not reported.
Northern county...............................	281	46	30	24	....
Country districts.............................	237	49	30	21	....
Villages:					
Resident physician..........................	35	20	29	46	6
No resident physician.......................	9	67	22	11	....
Southern county...............................	170	25	41	31	3
Country districts.............................	130	31	42	24	3
Villages:					
Resident physician..........................	22	9	36	55	....
No resident physician.......................	18	6	39	55	....

TABLE II.—*Infant mortality rates for each county, by nationality of mother, based on all births reported by mothers included in the study.*[a]

County, and nationality of mother.	Live births.	Infant deaths.	Infant mortality rate.
Northern county..........................	1,821	162	89
Nationality of mother:[b]			
American group [c]........................	298	29	97
German group............................	689	49	71
Polish group.............................	638	73	114
Miscellaneous and other foreign group......	185	11	59
Not reported.............................	11	....	....
Southern county..........................	415	34	82
Nationality of mother:			
American................................	213	15	70
Foreign born or of foreign or mixed parentage..................	202	19	94

[a] Except births occurring in the last year of the survey period.
[b] See p. 23 for discussion of nationality.
[c] Includes one Indian mother.

TABLE III.—*Stillbirth rates for each county, by nationality of mother, based on births in two years.*

County, and nationality of mother.	All births.	Stillbirths.	
		Number.	Per cent of all births.
Northern county........................	494	19	3.8
Nationality of mother:[a]			
American group.........................	99	2	2.0
German group..........................	180	8	4.4
Polish group...........................	157	5	3.2
Miscellaneous and other foreign group....	53	4	7.5
Not reported...........................	5	......	......
Southern county........................	178	5	2.8
Nationality of mother:			
American..............................	98	4	4.1
Foreign born or of foreign or mixed parentage................	80	1	1.3

[a] See p. 23 for discussion of nationality.

91

TABLE IV.—*Stillbirth and miscarriage rates for each county, by nationality of mother, based on all issues reported by mothers included in the study.*

County, and nationality of mother.	Total issues.	Total births.	Stillbirths.		Miscarriages.	
			Number.	Per cent of total births.	Number.	Per cent of total issues.
Northern county............................	2,214	2,087	48	2.3	127	5.7
Nationality of mother: a						
American group..........................	370	350	3	0.9	20	5.4
German group...........................	840	792	21	2.7	48	5.7
Polish group............................	740	710	11	1.5	30	4.1
Miscellaneous and other foreign group......	250	221	13	5.9	29	11.6
Not reported...........................	14	14	....	....	....	....
Southern county...........................	522	504	9	1.8	18	3.4
Nationality of mother:						
American................................	267	260	6	2.3	7	2.6
Foreign born or of foreign or mixed parentage.....	255	244	3	1.2	11	4.3

a See p. 23 for discussion of nationality.

TABLE V.—*Per cent of infants breast fed and artificially fed, by mother's nationality, northern county.*

Nationality of mothers.	Per cent of infants exclusively breast fed during specified month.				Per cent of infants artificially fed during specified month.			
	1st.	3d.	6th.	9th.	1st.	3d.	6th.	9th.
All mothers.....................	89.3	75.5	48.9	14.2	5.6	9.4	15.8	22.8
American group.....................	90.2	77.1	49.2	13.0	3.3	7.2	18.5	25.9
German group.......................	89.0	75.3	42.5	12.4	6.7	12.7	16.5	20.4
Polish group.......................	90.1	74.6	62.4	22.2	5.6	9.7	14.7	24.4
All others and not reported...........	86.5	76.0	34.0	....	5.8	2.0	12.8	21.9
All foreign born.....................	89.9	73.9	58.7	19.5	5.9	9.0	14.1	19.5

TABLE VI.—*Comparison of feeding methods in Wisconsin with other rural districts and with four cities in which infant mortality investigations have been made.*

Locality.	Per cent of infants exclusively breast fed during specified month.				Per cent of infants artificially fed during specified month.			
	1st.	3d.	6th.	9th.	1st.	3d.	6th.	9th.
Rural districts:								
Wisconsin—								
Northern county..............	89.3	75.5	48.9	14.2	5.6	9.4	15.8	22.8
Southern county..............	92.0	81.5	51.2	12.5	5.6	11.3	15.5	20.2
Kansas....................	92.0	83.2	60.8	23.3	2.1	6.1	12.5	19.3
North Carolina—								
Lowland county a.............	90.4	74.6	50.0	17.0	....	....	1.7	3.8
Mountain county.............	73.5	62.0	34.1	15.9	....	....	....	0.9
Cities:								
Saginaw, Mich....................	87.8	74.5	53.9	28.1	9.0	15.6	24.2	29.2
Akron, Ohio....................	87.9	74.2	55.0	28.7	7.1	15.5	22.9	29.5
Manchester, N. H....................	81.2	62.4	37.5	18.4	15.0	28.8	42.5	51.0
New Bedford, Mass...............	83.4	66.0	44.9	26.0	12.3	24.7	37.2	46.8

a White infants only.

U. S. DEPARTMENT OF LABOR
CHILDREN'S BUREAU
JULIA C. LATHROP, Chief

Maternity Care and the Welfare of Young Children in a Homesteading County in Montana

By

VIOLA I. PARADISE

℞

RURAL CHILD WELFARE SERIES No. 3
Bureau Publication No. 34

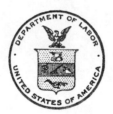

WASHINGTON
GOVERNMENT PRINTING OFFICE
1919

CONTENTS.

ILLUSTRATIONS.

LETTER OF TRANSMITTAL.

U. S. Department of Labor,
Children's Bureau,
Washington, July 5, 1918.

Sir: Herewith I beg to transmit a report entitled "Maternity Care and the Welfare of Young Children in a Homesteading County in Montana."

The study was made under the general supervision of Dr. Grace L. Meigs, head of the hygiene division of the Children's Bureau. The detailed direction was in charge of Miss Viola I. Paradise, who has written the text of the report. The special agents chiefly concerned in the field work were Miss Helen M. Dart, Miss M. Letitia Fyffe, Miss Dorothy M. Williams, Miss Janet M. Geister, Miss Stella E. Packard, Miss May R. Lane. The statistical material was prepared under the direction of Miss Etta F. Philbrook.

Acknowledgment is made of the valuable cooperation of Dr. W. F. Cogswell, secretary of the Montana State board of health, and Miss Margaret Hughes, director of the child-welfare division, State board of health, and the officials of the county studied.

As will be seen by the report, the facts as to maternity experiences were secured through home interviews with the mothers. Children's health conferences were held at several convenient centers, to which many well children were brought by their parents for examination and advice as to their general care. The conferences developed further facts as to the well-being of the children and gave a demonstration of practicable methods of child care, which served an important purpose in making the study of profit to the local community. Dr. Grace L. Meigs and Dr. Anna E. Rude conducted the conferences.

The infant mortality studies of the bureau show that the welfare of mothers and infants is fully safeguarded in none of the communities studied, whether urban or rural. In the rural studies new difficulties appear. And in the present study of a typical pioneer region the degree to which isolation intensifies both the need and the difficulties of safeguarding life is clearly indicated. The population is made up of young, vigorous, courageous, hard-working people who will ultimately succeed, yet the lack of agricultural development and of good roads makes it impossible for them to secure for themselves proper protection for maternity and infancy.

5

The safeguarding of human life and vigor is of national concern, and it is reasonable to invoke the cooperation of State and Nation to that end. We may, therefore, urge that the public protection of maternity and infancy should be accepted as a governmental policy, and that it be secured by such cooperation between the Federal Government and the several States and counties as has already been proved effective in the promotion of better farming, good roads, and vocational education.

The researches of students make clear that the loss of population in war time includes not only the deaths at the front but also a higher civilian death rate, especially affecting young children, and an inevitably lowered birth rate. Hence, this report, disclosing as it does an unnecessary waste of life, is of essential timeliness.

Respectfully submitted.

JULIA C. LATHROP, *Chief.*

Hon. W. B. WILSON,
　　Secretary of Labor.

MATERNITY CARE AND THE WELFARE OF YOUNG CHILDREN IN A HOMESTEADING COUNTY IN MONTANA.

INTRODUCTION.

THE NEED FOR RURAL SURVEYS.

In 1916 the Children's Bureau began a series of rural surveys of maternity care and child welfare. Letters coming to the bureau from women living in isolated districts, requests from State boards of health, and other public and private organizations in all parts of the country have urged a consideration of the problems confronting country mothers in childbirth and in the care of their children. The fact that the United States lost in a single year at least 15,000 women from conditions caused by childbirth [1] is even less well known than is the Nation's extravagant loss of infant life.

The important bearing upon infant life of the care a mother receives during pregnancy and childbirth is made clear by the fact that premature birth, injuries at birth, congenital weakness, and malformations were responsible for the deaths of over 55,000 babies, or more than one-third of the deaths of all babies under 1 year, in the registration area in 1915,[2] and that a large proportion of these babies could have been saved and many stillbirths and miscarriages not included in this toll could have been prevented had the mothers been properly safeguarded and adequately cared for in pregnancy and confinement. How many deaths the farm areas and small villages contribute to these statistics no one knows; but the isolation, the limited transportation and communication facilties, the small proportion of physicians and nurses to the population, and the lack of community and public-health activities over great areas of the country emphasize the need of such inquiries as these rural surveys.

The Montana survey is the fourth in the series, the previous studies having been made in typical districts in North Carolina, Wisconsin, and Kansas. The survey was made in the summer and autumn of 1917.

---

[1] Meigs, Grace L., M. D. : Maternal Mortality from All Conditions Connected with Childbirth in the United States and Certain Other Countries, p. 14. U. S. Children's Bureau Publication No. 19, Miscellaneous Series No. 6. Washington, 1917.

[2] Mortality Statistics, 1915, pp. 11 and 414. U. S. Bureau of the Census. Washington, 1917.

7

SCOPE AND METHOD OF THE MONTANA SURVEY.

The State of Montana, with its tremendous area, affords many types of rural country, ranging from rich and fertile irrigated farm valleys to uncultivated grazing plains and the dry farm land of the "homesteader's country." A newly settled county in the eastern part of the State was chosen for the survey because it presented the problems now encountered by pioneers in many recently occupied areas in the Great West. A little more than the western half of this county—approximately 5,500 square miles, or an area somewhat larger than the State of Connecticut—was covered by the survey. The greater part of this district is from 70 to 100 miles from a railroad. Agents of the Children's Bureau interviewed every mother [1] in the area who had had a baby during the five years preceding the study, provided that at the time of the baby's birth the mother was resident in the district. Four hundred and sixty-three mothers were so visited. A few who were not at home at the time the agent called were not revisited on account of distance, and perhaps a few others may have been overlooked. It is estimated that possibly 10 or 12 mothers were thus missed.

In no case was information refused. The quick appreciation of the purpose of the survey and the intelligent cooperation of the parents and of the whole community can not be too gratefully mentioned.

The work included also a series of children's health conferences. Parents were invited to bring their children to these conferences for a thorough examination by a Government physician who, though she gave no treatment or medicine, advised the parents about the care and feeding of the children and offered them the opportunity of discussing the many health problems which are encountered in rearing children. To these conferences the State board of health sent the public-health nurse who is in charge of its child-welfare division. Thus the conferences were a joint activity of the Children's Bureau, the State board of health, and the local neighborhoods in which they were held, where active committees did much to make them a success.

An investigation of the extent of birth registration, made jointly with the child-welfare division of the State board of health, was also a part of the survey. In addition, information was secured from State and county officials and from a study of available statistics and reports.

The great bulk of the information, however, was obtained from the interviews with mothers. Great care has been exercised so to present the material as not to abuse any mother's confidence. All the

---

[1] In a few instances when the mother was away or had died the father or another near relation gave the information.

stories cited represent or illustrate typical problems. Except where a mother's experience was generally known in a neighborhood and was not regarded by the mother as confidential, no examples have been cited which could in any way be identified.

The report includes a consideration of certain conditions at present inimical to the well-being of the homesteaders living in the area, especially of mothers and children. It should be borne in mind that practically all such unfavorable conditions are susceptible of change by concerted public action, and that such action, besides relieving present duress, would doubtless stimulate the development of this new homesteading country.

SUMMARY.

In this sparsely populated homesteading area of about 5,500 square miles the tremendous distances; the isolation; the inadequate means of communication; poor roads; total absence of telephones; inaccessibility of the railroads; the often hostile weather; the lack of hospitals, physicians, and nurses; and the agricultural and economic status of the community—these conditions made it, at the time of the survey, impossible for mothers to be provided with the kind of maternity care before, at, and after childbirth which they should have.

More than three-fourths of the 463 mothers visited by the agents of the Children's Bureau had no prenatal care whatever; 22 mothers had care which could be classified as fair; and 86 received only inadequate care. One-third of the mothers had attempted to get information about prenatal care from books or magazines.

One hundred and four mothers left the area for childbirth. Of the 359 who remained only 129 were attended by a physician. In other words, almost two-thirds of these mothers had to meet the ordeal of childbirth without competent medical care. Forty-six, or more than one in eight, were delivered by their husbands. Three were quite alone.

Very few received after care by physicians, and nursing care was largely unskilled, though 14 mothers had trained nurses and 113 had partly trained nursing care.

Many mothers suffered serious complications of pregnancy or confinement and eight died—a very large proportion of losses compared with other rural areas. The State of Montana, like the area studied, has a very bad record for maternal losses.

More than one-fifth of the mothers left the area for confinement. For the most part they succeeded in getting better care than they could have had at home, but to many in the last months of pregnancy or soon after childbirth the long trip to and from the railroad, often in bad winter weather, was exhausting.

The mothers who went away from home, as well as those who stayed in the area and were attended by physicians, found childbirth very expensive. Of the 219 attended by physicians, only 14 per cent paid less than $25, and for 22 mothers the physician's charges amounted to $50 or more. Many mothers were attended free of charge by relatives or neighbors, and much free nursing service and help with housework was given; yet nearly three-fourths of the 327 mothers reporting total immediate costs of childbirth—that is, the attendant's fees, nursing care, and help with housework—paid more than $25, and 28 mothers paid $100 or over.

For mothers who went away for confinement these costs, plus the cost of the trip, board while away from home, etc., were very large. Reports of the aggregate costs were secured for 19 mothers, for whom these aggregate costs, in all but four instances, were $150 or more, and in two instances $700 or more.

Certain forms of housework, chores, and farm work which countrywomen do before and after childbirth may be hazardous. Most of the mothers worked up to the time of confinement. Sometimes, because of the lack of conveniences and labor-saving devices, the difficulty of securing help with housework even at confinement, they performed very heavy tasks. The carrying of water was particularly difficult. As a rule, mothers resumed their work much too soon after childbirth. Nearly one-fourth of the women were doing all their housework, except washing, before two weeks had elapsed, and nearly half were doing their housework, washing, and chores within four weeks after parturition.

One of the most serious problems found in the Montana survey was housing. Seven out of 10 families·were living in one or two room houses, and the crowding was very great. In 57 per cent the rate of congestion was two or more persons per room. The sleeping-room congestion was even worse. Nine out of 10 families slept two or more persons in a room, and in slightly more than half the homes the rate was three or more persons to a room. In 27 instances seven or more persons slept in one room. The prevailing types of houses were the log house, the sod house, the tar-paper shack, and the dugout.

Two hundred and sixty-two homes, or well over one-half, were adequately screened; but even in most of these homes and in practically all the others flies were a great nuisance. Unscreened privies or lack of privies and inadequate disposal of waste water were doubtless partly responsible for the flies. Although the prevailing type of privy was the deep-pit privy, closed in back, and so built that the excreta were not accessible to the larger farm animals; nevertheless privies were unprotected against flies. A large number of families, nearly one-fourth, had no privies at all.

The water supply is a most important factor in sanitation. Only 54 families had drilled or driven wells. The prevailing type was the dug well, usually unprotected against surface drainage. Many of these wells were shallow and in hot weather they would dry up. The families living along the rivers used the raw river water, some of them cutting ice from the river in winter, storing it, and using the melted ice as long as it lasted. The use of melted snow in winter was also common. Often several sources of water were used for different purposes or at different times of the year. The high alkaline content of the water all through the area often led people to choose their source of drinking water by the taste rather than by the freedom from contamination.

As the county becomes more thickly settled the water supplies, if they remain unprotected, will doubtless cause much sickness. There had already been a few recent cases of typhoid fever.

Most of the infants and young children impressed the agents making the inquiry as unusually healthy and sturdy. Nevertheless the minimum infant mortality rate[1] of 71 per 1,000 live births was nearly twice as high as the rate of 40 for the area studied in Kansas and was 17 per 1,000 higher than the rate of 54 found in the Wisconsin area. Inasmuch as it is now known that many infant deaths can be prevented the inadequate prenatal and confinement care provided for the mothers in the area takes on an added significance.

On the whole, the mothers in the area are very careful about the feeding of their babies, practically all of them having given their children breast feeding. Only 21 per cent of the babies had been weaned before their ninth month.

The birth-registration test made in cooperation with the State board of health revealed that only 31 per cent of the live-born children born in the area covered by the survey had the advantage of a birth certificate, and that, though the children born within a year of the agent's visit had a slight advantage over the other children, only 39 per cent of these later births were registered.

Although the State has an excellent law permitting counties to use public funds to employ public-health nurses, advantage has not been taken of this law in the area studied. Indeed, there were practically no State or county activities which directly touched the welfare of mothers and young children in the area.

Before proceeding to a more detailed discussion of the chief findings the reader will wish to know something of the country in which the survey was made and of conditions there which affect the well-being of mothers and babies.

---

[1] See p. 70.

ECONOMIC AND SOCIAL CONDITIONS IN THE AREA STUDIED.

HISTORY AND POPULATION.

The history of the county has been the story of Sioux Indians and early explorers; of hunters and fur traders in the days not so very long ago when the bison ranged the prairies; then of a few ranchmen, scattered at great distances; of great herds of cattle and sheep, succeeding the wild buffaloes; and of the famous cowboy; then of the coming of the dry farmer with his hated fences; and of the crowding out of the open-range cattlemen and the substitution of the homesteader.

The country is still very young. A man who herded sheep here 20 years ago said that at that time he knew of only three families in the whole area studied and in hundreds of square miles besides, and that these lived over 50 miles from one another. Although there are a few families of over 12 or 15 years' residence, the district has been settled mainly within the past 5 or 6 years. Of the families visited, 56 per cent were still " squatting " or homesteading at the time of the birth for which a schedule was secured. The " squatters " are those who live on land on which claims can not be filed because it is still unsurveyed or the survey of the land is unaccepted. There are still over 1,400 miles of unsurveyed and unaccepted land in the area.[1] In some cases families were " squatting " after 10 years of residence. Taking the area as a whole, however, people who have lived here 5 or 6 years are regarded as old settlers.

The story of one successful family of these " old settlers " is typical of many others who have come to settle in the county. The family is exceptional in that it has been in the area longer than the great majority of the homesteaders. Five years ago the father bought a " relinquishment " from a homesteader who had become discouraged before the end of his first year on the homestead, and who had made practically no improvements on the land. The new homesteaders, who came in the late spring, at once put up a one-room sod house, 12 by 14 feet, in which they lived for four years.

The father cultivated a little land. The first crop consisted of five rows of potatoes, which by the exercise of great economy " took

---

[1] Information given by the U. S. surveyor general for Montana.

the family through the first winter." Each year the father plowed and seeded a little more land, until now, at the end of five years he has 50 acres under cultivation. He bought stock, one head at a time. For nearly five years he hauled water in barrels over a mile, because he was unable, except by expensive drilling, to get water nearer the house. As the cattle increased he had to haul a barrel every day. Recently he has had a well drilled; this well, a windmill, several outbuildings, and a new house bespeak comparative prosperity.

The new house was built after the family had been on the homestead for four years, the old "soddie" having dried out until it was no longer waterproof. The lumber for the new one-room dwelling, though enough only for the roof, floor, doors, and window frames, cost $200. The sides of the house are made of stone which the father dug from the neighboring buttes. These stones are plastered together with a homemade gumbo cement. The wooden roof is sodded to make it waterproof and warm.

The house furnishings consist of two double beds at one end of the room, a kitchen range, a large table and several chairs, a cupboard, and an improvised wardrobe made by hanging a curtain from a high broad shelf. A sewing machine and a cream separator were recent acquisitions.

On all these homesteads the women share with the men the burdens of pioneering and the credit for success. In the present instance, the mother, in addition to her housework, helps care for the stock, raises a garden, keeps chickens, milks, separates, and churns. Indeed, it was largely the money she earned by the sale of butter which made possible the installation of the windmill and other improvements.

The homesteaders in the district have come from all parts of the United States, and for the most part they are Americans of native parentage. In many instances they are the children of parents who homesteaded in the Middle West and in the Southern States. A few Russian-German neighborhoods formed the only considerable foreign element in the area studied; 30, or 6.5 per cent, of the mothers visited were of Russian-German birth; 367 mothers, or about 8 in 10, were American.

In this predominantly American community illiteracy is only a slight problem, 95 per cent of all mothers and 86 per cent of the foreign-born mothers being literate. There were, however, eight mothers of foreign or mixed parentage who, though born in the United States, were illiterate—unable to read and write in any language. Six of these could not speak English. One of these women explained apologetically that there were no schools in the North Dakota neighborhood where she was reared. Of the foreign born, 22 were unable to speak English.

No recent official statistics are available either for the population of the county as a whole or for the western part covered by the Children's Bureau study. In 1910 the county had a population of 12,725 How new the county is is evidenced by the fact that this was an increase of 420 per cent over the population at the preceding census. In 1910 the area of the county was 13,231 square miles, and on the average there was more than a square mile for each dwelling. The area has recently been reduced by the formation of new counties to 9,259 square miles [1]—an area somewhat larger than the State of Massachusetts. It is doubtful if the western half of the county, which was so much more recently settled, has even at the present day a much greater density of habitation than one dwelling per square mile.

DESCRIPTION OF THE COUNTRY.

The country varies greatly in appearance, but always there are tremendous, almost incredible distances. The great, wild, rugged, sweeping plains—broken by buttes of many shapes and by sudden gray cut banks—were at the end of a cruelly dry season burnt dun and brown and yellow. Occasionally, a bright green flax field or a small field of corn, looking almost as if painted on the landscape, gave a startling contrast; but such contrasts are rare, for the country has been used almost exclusively for grazing, very little of it being under cultivation. Frequently there are outcroppings of rock, fantastic in shape, the result of erosion or of wind sculpture. Scrub growths of bluish gray-green sagebrush mottle the prairie and occasionally cover whole fields; again, there are stretches with no grass but the sparse, sear wild hay, or buffalo grass. A low cactus grows in quantity here and there. Some Russian thistle, which at the beginning of the investigation was a dull unobtrusive green, changed to a glowing copper-red in the autumn. Indeed, this change and the yellowing of the few cottonwoods which grow along the Big Dry and other stream beds were almost the only changes of color brought by the autumn. The country, except for these cottonwoods and except in the "breaks," is treeless. An occasional little tar-paper shack or "soddie" of some homesteader, or a log house, or a sheep herder's white covered wagon on these sweeping plains and hills accents the wild vastness of earth and sky. Indeed, everything seems to emphasize this vastness, whether it be a small herd of cattle or a large, a great flock of sheep or a single grazing horse on the top of a distant hill silhouetted against the sky. Sometimes one can drive great distances and see no sign of human habitation and no sign of animal life

---

[1] Information given by the county surveyor.

except a flock of sage hens, or a prairie-dog town, or a coyote, or, less often, a bobcat, or some antelopes.

But of all the features of the landscape the most compelling are the buttes. These strange hills vary in size and shape and color. Many of them are classed as bad lands. Often they spring up out of a comparatively smooth plain and look like a child's drawing of a mountain; again, they heap themselves together in ranges of hills, giving a jagged, almost grotesque sky line. Sometimes they are covered with wild hay and sometimes they are bare; often they are streaked with lignite coal; often they are heaps of shale rock. Their colors vary from the tan of the prairie to a rare pastel red or orange. Most often, perhaps, the butte is the somber purplish gray of gumbo.

As one approaches either of the two rivers which bound the county on the north and west, the land becomes very much rougher and is known as the breaks. Here the many creeks and streams on the way to the rivers have cut deep twisting gullies; and here for the first time one sees trees in some abundance—abundance only by contrast with the county's treeless prairies, for the breaks are but sparsely dotted with pines, cedar, and juniper. In some places the hills are quite barren, except for a few gnarled and scrubby cedars. The ground is here and there covered with creeping juniper and creeping cedar.

The large areas of bad lands (really a part of the breaks, though not so considered locally) are weirdly picturesque. They are high, bare buttes of rock or gumbo, varying in color through all the shades of gray to the rarer brick red or orange. The sides of the canyons show the formation of the rocks in horizontal streaks of many different colors. The breaks and bad lands extend back from the rivers some 15 or 20 miles and are especially rough along the creeks. This rough land (excepting that which is absolutely barren) is much prized for grazing, because it affords protection for the stock in bad weather.

Along the two rivers cottonwood trees abound. The strips of river-bottom land are fertile and valuable for farming. This land was the first to be settled, and the comfortable log houses of the ranchers, the high hay stacks, the large corrals, the frequency of cultivated fields, bear witness that the settlers have prospered.

The river-bottom district comprises only a very small part of the area studied in the Children's Bureau survey. For the most part, the country consists of the rolling prairie and breaks and bad lands, which have been described.

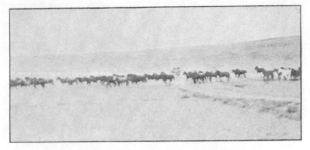

HORSES BEING DRIVEN TO MARKET.

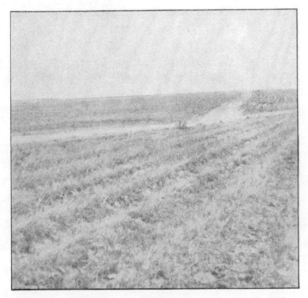

NOT A PLOWED FIELD BUT AN OLD TRAIL FUR-
ROWED BY WAGONS AND ESPECIALLY BY FREIGHTING
"OUTFITS."

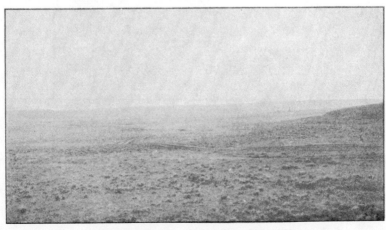

WINDING TRAIL ACROSS THE PRAIRIES.

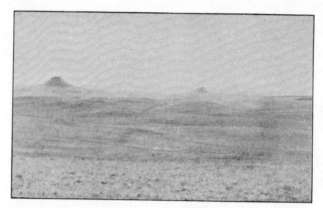

TYPICAL BUTTES.

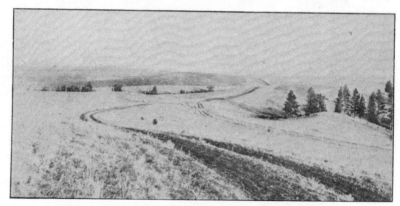

WINDING ROAD NEAR THE BREAKS.

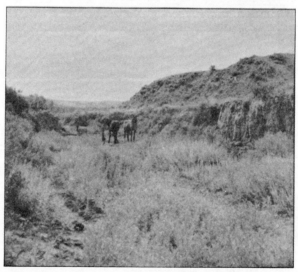

A COULEE.

ROADS AND MEANS OF COMMUNICATION.

In this area, the greater part of which is from 70 to 100 miles from a railroad and where even the telephone has not yet become a means of communication, one looks with interest at the roads, or rather at the trails, for they are seldom referred to by the people of the county as roads.

Needless to say, there are no hard-surfaced roads. Very little work had been done on the trails until recently, when the county took advantage of the new Federal road bill in accordance with which the Government contributes a sum equal to a county's appropriation. The county studied was among the first to take advantage of this offer and appropriated for 1917 $20,000, none of which, however, is to be spent in the area covered by the Children's Bureau investigation.[1] Work had already been begun at the time of the survey.

In this country work on a road consists of straightening, now and then digging out a hillside, filling in a gully, installing a culvert, building a wooden bridge over a stream, and grading and surface dragging. This work is confined to the "main traveled trails" and has not by any means covered all these; about 70 miles have been worked on in the area studied. It is impossible to get any figures for the total road mileage in this area, but it is safe to say that the improved road mileage is a very small fraction of the whole.

For the most part the roads are nothing but wagon trails, in some instances following the old buffalo trails to water. As soon as the ruts get so deep that the bodies of vehicles are endangered by the high centers, a new trail is started by the simple process of moving over a little, one new rut being started between the two old ones, and the other to the right or left of the old ones. After this process has gone on for some time, the ground looks, sometimes for a width of 50 feet, as if it had been plowed.

The less traveled trails, except where they are too faint, are often the best, for wagons and automobiles have not yet gouged them out. However, as they twist tortuously up a cut bank or down a coulee, or around the side of a butte, they test the skill of a driver, whether of a team or of a machine. There are many stretches of gumbo road which in wet weather are impassable on uneven ground; and even on comparatively level ground a car or wagon slithers around dangerously.

Many of the trails were established before the county was surveyed. As people have taken up homesteads or squatted on the land they have built fences across the casual trails, hence the traveler has many

---

[1] Information given by county commissioners.

gates to open. When he finds a rag tied to a barbed-wire fence he knows there is no thoroughfare and he must go around.

There are so many cross trails and branching trails and so few landmarks that to find one's way is difficult. A typical direction, "down Buffalo Hill, between Hell Creek and Crooked Creek on Beebee Bottom; you can't miss it," might be easily followed by one who knew the neighborhood well, but is almost baffling to an outsider who does not know where all the faint trails lead.

The transportation problem is complicated by the fact that many homes are far off the traveled trails. A neighbor will say in giving directions, "Just keep going in that general direction; you'll lose the trail and find yourself in the midst of some pretty rough sagebrush, but if you keep due west you'll find it again." The intricacies of travel are also illustrated by another direction, "Go to the top of the next hill where you see a gray horse. Follow the lane till you pass the horse, and farther on you'll come to some plowed ground. There you turn to the right and follow the fence a ways. You'll go through a coulee and you'll see a butte ahead. Climb to the top of that, and a mile or so beyond you ought to see the dugout."

Automobiles are becoming fairly common, though the great majority of people still must depend upon horses. Of 463 families visited in the investigation, 59, or about 1 in 8, owned automobiles. Frequently cars are purchased before other necessities. Sometimes a family of five or six will postpone adding a room to a one or two-room shack in order to use the money this would take to buy a car. The car is a business investment, and the well-being of a family is greatly enhanced by its possession.

Some homesteaders, just starting out, had neither team nor car; a few had not even a saddle horse. They were obliged to depend entirely upon neighbors for transportation.

In the breaks the roads are very much worse than in the rest of the area studied, though the oldest and most prosperous settlers live there. Some well-to-do families living in this part of the district do not own automobiles because it is impossible to drive them on the steep, narrow, winding trails of the breaks. Indeed, it is impossible to drive even a team on many of these trails. One father owns a car which he keeps with friends at the end of the roughest land. When he and his family wish to use it they walk or ride horseback to the car and leave their horses until they return. Another family lives 8 miles from the most accessible road which can be used by any vehicle. A very rough bridle trail leads from the road to the comfortable little log cabin. This trail can be traveled only on horseback or on foot; no supplies can be carried along it; and the family must get its supplies from across the river.

In the breaks the only practical way to get about is on a sure-footed horse, one capable of swimming the creeks when the water is up in the spring. Often, however, the water is so high and swift that it is dangerous to swim the creeks on horses, and families are cut off, sometimes for a week at a time, from their nearest neighbors. One father, in discussing the need of better maternity and infant care, remarked, "First get the county commissioners to put in roads that would make it possible for the doctor to arrive here if we did have him within calling distance. In the spring, when the water is high, and we can not cross, we are cut off from the world as effectually as though we were on an island."

People in cities usually think of every country family as having its mail box, with mail delivered daily to the door by rural carriers. In the area studied only a few families living along the " star routes" (on which the carriers bring mail to the post offices) are so fortunate. Nearly everyone must go to the post office, often many miles away, for mail which is delivered there once or twice—in some rare instances three times—a week. No post office had daily deliveries and the largest center in the district had only two deliveries a week. All the mail must be brought from railroad towns in other counties, and in some cases it is relayed to several carriers before reaching its distribution point. Bad weather, of course, complicates the service. During the winter preceding the survey first-class mail was delayed for a week or two at a time, and in parts of the area for much longer periods, while the parcel post was in many instances held up for months. "People had Christmas till Easter," said one woman describing the difficulties of getting mail.

The delay of the parcel post is very serious in a country community where the mail order is the predominant manner of purchasing. There were several complaints from persons whose winter underwear, ordered in the autumn, did not reach them until spring. In one instance a child was without shoes because the mail was delayed. A more serious case was that of a mother who, feeling ill during her pregnancy, consulted a physician. He gave her a prescription, which she sent to the nearest railroad town to be filled; but the roads were so bad that the medicine did not get through for two months.

Often long delays in the first-class mail create very difficult situations. In one instance a mother decided to go for her confinement to the home of her sister, 25 miles away, but within 2 miles of a physician. The mother wrote to the physician three months in advance to engage him. When she went at the appointed time the physician was away and she was confined without a doctor's services. He did not receive her letter until a week after the baby was

born. This delay of over three months was due to the winter weather
and bad roads.

The four or five villages had post offices. In addition to these,
there were about 35 scattered about in country stores and in some instances in private houses.

The stage, which runs daily in the open weather from the railroad
to the largest " inland " village, makes possible the delivery of tele-
grams for a limited area and for part of the year. However, one
woman who lives 74 miles from the railroad reported that last winter,
when the stage was not running, she had to pay $40 for the delivery
of a telegram three or four days late. There are, of course, many
districts to which it would be impossible to deliver a telegram during bad weather. An enterprising group had planned and purchased the equipment for the installation of a wireless service, but the
installation of all private wireless service was forbidden by the
Government on our entrance into the war.

The rivers which bound the county on the north and west are
further impediments to communication except in winter, when they
are frozen hard. The many families who depend for supplies, medical service, and mail upon towns across the rivers are often at the
mercy of the coming in or breaking up of the ice, the dangerous
spring floods, and the eccentricities of the ferry.

The telephone has not yet become a means of communication in
the community studied. No home was equipped with one. Only
26 families lived under 25 miles from a telephone and to many of
these the telephone, being across a river, was much more inaccessible
than the distance would indicate. As far as the people in the area
studied were concerned, this convenient tool which we have come to
consider indispensable might never have been invented. Nearly 7
families in 10 lived 50 miles or over from a telephone and 32 families
had no telphone within 100 miles.

Many of the problems of communication will be solved when a
proposed railroad which will run through the area studied is actually built. The people of the communities are looking forward to
this railroad with great eagerness. The phrase " When the railroad
comes " has to many the same connotation as " When our ship comes
in." Characteristic of the enterprising nature of the homesteaders
was a volunteer census which they made, covering many parts of the
county. A committee divided the county up into districts and persons were selected in each district to canvass the population to learn
the amount of acreage at present in crops in these areas and to get
a statement as to the amount which each farmer would plant if a
railroad were built. These statistics were incorporated into a petition, which was sent to Congress, for a Government railroad.

CLIMATE, LIVE STOCK, AGRICULTURE, AND MARKETS.

Climate.

The weather competes with the tremendous distances, the inaccessibility of markets, and the poor roads for the place of dominant factor in the economic and social life of the people in the area. The land lies at an altitude of 2,500 to 3,000 feet. The dry, clear atmosphere is very invigorating except in the extremely hot or cold weather, and even in such weather the heat and cold are not felt as much as they would be in a more humid climate.

At the two observation stations of the Weather Bureau in the area the mean temperatures for January, 1917, were 11.6° and 13.2° above zero, respectively; and the minimum temperatures for that same month were 38° and 42° below.[1] The maximum for August of the same year was 94° at one station,[2] but three stations near the area studied (indeed, nearer to some parts of it than the station within the area) reported maximum temperatures of 98°, 99°, and 110°. These figures scarcely begin to give the reader a correct impression of the weather, because the high winds and the cumulative effect of a long dry spell or a long cold spell can not be told in figures. The effect of the past hot, dry summer upon agriculture will be discussed.[3] Crops failed, and wells and streams dried up; automobiles trying to cross the Big Dry River near its mouth had to be hauled through the deep sand by teams. Now and again one finds a dry stream bed white with alkali deposit. In parts of the area studied the saying, " It hasn't rained since it snowed," was current. It had snowed on Decoration Day, and except for one or two negligible local showers there had been no rain up to the middle of October, when there were both rain and snow.

People were looking forward with misgiving to the winter and hoping fervently that it would be " open." Otherwise, with very little feed raised for the animals, many families expected losses as disastrous as those of the previous winter, when thousands of sheep and cattle had died in the cold. During that winter, one wealthy sheep raiser lost 5,000 sheep, though he herded them himself, thinking that he could care for them better than would a hired employee. What little hay there was in the neighborhood sold for $40 a ton, over twice as much as it had ever brought before; some persons reported that they had paid $75 a ton. In parts of the area hay could not be obtained for any price; and there were no means of getting it hauled from the railroad because of the snow. The animals suffered greatly,

---

[1] U. S. Dept. of Agriculture, Weather Bureau, Climatological Data, Montana Section, January and August, 1917.

[2] No figures for the other station are given.

[3] See discussion of agriculture, p. 22.

and many of them died of hunger after staggering around for weeks in the snow and bitter cold. The icy crust which formed over the snow made it impossible for them to get feed from the ranges. The autumn of the survey many of the farmers were selling much of their stock, because the risk of a bad winter was too great to take.

Isolation, of course, augments the distress caused by the winters. One mother's statement summarized the attitude of many: " It is maddening to be tied up the six long months of winter, day after day, with no break, and always in fear that the baby will be taken sick and we would be unable to get her to a doctor. It is dangerous to go after coal because storms come up suddenly, and then the men get lost easily. Last winter we ran out of coal in January, and we ran out of feed in April, and 70 cows perished from hunger."

Many terrible stories were told about the winter preceding the survey, in and around the area studied. For example, a woman and her three children left a neighbor's house, where they had been visiting, to return to their own home about half a mile distant. The husband, who had been away and was delayed by the storm, returned a few days later. When he was about a hundred feet from his house, his horse stumbled and shied, and the man, dismounting, found his wife in a snowdrift, sitting upright holding one child—both frozen to death. The two other children he found near by, also frozen.

Another story was told about two school-teachers who were homesteading and whose matches gave out during a blizzard. After waiting in vain for help, knowing that it was useless to go out into the storm, they wrote farewell letters and went to bed. They were found, some time after, frozen to death.

Such harrowing stories of the winter as these, and the accounts of the crop losses of the summer, strike the imagination so vividly that one is likely to forget the long, beautiful autumns with their bracing air and the pleasant weather in the late spring and early summer.

Live stock, agriculture, and markets.

Until very recently, the county was used entirely for grazing. The wild hay, or buffalo grass, which grows so hardily in spite of the worst droughts, is more highly prized by cattlemen than any crops at present cultivated. It is not many years since cattle were driven up from Texas to graze hereabouts.

The county agriculturist estimates that about half the land is tillable, having as the predominant type of soil a clay loam which would produce gratifying crops if it could get enough moisture, and, even with limited moisture, would produce an excellent yield of cereals if properly tilled and cultivated. The frequent long, dry summers,

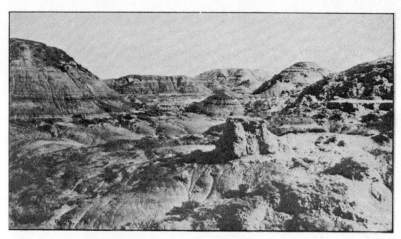

TYPICAL BAD LANDS NEAR HUNGRY CREEK.

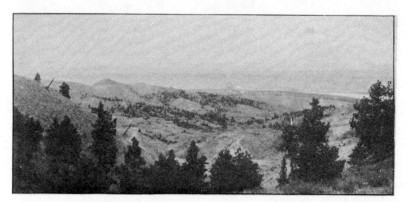

THE BREAKS WITH A GLIMPSE OF RIVER.

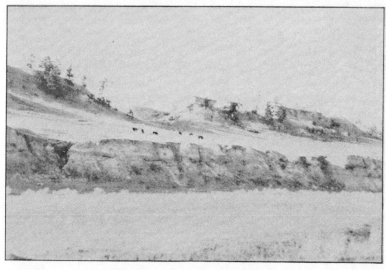

CATTLE GRAZING ALONG A CREEK BED.

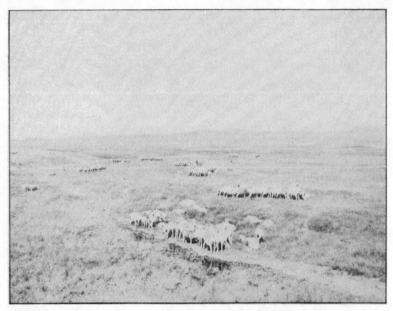

GRAZING SHEEP.

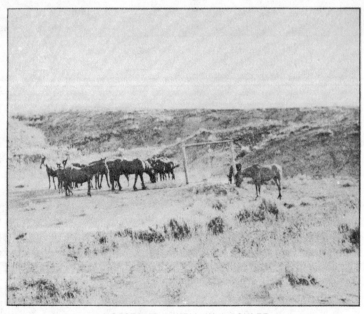

HORSES AT A WELL IN A COULEE.

however, with no means of irrigating the land[1] make farming a hazardous occupation. People are dependent upon the weather. The year of the Children's Bureau survey the crops were almost a total failure. The dry farmer, in answer to the country's demand for wheat, had endeavored to seed as much land as possible. Although a comparatively small acreage was planted (39 per cent of the farmers questioned having less than 50 acres each under cultivation), nevertheless, it represents a great effort on the part of these settlers who have come to their homesteads with little capital, slight equipment, and, not owning the land, with no opportunity to get credit. The loss of stock and the crop failure this year has meant financial ruin to many. The county agriculturist and others in the community think the land should remain for many years—at least until a railroad is secured—chiefly grazing land, with corn and other feed grains raised for home consumption. They think that, though the large-scale stock raising, possible only with the " open range," will be farther and farther crowded out, cattle will continue to be the chief product, with many small herds owned by many homesteaders instead of great herds owned by a few ranchers. This is indicated by the present tendency. As soon as possible after filing on his land the homesteader buys a few head of cattle. The number of cattle owned by the families included in the survey ranged from 1 or 2 head to 600; most of the homesteaders had under 20 head of cattle and horses, and only a few had over 100. A very few families had large herds of sheep, in some instances over 1,500.

The cattle are bred only for beef, there being practically no dairying. Only a small proportion[2] of the families who have cattle milk even one cow for their own use. The stores in the towns report that they sell hundreds of wagonloads of canned milk. This situation is hard for an outsider to understand even if he is told the difficulties of keeping a milch cow. Such a cow ought not to be allowed to range with the herd, because the calves would milk her; she would, therefore, have to be kept in a separate field; this would entail the expense of fencing and also of buying feed. At present, with markets so far away, there is no outlet for a surplus of dairy products, and many families feel that they can manage without milk and butter for a few years until the longed-for time " when the railroad comes." This is unfortunate, for fresh milk and dairy products should be important items in the diet of children.

---

[1] One or two farmers had built reservoirs in which they had saved some of the water from the full creeks of the spring season. Such reservoirs are very expensive and it is doubted by many local experts whether the results pay for the cost of such irrigation.

[2] Only 133 mothers, or a little over one-fourth, reported milking as part of their work.

The distance from markets and even from the means of getting to the market—i. e., a railroad—has a stunting effect upon many kinds of agricultural activity. Practically the only crops attempted are flax and wheat (the chief grain crops), and corn, oats, and barley (the important feed crops). Even these are undertaken on a very small scale, though enough wheat is raised to keep busy the two little mills in the area. Even garden products are few, for where water is scarce gardening is very laborious. A few gardens, however, which produced excellent vegetables, were found. In one of these rare cases the woman had achieved her successful crops by utilizing the waste wash water. If markets were available for garden surplus over what a family could use, probably many farmers would increase their garden space, and many more would undertake raising garden produce in spite of the scarcity of water.

The four or five villages in the area are not markets in any real sense. The only considerable product of the country is live stock, and that is "rounded up" in the spring and autumn and driven direct to the railroads. The villages are chiefly distributing centers for food, clothing, etc., brought out from the railroad to be purchased by people living in the country. For the most part they are small—often less than a dozen houses and stores altogether—sometimes only four or five buildings. The largest village has a fluctuating population reaching about 250 or, according to the most liberal local estimate, 300 inhabitants in winter, when people come into town from their homesteads to send their children to the town school or for other social reasons. Nearly every family in the town has a homestead, and during the spring and summer the population dwindles. This village and one of the others have each a small mill, from which flour is supplied to local stores.

Except this flour, the soft coal, which people can dig for themselves out of the sides of hills, and a little lumber from the breaks, practically everything must be "freighted" from the railroad. Some families, especially the large ranchers who have the horses and equipment, do their own freighting, going to the railroad and buying supplies for a season and in some instances for a whole year at one time. Often they have in their cellars and dugouts larger stocks than those kept by many of the country stores. Some men make a regular business of hauling. In addition to an auto stage, which drags "a trailer," the long freighting outfits with four or six horse teams, a string of wagons, and a white covered wagon at the end, are common sights on the long trails. This hauling, of course, makes the cost of living high. The freight rates from the railroad to the chief inland village range from $1 to $2 per 100 pounds in summer, and from $2 to $5 in winter.

One of the most expensive items is lumber, whether it is hauled from the breaks or from the railroad. In one country store fence

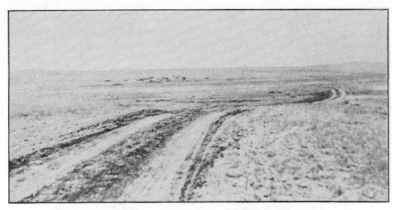

A VILLAGE ON THE PLAINS.

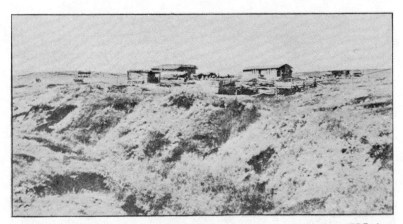

DWELLING AND COMBINATION POST OFFICE AND STORE WHERE A CHILDREN'S HEALTH CONFERENCE WAS HELD.

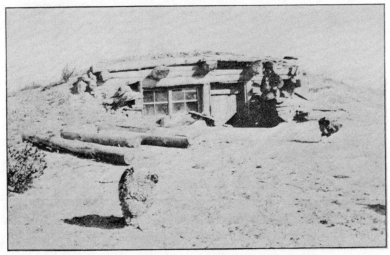

THIS DUGOUT SERVED AS A HOME AND POST OFFICE.

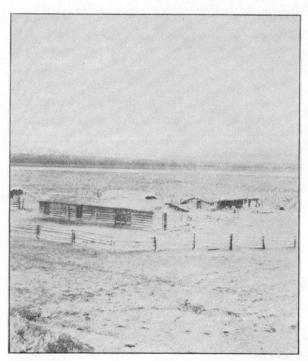

A PROSPEROUS RANCH ON THE RIVER BOTTOM.

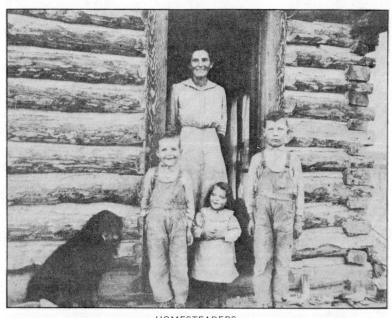

HOMESTEADERS.

posts, which sell for 25 to 35 cents apiece, supplement silver as a medium of exchange. The storekeeper takes pay for commodities in fence posts and then sells them or buys more stock with them.

Although the stores in the villages distribute large quantities of food and merchandise, nevertheless mail-order buying is the favorite method of purchasing, and the large catalogues are referred to with local humor as "homesteader's Bibles." It was interesting to learn that some families sheared their sheep and sent the wool to a mail-order factory in the Middle West, which made all their clothing, from underwear to overcoats, using the family's own wool and taking part of it in payment for weaving the cloth and making up the garments.

ECONOMIC STATUS OF THE FAMILIES VISITED.

In the infant mortality investigations which the bureau has made in cities, the coincidence between a high infant death rate and poverty has been conspicuous. In cities the economic condition of a family can as a rule be measured easily by the money income. In rural areas, however, the money income means very little because the farm contributes largely in produce instead of money to the family living. In an area like the one surveyed, where nearly all the farms have the same acreage, where tenancy is not a problem, and nearly everyone is either squatting or homesteading, or has just proved up on his homestead, it is impossible to classify the families visited into any income or economic groups which would be significant in regard to the care of the women at childbirth and the well-being of their children.

There is not a wide variation in the financial condition of the people; the whole area is young and struggling. There were perhaps 20 or 30 wealthy ranchers owning large herds of cattle or horses or large flocks of sheep. On the other hand, there were some who were having an especially hard struggle. The earliest years on a homestead are, of course, the hardest; and they are especially difficult if they include a drought. But even after several years of homesteading many families were having a difficult time.

A typical instance was one family which had proved up on its 320 acres, but had had "bad luck," as they expressed it, with the farm. The crops failed and two cows died with calves. Last year they borrowed over $1,000 on a mortgage at a 10 per cent interest rate, and they did not know how they were going to meet the interest due. The mother said, "We have nothing to sell but our milch cows, and that is my children's food." Doubtless many other families, and among them some who have the title to their land, have found themselves as hard pressed as this since the winter set in.

In another family the mother complained that the crops the previous year had been so poor that the father " had to go away last winter to earn money enough to keep us going." This winter, again, he had gone to get work elsewhere, and there was little prospect that the mother would be able to join him, for he was over 125 miles away and the trip was expensive. She had sent the oldest daughter to her grandmother in another State that the child might have the advantage of a good school. Her nearest neighbor and a family of relations who had come out to homestead when she and her husband came had both gone for the winter, and the mother had a very lonesome season in prospect.

One hundred and twenty-nine fathers had to supplement their incomes by a secondary occupation, in 38 cases by farm labor, some fathers " hiring out" only at seeding or harvest time. Twenty-two gave farming as a secondary occupation, having for their chief employment farm work not on their own homesteads, storekeeping, carpentry, well drilling, etc. They were holding their homesteads chiefly as investments, or postponing work on them until they could save a little capital for implements, seed, etc.

On the whole, neither the care of the mother at childbirth nor the family living conditions were dependent wholly upon the prosperity of the individual family. The problems which this report represents are not of any one economic group, but are problems of the whole community.

MATERNITY CARE.

INACCESSIBILITY OF MEDICAL CARE.

The inaccesibility of medical care in confinement was the most striking finding of the inquiry. The great area of 5,500 square miles had not one hospital. And in the period covered by the inquiry there were only three physicians in the area registered in the State of Montana, and two or three others, not registered, who said they came to the county not to practice medicine but to homestead. They were drawn into practice, however, because in emergencies their neighbors called upon them and they could not refuse to go; one or two reported that they did refuse unless it was a matter of life or death.

Less than one-third of the mothers lived within 10 miles of a physician and more than one-third were 20 miles or more away, 10 of these being from 50 to 100 miles from a physician.

The country does not invite physicians, because, as the agents making the inquiry were told again and again, "There is almost no sickness here except confinements and accidents." One result of this state of affairs is that when the importance of good confinement care is realized, and when the family can afford it, the women go away for confinement—sometimes to a hospital in one of the nearest cities, sometimes "back home," sometimes to friends or relatives in another rural district where medical care is more easily obtainable.

ATTENDANT AT BIRTH.

Of the 463 mothers, 104, or over one-fifth, left the area for confinement, 27 of these going to hospitals.

Of the 359 [1] who stayed in the area, only 129 were attended by a physician; in other words, almost two-thirds of these mothers had to meet the experience of childbirth without the safeguard of competent medical care. Three were entirely alone and delivered themselves, even tying and cutting the cord. Forty-six, or more than one out of every eight, were delivered by their husbands. Neighboring

[1] Including 13 who went away from home to friends or relatives elsewhere in the area for confinement. They are not discussed separately because conditions in the homes to which they went were not very different from those affecting the other mothers who stayed at home, excepting for five of these mothers who went to the house of a physician for confinement.

27

women—in a very few instances trained nurses, in a considerable number of cases practical nurses, but for the most part women quite untrained in obstetrics—attended 181, or over half the mothers who remained in the area for confinement.

Although in a few families childbirth was regarded as a simple and natural process, requiring no special care except what any neighbor could give, in the main the dangers of the lack of medical care were more or less realized. Nearly every neighborhood had known of a death or a narrow escape from death on account of childbirth. Five mothers had taken the precaution of going to the house of a physician in the area for confinement. Preference for an untrained attendant was seldom responsible for the lack of medical care. " We had planned to have a physician, but the snow was so bad it was impossible to send for him." " We were all packed ready to go to the city for the confinement, but storms came up, and the creek was so high we couldn't get away." " My husband rode horseback 12 miles in a bad snowstorm for the doctor, but he was away." " The roads made it impossible to get a doctor." " We intended to go to the city, but the baby came a few days before we expected him." " We couldn't get away on time, because all the autos in the neighborhood were being used for sheepshearing." These were typical reasons given why no physician had been in attendance. One mother had packed her belongings and was ready to start for the city when labor set in unexpectedly. The father left her to get a physician and some neighbors, but the baby was born while the mother was alone before anyone arrived. The physician was eight hours late.

In another case where the mother had expected to go away for confinement labor came on suddenly. Unfortunately her husband, who had delivered her first baby, was away on business across the river and could not get back because the ferry was not running. The mother was alone except for the grandmother, who was panic-stricken and could be of no help whatever, and who frightened the mother and made her nervous. The mother, however, was a very competent person, had always been interested in nursing, had delivered several of her neighbors, and knew what to do.

In another instance a young mother whose confinement came before she expected it found herself absolutely alone at childbirth and for two days after. The father, who had gone on business to the railroad a few days earlier, had arranged for a neighbor to stay with his wife. At the last minute the neighbor was unable to come, and the mother, having no one to help her, to give her nursing care, or to do her housework, had to cut and tie the cord, care for herself and the baby, and get what little food she ate for two days, at the end of which the husband returned and summoned a neighbor. This experience, which would have been terrifying at any time, was especially hard because the mother, who was only 19 years old, was having her first baby. Fortunately she suffered no permanent ill effects, but she was weak for about six months after childbirth and did practically no work during that time.

Another mother was all alone when her first baby was born. Her husband left at noon to go for a physician, but was lost in a storm and did not get back until 6 o'clock the next morning. This was in March. The baby was born at 9 in the evening. The mother cut and tied the cord herself. She was alone through the night, the fire went out, and she had no food. She was obliged to get out of bed in the cold room to get more coverings. This was her first child and she was badly torn. A physician whom she has seen recently says that she needs an operation.

In another case a father, who could not reach a doctor, delivered his wife with the assistance of a 19-year-old girl who was living in the household. They said that they did not feel entirely helpless, because they had had some instructions from the father's brother, whose wife had had a trained nurse during a confinement in the Philippines.

Often a physician had been sent for but did not arrive on time. Such a delay is disturbing enough to a mother who has no reason to expect complications, but it is especially distressing to a mother whose pregnancy has been complicated. This was the experience of one mother, who reported that the membranes had ruptured three days before delivery, and the physician who had been called at that time was unable to tell whether the fetus was alive or dead, but feared that it was dead. At the birth, therefore, the mother, who with her two previous children had had a physician and trained nurse, was much frightened and worried when the physician did not arrive on time. A neighbor who was not even a practical nurse was with her at confinement. A woman who had had more experience with confinement cases was sent for and arrived 20 minutes late, but in time to cut and tie the cord. The physician did not reach the mother until five hours after the baby was born, but came in time to deliver the afterbirth. Fortunately the baby was in good condition, and, though it was a dry birth, the delivery was not difficult.

In 30 instances, the physicians arrived late but in time to be of some service, either in cutting and tying the cord, delivering the afterbirth, or in looking after the mother. In a few instances, they arrived within an hour after the birth, and in others their tardiness ranged from 1 to 24 hours. In 56 additional cases unsuccessful attempts were made to secure a physician. In 12 of these the physicians did not answer the calls at all, for one reason or another— sometimes, doubtless, because they knew they could not reach their patients in time. In 44 instances they arrived too late to perform any service for the mother.

Many families who live great distances from a physician know in advance that it would be little short of miraculous if he should arrive on time; occasionally, in such cases, the father will send for a physician for the reassurance which even a late visit may give; but usually when the physician is so inaccessible the family can not afford to spend the money. " There was too little chance of his getting here on time; and besides it would have cost $50." " The ice was coming in the river, and the ferry couldn't get across; so we decided not to try to get a doctor; and it's very expensive; the doctor charges $75 to come here." Such were the usual comments.

Bad weather, swollen rivers and creeks, impassable roads, which make it hard or impossible to secure a physician at certain times of the year, also complicate the obtaining of less skilled care, such as a midwife or practical nurse. One family's experience illustrates several of the problems of securing even such care as a mother would consider second best. Knowing that it would be impossible to secure a physician (the nearest one being 40 miles away and across the river, which at that time was not navigable because of the ice), the mother had engaged a neighbor who was looked upon in the community as a midwife. However, labor set in at midnight a few days before the confinement was expected. The father, afraid to leave the mother, sent his oldest son, then 13 years old, out into the blizzard, for the midwife. The boy took a wagon and team, stopped to get a neighbor's boy of the same age to help him find the way, and together these two children set out. They soon were lost in the storm. Meanwhile, the mother was growing very anxious about the boys. " I was more worried about them than about my confinement," she said, in telling of her experiences. After a long while the father stepped outside and heard some one shouting near the house.

The two boys, after going a little distance, had got lost in the bad lands. They climbed out of the wagon to see if they could find a road, but the snow had covered every familiar landmark. They felt about for a while in the pitch dark and then could not find even the team and wagon. After wandering around for a long time, by great good luck they happened to stray near home. The next day, when they went out to look for the team, wagon tracks and their footprints were found on the edge of a 30-foot cut bank. " They escaped it by a miracle," said the father. " If we had been in the country longer we would have known better than to send them out on such a night. But our boy had always had such a good sense of direction and he thought he knew the way."

Meanwhile, the father, who knew nothing about the care of a woman in confinement, delivered his wife, with fear and trepidation. (Her previous confinements had all been attended by a physician.)

"Altogether it was a terrifying time," he said. The next day the midwife was sent for to see if the mother was in good condition.

Most of the fathers who had to deliver their wives felt that the danger of such lack of care was too great to be risked again if in any way it could be avoided. One father said he would never attend a confinement again, but that he would start to the hospital with his wife six months before confinement was expected. He feels that no price is too high to pay for adequate confinement care.

One local physician thought that the women, perhaps because of the character of their life in the area, had easier confinements and were less likely to suffer certain complications (such as might be expected to follow their poor confinement care) than would city women if the latter were subjected to the same conditions. However, there were many mothers and babies who suffered very serious results following the lack of good confinement care. Again and again mothers would say, "I've never been well since." Eight of the mothers covered by the inquiry had died as a result of childbirth, 10 babies had been stillborn and 12 had died under 2 weeks of age, and there were 39 premature deliveries.[1]

Women attendants.

One hundred and eighty-one of the mothers who remained in the area for confinement were attended by women who in a few instances were trained or practical nurses, but in a great majority of cases were only untrained neighbors or relatives. In many cases the attendant was a member of the household and in most of the others lived within 5 miles of the mother. Altogether, 122 women attended these 181 confinements. The question naturally arises as to how these attendants were equipped for the care of mothers at childbirth.

There are no licensed midwives in the area. When a doctor can not be secured, a neighbor is usually called in to care for the mother through her confinement. As a rule, she attends as a favor, often going with fear and misgivings, and only because no one else can be found and "a woman can't be left alone at such a time." She seldom charges for her services. "One neighbor does it for another out here," one mother remarked. Gradually some of the more self-reliant women acquire a reputation for skill in such cases and are called upon so often that they become the main reliance of a neighborhood and decide to consider their services as at least professional nursing and to charge a fee. This fee usually ranges from the most common charge of $1.50 or $2 a day, with no charge for delivery, to $25 a week or, in a few instances, $25 for the delivery alone.

---

[1] See discussion of Complications, Maternal Mortality, and Infant Mortality, pp. 39, 41, and 70.

Of perhaps 25 or 30 women who in the various neighborhoods had the reputation of caring for confinement cases, 10 were visited by the Children's Bureau agents and questioned about their work. Few had attended more than 2 cases in the past year, though 1 reported 22 cases in the past five years, of which 2 had been attended by a physician also; and 1 reported 5; 1, "about 6"; and 1, 7 in the past year. Several had had some training in a hospital or as practical nurses before they moved into the area studied. One was a graduate trained nurse (she had, however, attended confinements without a physician only twice in her three years of residence in the district). Those who had practiced before coming to the area studied had almost never cared for a mother at confinement, except as a nurse where there was a physician in attendance, and they all preferred to work with a physician. The trained nurse refuses to care for a case unless a physician is in attendance except in an emergency—where the physician does not arrive in time or for some reason can not be secured.

Even when a fee is charged the service is performed as an accommodation, and in many other cases with reluctance, especially where an attendant realizes the dangers of childbirth. One woman, who does not wish to attend confinement cases and does so only when no one else can be secured, said she knew what to do if everything went right, but would not have the least idea how to proceed if anything were abnormal. She had once had an abnormal case and the baby had died, partly on account of the mother's condition and partly because a physician could not be secured in time and she had not known what to do. This woman attended five cases in the year preceding the inquiry. When her own baby was born she went away for confinement because there was no one in the neighborhood whom she could trust to deliver her. Another woman said, "At first I used to be very much afraid, but since I've watched the doctor and have delivered a few cases myself I'm not afraid any more."

In every instance but one these women said that in addition to giving nursing care they did the housework in case the mother had no one else to do it; and a few of them considered the housework part of their regular duties. The majority remained with the mothers from nine days to two weeks, though several reported that they stayed only a few days, as short a time as possible, in order to get back to their own households. Several of the women limited their practice to their own children, grandchildren, and other near relations.

Most of these attendants do not feel competent to give advice on infant care, except such advice as one neighbor will give another. Several were very eager to get the Children's Bureau pamphlets on Infant Care and Prenatal Care that they might answer the many

questions which are often asked them. None of them gave any prenatal care or advice, except occasionally to tell mothers what supplies
to prepare for confinement, and in one instance to urge mothers to
have a physician make urinalyses.

Nearly all the women interviewed realized the need, if not of complete asepsis, at least of cleanliness in caring for their patients.
Antiseptics such as boric acid, carbolic acid, lysol, and mercury
bichloride were reported. One woman had persuaded a little country store to keep bichloride tablets in stock. Nearly all used scorched
linen and boric acid on the cord and a boric acid solution to wash the
baby's eyes. None of them, however, reported a regular equipment; and, though they usually carried antiseptics, nearly all depended for other supplies on what their patients had in the house.

It is obvious that these women occupy a very different position in
their neighborhoods from that of a city midwife, or the midwives of,
let us say, a southern rural community. For the most part they realize their limitations, and do not attempt to interfere with the natural
course of delivery or to " doctor " their patients with herbs and such
multitudinous home remedies as, for example, were reported by the
midwives in the North Carolina study. Only one woman reported
the use of any but the most common home remedies. In addition to
the use of boric acid she washes the eyes of new-born babies with a
rag soaked in honey and sage; in case of a laceration she applies an
egg fried in lard without salt, and for sore breasts she advises the
application of hot pancakes.

Almost all these women realized that maternity care was a great
problem in their neighborhood, and they approved of the idea of
county public-health nurses as a first step at least toward the solution
of the problem.

AFTER CARE BY A PHYSICIAN.

When a woman secures a physician for confinement in the area
studied of how much oversight and protection is she thus assured?
Except when the physician is late (there were 30 such cases) her
actual delivery has the advantage of medical attention. In this study
all mothers whose doctors arrived in time to perform any service have
been counted attended by physicians. It is possible that before the
physician arrives unskilled handling may have brought about infection or other complications, but at any rate even a late physician is
often a great safeguard.

After care by a physician, which in standard practice in cities
is considered a part of confinement care and consists of at least from
4 to 10 postnatal visits, is nonexistent in the area studied, except
for the six cases where the mother stayed, at the time of confine-

ment, in the house of the physician.[1] Indeed, except in 12 cases where complications developed and 32 cases where the mother lived or was staying within 5 miles of the physician, only 8 mothers were visited after confinement, and each of these women was visited only once. The tremendous distances and the small number of physicians for a great area would in themselves explain the lack of postnatal care. When it takes the greater part of a day and sometimes longer for the physician to reach his patients, fees are naturally high.[2] A physician would not make so expensive a visit unless called by the family; most homesteaders are by no means well-to-do and find it hard to meet the expense of the original confinement visit, much less any postnatal visits which do not seem to them absolutely necessary. Even if the importance of postnatal care were realized its almost prohibitive expense would lead many families to take the chance that the mothers would recover without complications, provided the birth had not been difficult.

NURSING CARE.

It happened that among the homesteaders there were several graduate nurses, and several other nurses who had had some training in hospitals but who had not graduated. Although most of these women were married and had families to care for, and none of them had come to the area to practice, they were, nevertheless, usually available in cases of emergency in their various neighborhoods, and practiced now and then, either as an accommodation to their neighbors or because they needed money. In addition to these, there were a number of practical nurses[3] whose experiences had in many cases made their services more valuable than those of persons quite untrained.

Of the 359 mothers who remained in the area for confinement,[4] 14 had been cared for by graduate nurses and 113 others by women who may be considered partly trained. In other words, over one-third of these mothers had had trained or partly trained nursing care—a rather unexpected showing, considering their lack of other items of maternity care. Indeed, a larger proportion of the mothers in the Montana area received trained or semitrained care than of the mothers in the Kansas study, though the latter had on the whole much better maternity care.

However, nearly two-thirds of the mothers did not have the safeguard of even semitrained care. Fifty-five women relied entirely upon the members of their households—very often only their hus-

---

[1] Including one in which the mother was the wife of a physician.
[2] See section on Cost of Childbirth, p. 49.
[3] See discussion of Women Attendants, p. 31.
[4] See discussion of Mothers Who Left the Area for Confinement, p. 47.

bands. In busy seasons, especially during harvest or at lambing time or during a round-up, it is often impossible for the neighbors to leave their work. Usually, however, the kindliness of neighbors is depended upon. The great majority of the mothers (176) were nursed by neighbors, friends, or relations who were not members of their households. One mother, whose husband was away on a freighting trip, was quite without nursing care. The neighbor to whose house she had gone for confinement was suddenly bedridden by an accident, and the mother had to leave her bed to get food for herself and the other woman for the first two days, after which she got up. She said she had such a hard time that she has never been well since. Several women were practically alone for the first day or two after confinement; consequently their nursing care did not begin when it was most needed.

Very frequently the care given by the father or another member of the household consists only in the bringing of meals to the mother and can hardly be considered nursing care. Thus one mother reported that her baby was born at lambing time, and on the third day after her confinement a crew of five men came to help with lambing and stayed 10 days. The father had to work night and day during this time, doing what housework was done and cooking for the lambing crew in addition to his farm work; and so the mother had only occasional attention. The mother bathed the baby and cared for herself. On the twelfth day she tried to get up, but had fever and had to go back to bed.

Often the neighbors who are kind enough to nurse the mother, and even some of the practical nurses, are quite unskilled. While they may perform such simple services as bathing and dressing the baby or preparing the mother's meals, they would be unable to recognize as important many symptoms of complications which a trained nurse would immediately know needed a physician's attention. Moreover, in many instances the neighbors do not stay at the mother's home, but come in for a few hours each day and combine a little nursing care with a neighborly visit. Thus, if a mother should develop some serious symptoms before or after the neighbor called, or, worse still, in the night, the father would have to leave her by herself while he " wrangled " and saddled a horse, rode a long distance to the nearest house where there was a woman, waited for her to get ready to come back with him, and rode back home, or perhaps left the neighbor to go to his wife alone while he rode for the doctor.

The importance of good nursing care in any community during the confinement period can not be too forcibly emphasized. But in such a county as this one in Montana how such care can be made accessible to every woman in childbirth is an especially importunate problem.

PRENATAL CARE.

The urgent need for prenatal care has been emphasized in previous publications of the bureau. Dr. Grace L. Meigs, in Maternal Mortality,[1] states in regard to complications of pregnancy and childbirth:

A large number of these complications can be prevented through proper hygiene and supervision during pregnancy and through skilled care at labor. Certain other complications which can not be prevented can be detected before serious harm is done, and treatment can be given which will save the mother's life. We can see this more clearly if we consider as examples two of the most important complications.

Puerperal albuminuria and convulsions, called also eclampsia, or toxemia of pregnancy, is a disease which occurs most frequently during pregnancy but may occur at or following confinement. It is a relatively frequent complication among women bearing their first children. When fully established its chief symptoms are convulsions and unconsciousness. In the early stages of the disease the symptoms are slight puffiness of the face, hands, and feet; headache; albumen in the urine; and usually a rise in blood pressure. Very often proper treatment and diet at the beginning of such early symptoms may prevent the development of the disease; but in many cases where the disease is well established before the physician is consulted, the woman and baby can not be saved by any treatment. In the prevention of deaths from this cause it is essential, therefore, that each woman, especially each woman bearing her first child, should know what she can do, by proper hygiene and diet, to prevent the disease; that she should know the meaning of these early symptoms if they arise, so that she may seek at once the advice of her doctor; and that she should have regular supervision during pregnancy, with examination of the urine at intervals.

Some obstruction to labor in the small size or abnormal shape of the pelvic canal causes many deaths of mothers included in the class "other accidents of labor" and also many stillbirths. If such difficulty is discovered before labor, proper treatment will in almost all cases insure the life of mother and child; if it is not discovered until labor has begun, or perhaps until it has continued for many hours, the danger to both is greatly increased. Every woman, therefore, should have during pregnancy—and above all during her first pregnancy—an examination in which measurements are made to enable the physician to judge whether or not there will be any obstruction to labor. A case in which a complication of this kind is found requires the greatest skill and experience in treatment, but with such treatment the life and health of the mother are almost always safe.

These two examples will suffice. In the same way it could be shown, with regard to all the other complications of pregnancy and labor, that those which can not be prevented can be treated successfully in most cases if detected in time.

It can be regarded, then, as a generally accepted fact that all illness and death connected with childbearing is, to a certain and

---

[1] Maternal· Mortality, pp. 12–13.   U. S. Children's Bureau Publication No. 19.

large degree, preventable through the application of the scientific knowledge which is now well established.

Even in cities where there has been active propaganda on behalf of prenatal care the importance and necessity of such care is not generally realized. Therefore it is not surprising that in the remote area studied where there has been no such propaganda more than three-fourths of the mothers had no prenatal care whatever—saw no physician, had no physical examination, measurements, or urinalysis.

Several mothers expressed surprise at being asked whether they had seen a physician or had any prenatal care. "No; why should I? I was feeling all right."

Indeed, considering the inaccessibility of medical care, the difficulties imposed by weather, roads, distances, and expense, it is surprising and encouraging to learn that nearly one-fourth of the mothers had secured at least a little prenatal care. However, when the extent and quality of this care is analyzed, the showing is not so favorable.

In order to measure and compare prenatal care in different communities, certain standards of what constitutes adequate and fair prenatal care have been drawn up by the bureau, after consultation with Dr. J. Whitridge Williams, professor of obstetrics at Johns Hopkins Univeristy.[1] By these standards, adequate care—which would include as a minimum an obstetrical examination; continued supervision by a physician through at least the last five months of pregnancy; monthly examination of the urine at least through the last five months; and, in case of a first pregnancy, measurement of the pelvis to determine whether any structural deformity exists which is likely to interfere with birth—was afforded no mother in the area studied. Twenty-two mothers received what is classified as fair care—which includes an obstetrical examination; from one to four urinalyses at monthly intervals; some supervision by a physician; and, in the case of a primipara, pelvic measurements. Anything less than this is considered an inadequate protection for the mother against those complications of pregnancy and childbirth which are preventable. Eighty-six mothers received only inadequate care, which in a great many instances consisted of a single visit to the physician and sometimes of submitting one sample of urine during pregnancy—a dangerously inadequate protection.

Of all the mothers, less than 1 in 4 had consulted a physician, and over three-fifths of these had consulted him only once; about 1 in 10

[1] Moore, Elizabeth: Maternity and Infant Care in a Rural County in Kansas, p. 28. U. S. Children's Bureau Publication No. 26, Rural Child Welfare Series No. 1. Washington, 1917.

had had an obstetrical examination; and only 1 in 7 had urinalysis. Of the 127 primiparæ,[1] only 3 reported pelvic measurements.

Instances in which a mother was ill, but, even so, secured no prenatal care were not uncommon. In this group, for example, was one who had had many slight uterine hemorrhages all through pregnancy; another mother, whose previous pregnancy had resulted in a miscarriage, had had such pain in her limbs that for several months before the baby's birth she could hardly walk. This mother was again pregnant at the time the agent from the Children's Bureau visited her and was again suffering from badly swollen limbs, but had had no medical treatment nor advice.

Another mother who throughout pregnancy was very ill, weak, and listless, and who suffered from headaches, swollen hands and feet, and numbness, had no prenatal care. She was again pregnant at the time of the survey and was suffering from the same symptoms, and, though eager to consult a physician, felt she could not do so because there was none within 35 miles, and the trip would be both difficult and expensive beyond the family's means.

Another woman, who reported an " extremely nervous " pregnancy, took " spikenard," on the recommendation of a neighbor, but had no prenatal care.

Sometimes mothers reported the use of patent medicine which they saw advertised in newspapers. Thus, one mother who had had kidney trouble before her marriage and was ill throughout her pregnancy, had no medical care, but bought some " Easy Childbirth Tablets." Another, who had suffered much from nausea, secured no prenatal care, but wrote to a Texas physician who advertised in a foreign newspaper and who sent the mother some pills. On the whole, however, comparatively little " home doctoring " was reported, only 46 mothers, or 1 in 10, having used any home remedies. Such as were used were for the most part olive oil, either taken internally or applied externally, and simple cathartics, though several patent medicines—whose value was, to say the least, doubtful—were reported.

Several mothers whose pregnancies were complicated made only one or two visits to a physician, in spite of their dangerous condition. Thus, one woman who began to have profuse hemorrhages at six months consulted a physician and had a urinalysis only shortly before her baby—born prematurely at seven months—was delivered. She did not realize the importance of the doctor's advice to rest, and continued her work up to the day the baby was born. The prematurity of this baby and its death at the age of 7 hours could probably have been prevented had the mother had good prenatal care throughout her pregnancy, and had she followed the doctor's advice.

---

[1] Excluding three about whom no reports were available.

It is significant that of the mothers who obtained prenatal care, only 21 sought it because of discomforts or complications of pregnancy. And often women who had no prenatal care realized its importance, but had been unable to secure it, sometimes because of its inaccessibility, again because of its expense. One mother, who with her previous children had had good prenatal care, including monthly urinalysis, was much disturbed because she could not protect herself and her last child with the safeguards such care would have provided.

A fairly large proportion of the mothers had realized their need of instruction about prenatal care. One hundred and fifty-five, or one-third, reported that they had read books or pamphlets on this subject, sometimes borrowing such reading matter from their neighbors. A list of literature made up from the mothers' reports, contained such standard books as Slemmons's The Prospective Mother; Practical Nursing, by Pope and Maxwell; the Children's Bureau publication, Prenatal Care; and others. Several women's periodicals having "Advice to Mothers" departments were read by many of the women. "Doctor books," the names of which the mothers had forgotten, were frequently reported. There were also some books, standard in their day, but not containing the latest findings of medical science on the subject of prenatal care; and there were a few fairly good pamphlets, published as advertising matter. On the other hand, publications advertising patent medicines were common, and many books which gave dangerous advice—one of them, for example, advising mothers to get up on the second day after confinement—were for several women the only available sources of information.

However, even though much of the reading was indiscriminate and ill-chosen, the very fact that the printed page was sought by one-third of the mothers as a guide is an index to the intelligence of the community. The eagerness of the mothers to secure the Children's Bureau publication on this subject presages well their acceptance of further instruction in prenatal care, if such should be offered by county public-health nurses.

COMPLICATIONS.

It is never possible to get complete data on the complications of pregnancy and confinement in a community, and it is especially difficult in such an area as the one studied, where many mothers had secured no medical attention and no accurate diagnosis had been made. Unless a physician had informed her, a mother might not know of a laceration resulting from confinement; might not know of puerperal fever; and might accept as a normal part of childbearing many symptoms which, with good prenatal and confinement care, she might have been spared.

However, there are several complications which any mother having experienced them would recognize. These are Cæsarean section, convulsions, premature delivery, stillbirth, and instrumental delivery. Seventy-four, or almost one-sixth of the women, reported at least one of these complications, nine of them reporting two and one reporting three. There were 39 premature deliveries, 10 stillbirths, and 7 cases of convulsions. Twenty-nine instrumental deliveries were also reported. That one-sixth of the mothers should have suffered these complications at childbirth is bad enough; yet this statement does not even begin to tell the whole story. These complications are the most easily recognized, and are very serious, but not necessarily the most dangerous. The greatest single cause of death in childbirth—puerperal septicemia—is omitted.

Although, as has been said, no attempt was made to secure statistics on any complications except the five already listed, many mothers reported symptoms of very serious diseases, either in addition to those listed above or separately. The significance of the dreary reiteration of such statements as "I have not been well since" can not be conveyed by statistics. Difficult presentations, prolonged labor, and lacerations were among the most common complications reported. One mother reported labor that lasted three days, after which she had fainting spells for one hour. Another mother was badly lacerated and the laceration was not repaired. She was unable to get out of bed for two and a half weeks, and it was many weeks before she could walk even around the house.

Many women had had severe hemorrhages. One mother, whose baby was born four hours before the physician arrived, was attended by a neighbor who had never had any previous experience in confinement cases. A hemorrhage followed the delivery and the mother said she nearly bled to death before the physician reached her. Several mothers had had chills or chills and fever after confinement, and one, whose delivery had been a shoulder presentation, developed a chill two weeks after confinement. The practical nurse who delivered her had told her that this was "a sure symptom of blood poisoning." No physician was engaged even then, and douches were given for several days without a physician's supervision. The mother remained in bed for two days, but was ill for two weeks. At the time of the Children's Bureau inquiry, over a year later, she was still in poor health.

"Blood poisoning" was frequently reported. One mother said she almost died; another, who did not consider a physician necessary at childbirth, felt very ill three days after delivery. Only upon the urgent advice of the nurse who had attended her, however, did she finally send for a physician who diagnosed " blood 'poisoning, due to retention of part of the placenta." She was confined to her bed for 21 days and unable to resume her housework for over a month. Another mother who had had no prenatal care had three convulsions just preceding delivery, before the physician reached her, and four after he arrived. She realizes now how dangerous her situation was and that it probably could have been avoided had she secured good prenatal care.

Another mother, who said she had " kidney trouble " during pregnancy and had suffered from vertigo, had had no prenatal care. Her baby was born prematurely at seven months. Two hours after labor began a physician who lived over 20 miles away was sent for, but he did not reach the house until after the mother had had seven convulsions and the baby had been born, the father having performed all services. The mother was confined to her bed for three weeks afterwards.

Still another mother—a primipara—had an even narrower escape from death. During her girlhood she had had kidney trouble, and, though she was ill throughout pregnancy, she, nevertheless, had secured no prenatal care. Just before labor she suffered with severe nausea and vertigo and became blind. As soon as labor set in she began having convulsions. The father summoned the neighbors— one of whom was a practical nurse—and then went for the nearest physician, who lived 25 miles away. When the father reached his house the physician was out on another case. The mother had been in labor and had had convulsions for 36 hours before he arrived. The practical nurse had administered chloroform several times, but was afraid to continue on her own responsibility. The physician immediately delivered the baby, which was stillborn, with instruments. The blindness, convulsions, and an unconscious condition continued until the fourth day, but the doctor made no postnatal visits, nor did he repair a severe laceration which occurred during the birth. The neighbors took turns nursing the mother for the first four days. On the fifth day a graduate nurse was secured. The mother's sight gradually returned, but at the time the information was secured by the Children's Bureau agent, over five months afterwards, the mother reported that she had " not had a well day since."[1]

MATERNAL MORTALITY.

It is important to know what proportion of mothers in a given community die as a result of childbirth. The maternal mortality rate is commonly stated as the number of such deaths compared with the number of live-born infants in a given period.

---

[1] See also discussion of Prenatal Care, p. 36.

During the five years covered by the Children's Bureau survey there were 628 live births in the district, and 8 mothers died from diseases of pregnancy or confinement.[1]   In other words, the "cost" in maternal deaths for this number of live-born infants was 12.7 per 1,000.

Although the figures on which this death rate is based are small, it may, nevertheless, be worth while to compare it with other available statistics. The corresponding maternal mortality rate for the United States birth-registration area in 1915 was 6.6,[2] a rate only about half as high as that of the Montana area studied. And this rate for the United States birth-registration area is higher than the rate of any one of 15 foreign countries for which the figures for the year 1910 were secured.[3]

Of these countries, Scotland has the highest rate, 5.7, and Italy the lowest rate, 2.4 per 1,000 live births. The Montana district's shockingly high rate of 12.7 is more than five times as high as Italy's.

The risk to the mother may be stated as the number of maternal deaths in relation to the total number of pregnancies resulting in live or stillbirths. During the five years covered by the survey the total confinements to all mothers numbered 634. Seven mothers died, excluding one whose death followed a miscarriage.[4] This gives the high mortality rate of 11 per 1,000 confinements.

A comparison with other rural areas where similar studies have been made by the bureau is significant. In the Kansas area only 1 in 349 confinements terminated fatally,[5] a rate of 2.9 per 1,000; in the Wisconsin areas only 4 out of 661, or a rate of 6 per 1,000. In other words, childbirth is nearly four times as fatal to mothers in the area studied in Montana as in the Kansas area, and nearly twice as fatal as in the Wisconsin areas.

These rates are especially illuminating when considered in relation to the proportion of mothers attended by physicians, taking attendance by physician as an index to the quality of care a mother receives. Nearly all the Kansas mothers—95 per cent—and 68 per cent of the Wisconsin mothers were delivered by physicians, whereas

---

[1] This does not include the death of one mother who did not recover after childbirth, but whose death certificate gave Bright's disease as the cause of death, and the death of another which occurred during the investigation, but after the period which the study covered, i. e., Aug. 1, 1912, to July 31, 1917.

[2] Computed from figures for the birth registration area of 1915, U. S. Bureau of the Census, Birth Statistics, 1915, p. 10 ; and Mortality Statistics, 1915, pp. 298–303.

[3] See Appendix A, Table I, p. 95.

[4] Owing to the fact that the reports of miscarriages were not complete they have been excluded from the number of confinements ; to secure a " probability of dying " to correspond, the death of the mother following the miscarriage must be omitted. This death was included above in the statement of the " cost " in maternal deaths corresponding to 1,000 live births.

[5] Excluding two deaths which followed miscarriages.

only 47 per cent of the 463 Montana mothers [1] had the advantage of delivery by a physician.

Because of the knowledge that deaths from childbirth are largely preventable it will be significant to consider the kind of prenatal, confinement, and postnatal care afforded to these seven mothers.

In one family the mother was confined in midwinter. No physician had been engaged, though after a previous confinement where there was no trained attendant the mother had suffered a serious illness of six weeks' duration. The night before birth the family and a neighbor sat up late reading a "doctor book." The mother had had no prenatal care whatever. When the baby was born the father and a neighbor cut and tied the cord. Half an hour after the delivery the mother began to feel very ill. She became rapidly worse, and the father, three hours later, started for the nearest physician, who lived 15 miles away. The snow was deep and it took two teams of two horses each to get the doctor and bring him to the home. But six hours before the father returned with the physician the mother died. The doctor could not be certain of the cause of death, but thought that it was internal concealed hemorrhage.

One mother had been seriously ill for several months before childbirth, with hemorrhages and weakness. A severe, unrepaired laceration due to a previous confinement added to her wretchedness. In her sixth month of pregnancy she consulted a physician, who examined her, made urinalysis, and pronounced her in a serious condition and in need of hospital attention. The husband, however, could not be persuaded that there was any danger in so natural a function as childbirth, and the mother received no further prenatal care. At confinement she suffered no labor pains but had excessive hemorrhages. The physician, who lived 35 miles away, was sent for but did not arrive for 24 hours. He diagnosed the case as placenta prævia and delivered with instruments a stillborn child that he said had been dead for at least four days. When interviewed by a Children's Bureau agent he stated that it was a case of placenta prævia; that he had thought the mother was in no danger after the child had been delivered; and that he was surprised at a later call. He believed that blood poisoning had set in because the fetus had been dead so long before delivery. The mother died on the seventh day.

Another mother, who in her previous deliveries had experienced much difficulty, did not wish to go away from home for confinement because it entailed leaving her children. She consulted a physician several times during pregnancy, and he felt that she could be safely confined at home, though he did not examine or measure her and

---

[1] Including those who left the area for confinement.

made no urinalysis. The mother had some instruction from a nurse. At the confinement—a breech presentation—the physician twice attempted to deliver her with instruments but did not succeed. After she had been in labor three days he realized that she could not be delivered at home, ordered an automobile, and took her to the nearest hospital, 115 miles away—a terribly long ride over rough roads— where she arrived thoroughly exhausted. The physicians called in consultation did not perform a Cæsarean section because of her condition. The following morning instruments were again applied, and a very large stillborn baby was delivered. The mother lived until the following day, when she died of exhaustion.

A young mother of 21 who was confined for the first time had had absolutely no prenatal care. Although she suffered from swollen ankles and what she believed to be kidney trouble, she had had no urinalysis and came to her confinement in every way unprepared, not even having read any instructive literature. The physician left shortly after the delivery, which had seemed to him quite normal. Six or seven hours later the mother developed convulsions. The physician lived only 10 miles away and was sent for again. He came and asked to have another physician called in, but the two physicians were unable to save the mother. She died 13 hours after the delivery.

Another primipara, who had been " ailing " all through pregnancy, attempted to relieve her discomfort with patent medicines—one a " womb and liver tonic." Three weeks before confinement she had a hemorrhage and went to a physician, who told her that she was all right, though he made no examination and gave her no treatment. The confinement was complicated, the physician said, by placenta prævia. He was with her while she suffered for three days and three nights, but did not interfere. Finally he said that another physician must be sent for. Two physicians were secured from the nearest city, 60 miles away, but the mother died just before they arrived. The child was never delivered.

Another mother, who had a history of Bright's disease, and whose death is, therefore, not included in the eight deaths resulting from childbirth, never recovered after parturition. She suffered from kidney trouble during most of her pregnancy, and in her sixth month consulted a physician. He made no examination or urinalysis, but advised that another physican be consulted. The family, however, did not follow his advice and neglected to engage a physician for the confinement, which an aunt attended. The child was stillborn. The mother did not recover, and her husband took her to the nearest city to see a physician, but " no medicine did any good." After suffering from severe headaches, temporary blindness, and swollen legs for eight months—a great part of the time confined to her bed—she died.

Two of the mothers went away for their confinements. One of these had had kidney trouble in her girlhood, and during her entire pregnancy had felt miserable, yet up to the time she went away she had not seen a physician, had had no prenatal care, no urinalysis, and no instruction about her diet or how to take care of herself. About two weeks before her confinement she felt very ill, and two days later her husband took her to her parents in another State. They also lived out in the country, 26 miles from the attendant physician, who in addition to the visit at confinement made only four later visits. The husband (who gave the information) did not know whether after reaching her parents' home the mother had seen a physician before confinement. Her baby, born prematurely, died at 2 weeks of age. The mother continued to grow worse, and about six weeks after childbirth was taken to a hospital, where, after another six weeks of suffering, she died.

The other mother who left the area for confinement was a primipara. She went to her parents in a city two months before her baby was expected. Her husband (who gave the information) did not know what care she had had, except that three physicians were present when she died of puerperal septicemia on the eighth day after childbirth.

Is the area studied in Montana exceptionally bad, or does the whole State share its deplorable rate? The available statistics are so limited that it is impossible to answer the question. Montana is not yet in the birth-registration area and was only in 1910 admitted to the death-registration area; therefore the most significant maternal mortality rate—the number of deaths per 1,000 births—can not be reckoned. However, the maternal death rate per 100,000 estimated population has been computed and can be compared with rates for other States and certain foreign countries, as can also the rates per 100,000 female population and per 100,000 female population of from 15 to 44 years of age.[1]

The death rates from diseases of pregnancy and confinement per 100,000 population in Montana, from 1910 to 1915, were:[2] 16.4, 19.9, 18.5, 19.1, 23.1, 20.4; the average[3] rate for these six years was 19.6. The Children's Bureau, in a study of maternal mortality,[4] compared

---

[1] See Appendix A, p. 95, for tables showing these figures and for notes on the possible sources of error. The estimate of population is based on the assumption of a constant annual increase equal to that between 1900 and 1910. In the case of a rapidly growing State like Montana these estimates may not correspond accurately to the true population. The error would be likely to increase the longer the period after the census of 1910.

[2] Based on estimated population (Bulletin of the U. S. Bureau of the Census No. 133) and deaths from diseases of pregnancy and confinement (Mortality Statistics, published annually by the U. S. Bureau of the Census).

[3] That is, the average number of deaths related to the average estimated population for the six years.

[4] Meigs, Dr. Grace L.: Maternal Mortality, Table XII, p. 56.; U. S. Children's Bureau Publication No. 19. See also Appendix A, Table I.

the average rates of 16 countries from 1900 to 1910.[1] This comparison showed Sweden with the lowest rate, losing only six mothers out of every 100,000 population, and Spain the highest, with a rate of 19.6. Montana falls to the level of Spain's unenviable place, and is one of several States that lower the rate for the whole United States registration area, which occupies the discreditable rank of fourteenth, or third from the last, in this vital international comparison.

Comparison between the maternal death rate per 100,000 population for a State which has so great a preponderance of males as has Montana, and the death rates of the New England States or of foreign countries where the preponderance is almost always female, may be misleading. But the comparison gains significance when it confines itself to the death rate per 100,000 estimated female population aged 15 to 44 years. Here Montana makes an even poorer showing. Montana's maternal death rates for the female population of the ages specified for the years 1910 to 1915 were as follows:

1910	78. 9
1911	95. 9
1912	89. 1
1913	92. 0
1914	111. 4
1915	98. 4

Statistics for 11 foreign countries upon which some corresponding rates could be computed are given in Table III.[2] Montana's lowest rate, 78.9, was 13.8 higher than the rate for Scotland for 1914, which was 65.14, the highest rate found for any of these countries. Her highest rate, 111.4, was nearly four times as great as the lowest rate— 29.3 for Sweden in 1911—found for any of the foreign countries.

When Montana is compared on the same basis—maternal deaths per 100,000 female population aged 15 to 44 years—with the other States in the death registration area, her showing is again unfortunate. Except for 1910, the first year after her admission into the area, she has had a higher maternal death rate than any other State. In 1910 Colorado exceeded the Montana death rate by 1.6. In 1911, 1914, and 1915 her rate was over twice as great as the lowest rates for States in the registration area for the corresponding years.[3]

That many of the deaths which go to make up such rates as these could have been prevented has already been emphasized. Significant as these figures are, they do not begin to indicate the sickness, invalidism, and misery which follow poor or inadequate care in childbirth. If some means could be devised to gauge these distressing

---

[1] Except where figures were not available for the entire period, in which case the averages for shorter periods were used.

[2] See Appendix A, p. 96.

[3] See Appendix A, Table IV, p. 96.

results, such statistics would be forthcoming as would compel the attention of the country and would give great impetus to the movement for the protection of the Nation's childbearing mothers.

MOTHERS WHO LEFT THE AREA FOR CONFINEMENT.

The purpose of going away for confinement is almost always to secure better confinement care than can be obtained on the isolated homestead. It is, therefore, not surprising that 63, or 6 out of 10, of the 104 women who went away were delivered by a physician, and that 27, or over one-fourth, of these were confined in a hospital or maternity home; whereas of the women who stayed in the county only 36 per cent were attended by physicians, and in 23 per cent of these cases the physician was late. On the other hand, that 14 women should have taken a long trip to get good confinement care and yet should have had no physician is a somewhat unexpected finding. One of these 14 mothers was attended at confinement by her husband on the way to the city; the others were attended by a midwife, a neighbor, or a relative in the places to which they went.

Just as the proportion of confinements attended by physicians is greater among the mothers who went away, so is the extent of after care by physicians. Only one-tenth of these mothers had no postnatal visits; whereas, in addition to the 27 who were confined in a hospital, 21 had over 4 visits, and of these, 7 had 10 or more such visits; that is, 48 or well over half the women attended by physicians had more than 4 postnatal visits, whereas of the mothers who stayed in the area only 7 of those attended by physicians, or 5.4 per cent, had more than 4 postnatal visits.

The mothers who went away had an added advantage in being relieved of their household and farm tasks for a longer period before and after parturition than the mothers who stayed at home and in the kind of nursing care they received. Fifty-three per cent had trained or partly trained nursing care, whereas of those who stayed in the area only 35 per cent had such care.

Often a great struggle is made and a large debt incurred in order that a mother may go away for confinement; frequently, however, the high cost of board and room, in addition to the expensive trip, is so great that the mother can not afford to be gone long; and often there are children whom it is difficult to leave. Therefore, it is not surprising that a large number of women who plan to go away are delayed by bad weather until the time for confinement is upon them, or that they do not allow enough time to take the long trip to and from the railroad in comfort.

One family started out in a sleigh at 7 in the morning on a 60-mile ride to the hospital. Toward evening the mother began having labor pains. They had gone too far to return home, and, deciding that it would be best to try to get to the hospital, they drove all night. The next morning at 10 o'clock the baby was born, in the snow, 10 miles from the city to which they were going. The father was the mother's only attendant, and he cut and tied the cord. They then borrowed a more comfortable vehicle from a family that lived near the road and continued their trip to the hospital, the mother carrying the baby on her lap.

A long trip over bad roads and often in bad weather is a great physical drain on a woman near the end of her pregnancy; and the return with a small baby before the mother has completely recovered her strength may be even more taxing. One mother who was feeling very ill drove into the nearest city—a five-day trip by wagon—about a month before her confinement. It snowed every day and she had a very distressing time. When she and her husband reached their destination they moved into a shack 1½ miles from town, where she tried to keep house until the time for her confinement. She was unable to do her housework, however, and had to engage help. She did not have hospital care, but a physician attended her. When the baby was 10 days old they started back on their five-day trip.

Another woman left home with her husband in November, two weeks before confinement, and after a 65-mile auto ride to the railroad went over 100 miles farther by train in order to get to a hospital. They started back before the baby was 1 month old, in some of the worst winter weather. They knew this was unwise, but the mother was so worried about the other children at home alone—who would have no way to get help if any of them should become sick—that she was unwilling to wait any longer. The 65-mile journey from the railroad took four days. One night they drove till 10 o'clock before finding a place to sleep, and they spent one whole day covering the 4 miles between two post offices, where the road, though fairly level, was so deep with snow that their car could hardly get through.

Several mothers felt that an arduous wagon trip of four or five days was fully repaid by the care which they received. " The doctor told me I could never have lived through this at home without skilled care " was a typical remark after a woman had told of a difficult instrumental delivery, prolonged labor, or some other complicated parturition in a city, where physicians, hospitals, and trained nurses were available. There were some instances, however, where a mother went not to a city but to a rural district less isolated than her homestead, or to a little town where a physician could be much more easily secured than at home, but where there was no assurance of having good confinement care.

In 14 instances mothers were not attended by a physician; in 4 of these a physician had been called but arrived too late to perform any services. In 3 cases, though the physician was late, he arrived in time to cut the cord or deliver the afterbirth. So far as the physician's attendance was concerned, most of these mothers had taken long and expensive trips almost to no purpose.

Sometimes the possibility of getting a physician is the only thing considered. One mother, three weeks before parturition, went to a little railroad village, where she lived in a shack near a physician. There was no trained nurse in the village, and when on the third day after confinement she began to have convulsions, the frightened father sent to a city 80 miles away for a trained nurse. Two days later the mother showed symptoms of returning convulsions, and the physician advised taking her to the city from which the nurse had come, where she could have hospital care. In her dangerous condition she was taken over 80 miles by train to a maternity home. She is one of many mothers who report that they have not been strong since confinement.

Obviously, when the mother goes away, the expense of securing good confinement, postnatal, and nursing care, of getting some one to do the housework and care for the children left at home is a great financial drain, possible only for families who have some capital, credit, or some means of raising money. A large percentage of the families studied were homesteading at the time of the mother's confinement. To most of these such an expense would have been very difficult if not impossible. Some means, therefore, must be devised by which good care can be provided for all childbearing mothers, whether or not they can afford to take a long and expensive journey for confinement.[1]

COST OF CHILDBIRTH.

Because a community, in any movement to supply itself with good maternity care must consider the expense in making its plans, it is very important to study the cost of childbirth, along with other problems of maternity.

Physicians' fees.

The mothers in the area studied found childbirth very costly, especially those who had a physician's service or who went away for confinement. The same conditions which make it difficult to get physicians increase the expense when they are secured. The distance, the poor roads, the fact that some of the doctors must hire automobiles to get to their patients, the time they must spend on the way to

---

[1] See Conclusions, p. 91; also discussion of Cost of Childbirth, p. 49.

and from patients when they ride horseback, or when a horse or team and wagon is sent for them—these things explain their high fees. Some physicians charge $1 a mile. Others charge 50 cents. The charge for confinement seems to depend chiefly not on the doctor's services but on the distance the family lives from the physician.

All cases in which it was impossible to distinguish between charges incidental to childbirth and for other illnesses; in which the mother or father had not yet received a bill; in which they had paid not in money but in produce or other gifts, the value of which they did not know, have been classified as not reported.

Of the 219 mothers attended by physicians, 5 received free care, and in 13 instances the cost was not reported. Of the remaining 201, only 30, or 15 per cent, paid less than $25; and 171, or 85 per cent, paid over this amount—22 paying $50 or more. In 18 instances the cost of prenatal care—which in most cases consisted of one visit to the physician—was included in the above figures, and also the cost of whatever postnatal care was given.[1]

The place of confinement—i. e., whether in or out of the area—seems not to affect the physicians' charges, though a slightly larger proportion of mothers staying in the area paid $25 or more; and this in spite of the fact that some of the mothers who went away had hospital care and that a much greater proportion of them had after care by their physicians.

Total immediate expenses of childbirth.

The physician's fee, though the most definite figure obtainable in an inquiry on the expense of childbirth, is only a part of the total cost. In the area studied this charge, in many instances, does not enter into the cost, because such a large percentage of mothers were not attended by physicians. Under the heading " Total immediate expenses of childbirth " are grouped the expenses for prenatal care, fees of physicians and other attendants, nursing care, and expenditure for household help on account of confinement. This, though a nearer approach to the real cost of childbirth, is still a gross understatement, because the cost of supplies, the cost of food for the persons giving nursing care or household help, the traveling expenses of those mothers who went away—all expenditures which should be charged against childbirth—are excluded.[2]

There were 44 instances in which the total immediate expenses of childbirth were not reported, and 92 others in which all the confinement and nursing care and help with housework was given free of charge, either by members of the household, or by other relatives,

---

[1] See After Care by a Physician, p. 33.
[2] See section on Aggregate Cost of Childbirth to Mothers Who Left the Area for Confinement, p. 51.

friends, or neighbors. When these are subtracted from the total of 463, 327 instances remain. The total immediate costs in only 94, or 28.7 per cent, of these were under $25. This is a striking contrast to the findings of the Kansas study, in which nearly half the families reported these costs as less than $25. Moreover, many of the Montana mothers in this group received care which was almost free; for example, in one instance the grandmother delivered the mother, and she and an aunt ·came in daily, waited on the mother, and helped her with housework. For these services each was given "a little pig worth $6." The total immediate costs for 134 women ranged from $25 to $49; for 71 women from $50 to $99; and for 28, or 1 mother in 12, $100 and over.

These figures include the expenses of mothers who went away for confinement and had hospital care; but even for them the cost of getting to the railroad, the railroad fare, and the mother's board while away from home, except board included as part of a hospital fee, are not counted in. In 5 instances the cost to mothers who had hospital care was not reported, but in the other 22 the cost of childbirth in every instance was $40 or over, and in 9 instances $100 or over. This does not surprise one; but it is surprising to learn that of the 243 mothers from whom reports were obtained and who did not go away for confinement or did not receive free confinement care, 59, or nearly one-fourth, paid $50 or more, and 15 paid $100 and over.

The figures for the total immediate costs are much lower than they would have been if in many cases some free service had not been given; for example, free attendance at birth, free nursing service, or free help with housework.

Aggregate cost of childbirth to mothers who left the area for confinement.

It was possible in 19 instances in which the mothers went away for confinement to secure statements or estimates of the aggregate costs, including railroad fare, board, cost of household help on the homestead while the mother was away, etc. In all but 4 of these the aggregate cost was $150 or over, and in 2 instances $700 or more. No attempt has been made to tabulate these estimates in detail because the items they include vary greatly with the individual families. Some mothers who went away for the purpose of getting better care than they could have had at home combined a visit to a relation with their journey to secure good confinement care. These mothers usually paid greater railroad fares than those who went to the nearest city; but, on the other hand, they often paid nothing for board. Some families had to pay transportation to the railroad; others used their own vehicles and made no money outlay for the trip. The length of time the mothers stayed away from home and the illnesses and complications of confinement were among the factors which made it impossible to give with accuracy the aggregate cost.

It is thought, however, that the following typical statements will show the great expense to which many of the parents were subjected. Each statement gives the items covered by the aggregate:

Aggregate cost at least $240. Of this, the "total immediate costs"—i. e., for attendant's fees, nursing, and housework—were $105. Besides this, the aggregate includes $35 for rent and $100 for housekeeping expenses for four of the five months the mother was away. The first four months were spent in the nearest city; during the fifth, the mother visited relations in Wisconsin. The aggregate does not include the cost of transportation to and from the nearest city nor, of course, the railroad fare to and from Wisconsin.

Aggregate cost $180. Of this, the total immediate costs were $100, and $80 covered the stage fare to and from the nearest city and board while in the city. The mother went to the city five days before confinement and stayed two weeks after. She then left for a near-by town, where she visited her parents for four weeks.

Aggregate cost $225. Of this, $60 covered railroad fare and board. The mother spent 11 days in a hospital, and then visited her parents, but paid board while with them. She was away from home for two and one-half months.

MOTHER'S WORK IN RELATION TO CHILDBEARING.

That healthy childbearing mothers during their entire pregnancy should keep fully occupied with work which affords them varied exercise, but which does not unduly tax their strength, is now the consensus of opinion among leading obstetricians. Ordinary housework and many of the chores on a farm afford mothers the opportunity for the necessary exercise; but some household tasks and many farm occupations demand heavy lifting or cramped posture or other excessive muscular exertion and entail hazards to the pregnant woman. This is at present too little realized by the women themselves, their husbands, and by the community as a whole.

In the area studied all the mothers but 2—of whom 1 was insane and the other a chronic invalid—did housework, and all except 11 reported washing as part of their usual work during pregnancy or after childbirth or both. In addition to their regular housework, more than half the mothers cooked or did other work for hired help. These services were, as a rule, of brief duration, but so arduous while they lasted that they deserve special mention. Nearly all the women—92 per cent—reported some chores, such as milking, churning, gardening, care of chickens, care of stock, carrying water, etc.; 76 women reported both chores and field work.

Perhaps no other occupation is so difficult to measure, either in regard to the effort it consumes or to its effect upon women as housework. The number of persons in a household; how many of them help the mother with her work; how many demand care; what hired help a mother can employ; the size and construction of the house; the conveniences and labor-saving devices; the location of the water supply; whether separating, churning, and butter making are among her undertakings—these are a few of the numberless factors in household labor. Indeed, even the weather and the season of the year affect women's work, especially in the country and in such an area as the one studied, where high winds and dust storms are to be reckoned with; and where in certain months extra tasks, such as cooking for a round-up, for a lambing crew, or for harvest hands are added to a mother's regular housework.

Again, especially among the older settlers, the "custom of the country" of hospitality to passers-by, whether friends or strangers, is a very considerable tax on a housewife's strength. One mother whose husband is fairly prosperous said that the first Sunday after she moved onto the homestead, before she was settled, 30 persons, all strangers to her, " dropped in for dinner." Now, she said, guests do not come as often as they did, for a road house has been opened near by; yet, she often has from 10 to 15 extra persons at meals. Another mother, who is also an " old settler," says that people frequently stop for meals and lodging. She sometimes has 12 or 14 to dinner. Nevertheless, though such large numbers of guests, or even smaller numbers, add materially to women's work, very few of the women in this western country would be willing to save labor by limiting their hospitality.

The regular housework as it is done by most of the mothers is in itself not very extensive. The houses are small, most of them one or two room cabins or shacks, with a minimum of furniture. When of sod, unless they are plastered inside, they are hard to keep clean, because the sod gets very dry and dust keeps dropping into the room. To minimize the dirt this creates many women line their walls and ceiling with cloth, gunny sacking, or newspapers. One woman said that for a while she had sprinkled the walls with water, but that she was obliged to discontinue this practice because the water had to be hauled a mile in summer and was too scarce and precious to be used in this way. This house was neatly lined with newspapers. The advantages, so far as work is concerned, which the mothers have in a small house and simple furnishings are offset by the difficulties which crowding entails, by the scarcity of water, and by the lack of conveniences or labor-saving devices.[1]

HELP WITH HOUSEWORK.

Only 10 mothers regularly employed hired household help. Nearly all did their housework alone, or with the assistance of their husbands or other members of the family. One hundred and fifty-three, or less than half the mothers who were confined at home, had hired help with housework at the time of confinement. In 75 instances members of the household did the usual work of the mothers, and of these, 45 fathers did what housework was done until their wives resumed the household tasks. In 48 instances a relation, neighbor, or friend stayed with the mother or came in daily to do all the work, and in 46 other instances neighbors came in to assist the father or other members of the household with the work.

Sometimes several persons helped a mother with her work at the confinement period. In one case a woman came when the baby was 6 hours old and stayed 28 hours, doing the housework and taking care of the mother and baby. When this neighbor left, a young girl

---

[1] See discussion of Housing and Sanitation, p. 61.

of 15 came and stayed one week, and she returned later for one day to do the washing. All this service was given free.

Even the women who were paid for their services performed them chiefly as an accommodation. In almost every case, the woman recorded as "hired help" also gave what nursing care the mothers received; or, to put it the other way around, the women who were hired for nursing care also did the housework, and in a large number of cases the same persons also gave the confinement care. For the most part, they stayed with the mother only a very short time, about half remaining less than two weeks. In about two-thirds of the instances their work was supplemented by a neighbor or a member of the family.

Even the well-to-do families and those who are very eager to hire some one to help with their work find it practically impossible to secure a servant, either at the time of confinement or at other times. One woman who was ill two months after childbirth had to get up out of bed to cook for 13 thrashers, who stayed four days. Most of the women in the area are homesteaders with households of their own to look after, and they would not have the time or inclination to supplement their income by domestic service for other families. In an emergency they will almost always "help out," occasionally accepting pay. This is usually in the form of a gift and not necessarily commensurate with their services. More often, however, they prefer a return service which is also given "as an accommodation."

CONVENIENCES AND LABOR-SAVING DEVICES.

Except for sewing machines, which were found in 322 households, or 7 in 10, there was a great dearth of conveniences. Even the families who are fairly well to do have very few labor-saving devices. One mother who lived on an exceptionally good ranch explained that, though she could afford some of the conveniences themselves, the prohibitive cost of their transportation from the railroad placed them beyond her reach. Another family tried to buy a high chair for the baby, but found that the carriage would cost more than the chair itself. Considering the transportation difficulties and that the great majority of the families were pioneering and by no means prosperous, it is noteworthy that 168, or over one-third the mothers, owned washing machines.

Two families were supplied with running water, which in one instance was piped into the house from a flowing spring, and in the other pumped in by a windmill, but no other family had running water, though 22 had windmills.[1] On 23 homesteads there were engines, but on 5 they were used only for farm purposes and not as a

---

[1] See discussion of Water Supply, p. 67.

help in the housework. Eighteen mothers, however, had the advantage of engines, usually applied to the washing machine or used to pump water for household use. Two hunderd and forty-three, or over half the families, had no pump, but were obliged to dip water from a spring or river or draw it from a well, often without the aid of a windlass or pulley.

Only a few women had sinks, all but 9 out of 463 having to carry their waste water out of the house. This is laborious at any time, but especially so on wash days.

Only one family had a furnace, all the rest depending for their heat upon stoves, which in most instances were used both for cooking and househeating. In 69, or a little over one-seventh of the families, gasoline or oil stoves gave comfort to mothers, especially during the hot summers when the heat from ordinary stoves aggravates the burden of housework. Many mothers took the heat as a matter of course and considered an oil or gasoline stove as an unnecessary or too expensive innovation. One woman said, " Oil costs money, but we can get coal for nothing." When a homesteader can dig coal from the side of a butte and can pull sagebrush, which makes a quick, hot fire and which is a grievous incumbrance to him so long as it grows on his land, it is not surprising that he does not buy a gasoline or oil stove.

Lighting, like heating, is still in a crude state. All the families depend entirely upon the kerosene lamp, except 15 who had gasoline lamps. There is no electric or gas lighting in the area.

Twenty-three mothers had bread mixers, four had fireless cookers, and one had a vacuum cleaner. No mother reported the iceless refrigerator—a very easily made and great convenience.

Various methods of keeping food cool were practiced. The dugout, cave, cellar, or " root house " were the most common, 8 out of 10 of the families reporting these. Often they are nothing more than holes in the ground or in the side of a butte, but sometimes they are fairly large. Sometimes a family living in a dugout will merely dig back a little farther into the hill and thus make their cellar or storeroom. Very often the cave or " root house " is some little distance from the house, and to take supplies to and from it adds appreciably to a mother's work. A cellar under the house is less common. None of the refrigerating devices is very cold, nor is any one of them an adequate substitute for ice. The fact that one mother kept her baby in the " root house " on hot summer days, because it was the only cool place she could find, may suggest the temperature of these cellars. Thirty-eight women kept their supplies in the well or spring, 11 had ice boxes, and 10 had ice houses. One father gets ice from the creek in winter and stores it in a dugout. In summer the family takes it out as it is needed and stores it in a box in the cellar which is used as a refrigerator. A few other devices were reported, while 35 women had no means of keeping their food cool.

CHORES AND FIELD WORK.

Four hundred and twenty-eight of the 463 mothers, or 92 per cent, reported chores as part of their usual work. Over two-thirds cared for a garden, and four-fifths raised chickens. Over one-fourth milked and two-thirds churned butter—usually for home use only, but occasionally for sale—and about one-eighth reported separating as part of their work. Nearly one-fifth cared for the stock; that is, fed and watered them.[1] Half the women carried water.

Carrying water is one of the most arduous of farm duties, especially in an area like the one studied where the water supply is often far from the house. However, when the supply is very far away the father usually hauls it by team in barrels, and the mother need carry it only from the barrel, which is usually kept near the house, into the kitchen. When the father happens to be away, however, if water is needed, the mother must attend to the hauling herself. One mother, who at the time of the investigation was in her fifth month of pregnancy, hauled practically all the water used for household purposes and for six horses, her husband being away a great deal of the time. She would hitch up, drive the wagon one-half a mile to the well, pump the water, and fill the barrels by the bucketful. The strain of lifting the heavy buckets to the top of the barrels certainly entails risk to the pregnant mother. The difficulty, whenever water is needed, of getting it from the barrels in the wagon can be imagined.

Of the 233 mothers who reported carrying water as a usual task, only 34 had the advantage of the barrels already hauled from the well or spring. In one instance the barrel was kept in the house. Of the other 199, only 26 had the source of supply within 25 feet from the house, and only 35 more had it within 50 feet. All the rest had to carry the water over 50 feet; and 96, or nearly half, had to carry it over 100 feet. Twenty-one mothers had to go a quarter of a mile or more, and in one instance over 2 miles for water.

Heavy lifting was frequently reported by mothers as the cause of a miscarriage or a stillbirth. One mother who lost a baby that was stillborn at seven months believes that the cause of this was the carrying of heavy pails of water from the well, which was half a mile from the house.

The use of melted snow or ice in winter saves[2] much hauling of water, but obviates only part of the labor of water carrying. One

---

[1] " Riding after cattle " on the range is classified with field work.
[2] See discussion of Water Supply, p. 67.

mother, whose husband was away much of the time, cut a large piece of snow and in lifting it in a pan to the stove strained herself and the next day had a miscarriage. This occured in the fourth month of pregnancy.

In addition to certain chores, 76 mothers, or about one-sixth, had also as part of their usual tasks field work, such as planting or helping with the planting of various crops, cutting and stacking hay, digging potatoes, plowing, harrowing, or riding after cattle. When the fathers are away—and many of them having supplementary occupations are away a great deal—the mother must bear the brunt of all the work on the homestead.

Of course, the harmfulness of any of these occupations—whether chores or field work—to a mother who is pregnant or who has a young baby depends upon the extent to which she does them and upon her strength. The facts that the great majority of the mothers had lived on a farm for at least 10 years before their marriage and that nearly half had done farm work in their girlhood are other factors which enter into the personal equation. Some mothers do very hard work and yet suffer no ill results. Others, as has been shown, after telling of some complication of pregnancy or of some serious condition after confinement, attribute the trouble to hard work during pregnancy.

CESSATION OF WORK BEFORE CHILDBIRTH.

The great majority (68 per cent) of the mothers continued up to the very day of confinement all their housework except washing, and over one-half continued even their washing. Practically the same proportion (one-half) continued their chores; 14 mothers did not cease even their field work before the day of confinement, and 24 performed some services for hired help. These figures would be even higher if cessation within one week of confinement were considered, but they are striking enough as it is. Moreover, the figures do not present a complete picture of the mother's work, because some mothers continued not one task, but several classes of tasks, up to the day of childbirth.

One mother, for instance, who, besides her housework, reported as her usual tasks milking, churning, care of chickens, gardening, and carrying water from a well over 300 feet from the house, continued all her work up to the day before confinement; and did a large washing on that day. Later in the day she walked 2 miles to a neighbor's, where labor suddenly began—all this in spite of the fact that she had not been well during pregnancy and that the membranes had ruptured five days before parturition. The father was away, "freighting," at the time of confinement, and consequently he could not relieve the mother of her work; moreover, she had the added responsibility of things which must be done on a farm whether or not a man is there to do them. The mother remained at the neighbor's for confinement and for six days following. The day she reached home her husband, who had returned, did her work for her; but beginning the next day—that is, a week after confinement—she resumed her chores, housework, and washing, in addition to the added care of the new baby, who was not very strong. When the baby was 4 months old the mother had to cook for three harvesters for one week, and a month later for six thrashers for one day.

Another mother, in addition to her washing, other housework, and chores, cooked three meals a day for six hired men for three days preceding confinement, including the day the baby was born. She felt very ill, but was so eager to have the men finish their work before the cold weather came that she did not let anyone know how she was feeling. Labor came on suddenly on the evening of the third day and, though she had intended to have a physician attend her and was much frightened at not having medical care, the child was born so soon after the pains began that there was no time to send for a physician, and her husband delivered her. She resumed her housework and washing a week after childbirth and her chores two weeks after. This same mother, in her seventh month of pregnancy, cooked for 18 thrashers for one day.

Another mother, who had six children, of whom the oldest was 12 and the youngest 3, and whose husband during the last three months of her pregnancy was over 5 miles away herding sheep, rode to see him once a week. She made this long trip on horseback two days before the baby was born. The next day she did a large washing, though she had no washing machine or wringer, and on the morning of the day on which her baby was born she moved a heavy piece of furniture down into the cellar. Besides her housework, this mother had continued up to the day of confinement all her chores. These included caring for the garden and chickens, milking, looking after the stock, and carrying water from the well, which was 60 feet deep and a quarter of a mile away. The only aid she had during her pregnancy was from her two older children—a boy of 12 and a girl of 11.

Her new baby was born prematurely and was very small. A neighbor came and did the housework for four days after the baby was born. The mother stayed in bed only five days, and at the end of the week she was doing all her housework except washing and at the end of two weeks had resumed her washing and chores.

RESUMPTION OF WORK AFTER CHILDBIRTH.

The instances cited in the discussion of cessation of work before childbirth include statements of the time after parturition when the mothers resumed their work. These instances are by no means exceptional. Although nearly two-thirds of the mothers stayed in bed 10 days or more, 57 got up on the seventh day or sooner. Nearly one-fourth of the women were doing all their housework, except washing, before two weeks had elapsed. Forty-eight, or over one-tenth, had also done washing within this time, and 62, even a larger proportion, had resumed their chores. Before four weeks had passed nearly two-thirds of the women were doing all their housework except washing, and nearly half were doing their washing and their chores.

Seven of the mothers did field work within four weeks after childbirth and 29 had to prepare meals for hired help. The time of the year at which childbirth occurs would, of course, affect the numbers reporting either field work or services for hired help.

These figures are especially impressive when one considers that the pelvic organs do not resume their normal condition until about six weeks after parturition. Obstetricians usually prescribe 9 or 10 days in bed and complete rest for two weeks and consider that heavy work within a month after confinement imperils a woman's future health.

Mothers frequently complained of the results of hard work after confinement. One mother reported a fallen womb as a result of hard work after childbirth. Another said that three weeks after confinement she milked the cows, and instead of opening a difficult gate which she thought was too heavy for her, she lifted the full milk pails over the fence and " tore and hurt herself internally." She has not been well since that time. During the pregnancy which began about two years later she felt very miserable, and after her second child was born she did not resume her washing or her chores for six months, though she did all her housework except washing two weeks after childbirth.

Another mother, whose duties included washing and cooking for several farm hands, complaining that she " hurt her back " from hard work after confinement, remarked, " The men expect work done up just as well at that time as at any other."

It must be borne in mind, in studying a mother's work after childbirth, that the added task of caring for a newborn infant is in itself a considerable labor.

HOUSING AND SANITATION.

HOUSE CROWDING.

In this country of tremendous distances and sparse population it would seem that everybody might have those health requisites so often urged by public-health experts—plenty of room and fresh air. Yet small and crowded houses are the rule rather than the exception in the area studied; and this despite the fact that the majority of the people have high standards in regard to housing and sanitation. The scarcity of lumber and the difficulty of getting building materials, the dearth of masons and carpenters, the great distances from railroads and markets, the high cost of transportation, the lack of ready money, and the pioneer attitude that to "do without" things is a part of the homesteader's lot—these factors combine to explain the small house and the inevitable crowding.

Seven out of 10 of the homes consisted of one or two rooms, 148 having only one room, and 178 having two rooms. Wherever a tent, dugout, sleeping porch, or an outbuilding, such as a granary, bunk house, or supplementary shack was used by the family for sleeping or general living purposes, it was counted as a room and added to the number of rooms in the main dwelling. Two hundred and sixty-two families, or 57 per cent, were living, at the time of the mother's confinement, two or more persons in a room.[1]

The full force of these figures is not appreciated until they are compared with conditions elsewhere. In the bureau's infant mortality investigation in Waterbury, Conn., a crowded industrial city with a large immigrant population, a special study was made of certain districts, selected because they were typical of the worst housing conditions in the city. That study revealed that in 32 per cent of the 742 households for which reports were secured the rate of crowding was two or more persons per room.[2] The rate for the area studied in Montana, where houses are frequently over a mile apart, was nearly twice as great as that found in the congested immigrant quarters of Waterbury. To be sure, the fact that in good weather the children

---

[1] In this discussion, except in the illustrative stories, the figures for the number of persons always exclude the " schedule " baby, partly because in some instances the babies died and partly because the period studied covered the mother's pregnancy as well as the baby's first year of life.

[2] Hunter, Estelle B. : Infant Mortality : Results of a Field Study in Waterbury, Conn.. based on births in one year. U. S. Children's Bureau Publication No. 28, Infant Mortality Series No. 7. Washington, 1918.

have all outdoors to play in, and that, except for the mothers, the members of the family spend much of their time out of doors, counteracts to some extent the evils of crowding.

The sleeping room congestion is even greater than the general house congestion. Nine out of 10 of the families slept 2 or more persons in a room; in slightly more than half the houses 3 or more persons slept in one room, and in 3 families out of every 10 the rate was 4 or more persons per sleeping room. In 27 instances there were 7 or more persons per sleeping room.

The number of persons per room or per sleeping room is only a rough index to housing congestion and offers no information about the adequacy of the cubic air space per person. Unfortunately this can not be given, since no attempt was made to measure the dwellings. The following few examples of overcrowded homes will doubtless give the reader a better idea of the house congestion than the figures convey (other examples will be found in the further discussion in this section):

A family of nine persons lived in two rooms. The main dwelling was a one-room frame house covered with sod. Three of the children slept in a dugout about 25 yards away.

Another family of seven persons lived in a one-room frame shack 12 by 14 feet. The two beds, a cookstove, and two chairs practically filled the room. The mother said that it was very hard to keep the house clean because it was so small.

In another family seven persons lived in a tiny frame house. A bed, a small table, a stove, and a few chairs entirely filled the main room, in which the whole family slept.

In another instance eight persons lived in a one-room house which was a combination of a tar-paper shack and a dugout. The room is very large. At the back were four beds; in the middle, a small cook stove. A table, some chairs and boxes used as chairs, and a shelf of dishes made up the chief furnishings of the room. 'There is only one window and so the back of the room is very dark. The outside of the house is picturesque, with a row of ears of red corn hanging across the front and some bright flowers in cans.

Another family, consisting of five persons at the time the baby was born, lived in a small one-room tar-paper shack. They have now moved to a " fairly large " frame house, which consists of two rooms and a pantry.

A very common arrangement in one-room houses and in larger houses where one room has to be used for many purposes or shared by many persons is a curtain hung on a wire across the middle of the room. Such a curtain can be pushed aside in the daytime and at night so drawn as to divide a room into two parts. This is a helpful arrangement, but of course does not relieve the crowding. The

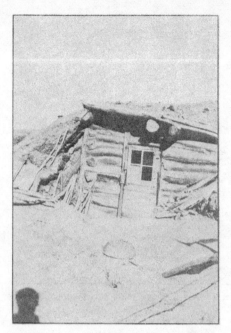

DUGOUT WITH LOG FAÇADE. NO OPENING
TO OUTSIDE LIGHT EXCEPT THE DOOR.

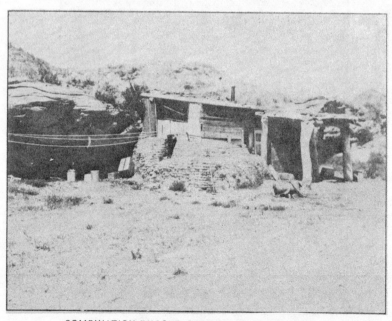

COMBINATION DUGOUT, FRAME, AND SOD HOUSE.

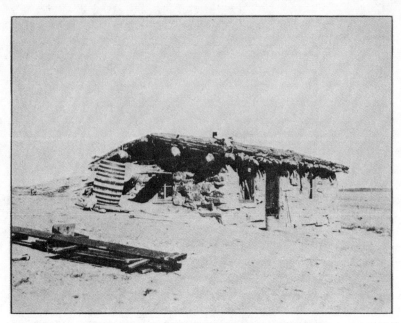

STONE HOUSE. NOTE BUFFALO SKULL ON ROOF.

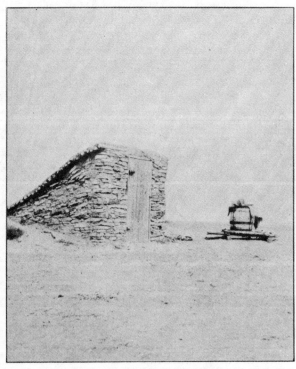

UNUSUALLY WELL-BUILT "ROOT HOUSE"; ALSO WATER
BARREL.

extent to which the overcrowding in the small houses adds to the difficulties and discomforts of confinement may be imagined.

CONSTRUCTION OF HOUSES.

The houses varied in type of construction and kind of building material much more than they varied in size. In the breaks nearly everyone lived in a log house. Elsewhere, the prevailing types were divided about evenly among the dugout, the tar-paper shack (a light frame structure covered with tar paper to keep the wind out), the sod house (made by cutting oblong chunks of sod and piling them on top of one another to form the walls), and the gumbo houses (made of the fine gumbo clay so common in the area and much like the adobe houses found farther south).

There were some houses made of stone, which in some instances had been quarried from the buttes on the homestead; and a few frame houses of the type common to the farms of the Middle West—plastered and ceiled inside and probably more comfortable than the other types, though not nearly so attractive in appearance. Often a house would combine several styles—would be part dugout, part sod, and part log; or a combination of stone and dugout; or part sod and part tar-paper shack.

Dugouts.

The dugouts, which are scarcely more than holes or caves in the sides of the hills, always have to be finished with some supplementary material, such as sod, log, or stone. Sometimes a home begins its existence as a sod, frame, or log house on the side or at the foot of a hill. Later, when the occupants wish to enlarge it, they dig back into the hill to make another room, and the house then becomes part dugout. In the main, the dugouts represent the crudest type of home, and the occupants usually regard them as temporary expedients to be given over for farm purposes or to be used only as supplementary rooms when better dwellings can be constructed.

A typical dugout, occupied by four persons is a small one-room home, almost inaccessible from the main road. To reach it, one must descend a steep, rough embankment and then climb another, equally steep and rough. However, steps have been cut into the hillside, and lead three-fourths of the way up the hill to the door. Only the front of the house protrudes from the hill. Two windows, each about 2 feet square, furnish all the light and ventilation for the home. A small bed, a stove, one chair, and several boxes constitute the furnishings and practically fill the little room.

Another dugout consists of two rooms, with a log front, on the side of a hill. Back of the kitchen a hole which serves as a cellar has been dug and provided with a ventilating flue. A family of eight occupies the house. It is unscreened, and the chickens take advantage of their free access to the dwelling. Across one window, a chair has been placed to keep the pig from falling off the hillside into the room.

Another one-room home is a frame shac κ half buried in the side of a hill. The front of the house, which protrudes from the hill, is poorly constructed, and great cracks let in the wind. The meagerly furnished room offers only boxes for seats, and the narrow bed, which apparently serves the four persons who live there, has scant covering.

Sod and gumbo houses.

The sod and gumbo houses are often much more comfortable and much more attractive than would be imagined by persons unused to them. As a rule the walls are thick and keep the houses cool in summer and warm in winter. Sometimes the interiors are plastered. A common and attractive plaster used for the interiors of gumbo houses is a mixture of lime, gumbo, and sand, which makes a fairly smooth sand-colored surface. The walls of some gumbo houses have been decorated by a sprinkling of laundry bluing, which gives a surprisingly effective "all-over" design.

A neat one-room house is built of gumbo mixed with straw, giving it a finish like that of a tinted concrete house. The walls are 18 inches thick. The roof of sod is reinforced with heavy timbers. Cross ventilation is secured by two windows, 2 feet square, in opposite walls. Both windows and the door are carefully screened. A family of five persons lives in this one-room dwelling.

Another sod house has two rooms in which nine persons dwell. It is built somewhat on the principle of the dugout; that is, though it stands on comparatively level ground, one has to descend four steps to enter the two rooms. The walls are decorated with an odd blue stencil. The house, though crowded with children and furniture, was clean and cool.

An exceptionally good two-room sod house has a very attractive exterior. The red, slanting roof and the bright-red broken shale piled up against the base of the house contrast pleasantly with the gray of the sod. The three short windows placed side by side, giving the effect of one broad, low window, carry out the horizontal lines of the house. Inside, the walls are a warm gray plaster. The main room is large. The floor is covered with linoleum, with rag rugs here and there. Under the broad windows on one side of the room is a long, low box used as a window seat; and on either side of this are bookcases full of well-worn books. There is no crowding in this house, for it is occupied by only three persons—a mother, father, and baby.

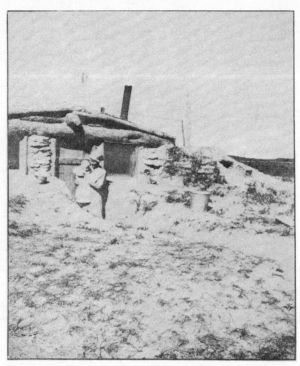

THE FATHER OF THIS BABY HAS TAKEN THE PRECAUTION
OF FENCING THE ROOF OF THE DUGOUT AGAINST
CATTLE.

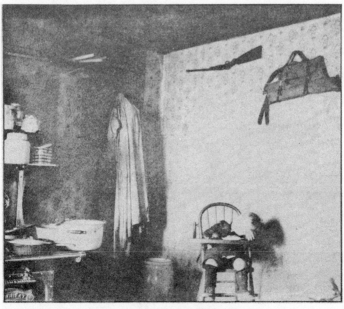

INSIDE A ONE-ROOM FRAME HOUSE.

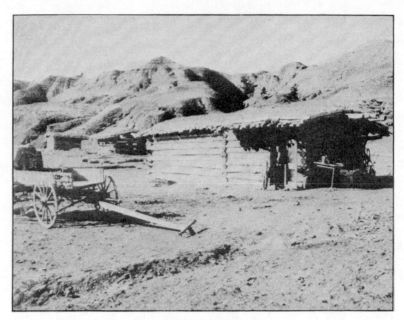

LOG HOUSE IN HELL CREEK.

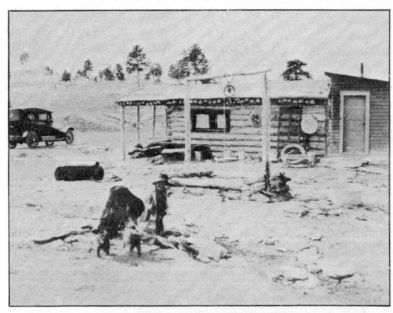

LOG AND FRAME HOUSE AND OPEN WELL.

Log houses.

In the breaks, where lumber can be found, most of the houses are made of logs. The breaks were settled before the other parts of the area, and most of the well-to-do ranchers lived there; it is, therefore, not surprising that some of the log houses are large and well furnished.

One ranch home, large in comparison with most of the homes in the area, has four well-furnished rooms, including a large kitchen and living room. Good porches, screened in, and a well-fenced yard add much to the comfort of the household of six persons.

Another home in the breaks is a broad, low, log house, nestling under a group of pine trees and facing a broad expanse of cleared land. The mother and father carefully selected the most effective location for the house. It has three large, comfortable rooms, well furnished and not crowded, though seven persons occupy them. There are plenty of broad, low, small-paned windows, with rows of plants on the window sills.

The majority of the homes—even in the breaks, where they are somewhat larger than those in the rest of the area—are small and crowded. One log house, in which live nine persons, consists of two rooms; the main sleeping room is the cellar under the house, though there is one bed in the upper room also. The interior walls of this house are painted white. The ceiling is papered with newspapers.

Log houses have certain structural disadvantages. They must be "chinked up" about twice a year with cement or mud. The logs contract and expand with the differences in moisture and temperature, so the chinking can not be permanent.

The interiors of the homes in the area represented many stages, from the crude and almost unfurnished to the plastered, ceiled, and well-furnished home. Many houses had no floors except the ground, and often a floor covered only one room or occasionally only part of a room.

FURNISHINGS.

Many families, either because of financial necessity or because of the difficulty of getting furniture from the railroad, were using various makeshifts and substitutes for regular furniture. The most common instances were boxes used for chairs. One family had no bed but used springs set on boxes. In another instance, where a family of seven lived in a one-room house, the mother and two children used a narrow bed and the rest of the family slept in a flax bin which occupied one side of the room.

Frequently very attractive homemade furniture was found. One family, for example, had a homemade cupboard, and a table so hinged that it folded up and served as the door for the cupboard; also a baby's high chair, ingeniously made chiefly of small boxes, which could be converted into a kitchen table.

Occasionally a family, realizing the need for recreation, purchases a phonograph, organ, or piano before ceiling or plastering the house or buying much needed furniture. Thus, a family of 11 lives in a one-room log house which is not plastered or papered. The room was not large, but it contained a wooden bed, an iron bed, a table, a range, a heating stove, a dresser, several open shelves, nine chairs, an empty box to be used as a chair, another box used as a soiled-clothes hamper, a board across some small wooden horses, a half dozen full gunny sacks, and a phonograph. The difficulty of house-keeping and caring for children in this house may be imagined. The home was not screened and chickens flew in and out at will.

SANITATION.

Flies.

Despite the difficulties imposed upon the housewife by the crowd-ing, the lack of a convenient water supply and of household con-veniences, the homes were on the whole clean. Two hundred and sixty-two homes, or well over half, were adequately screened against flies; that is, had screens in good repair at every door and window.

Unfortunately even adequate screening does not insure freedom from flies. Where there are children running into and out of the house, the screen door is only a slight protection. Moreover, when a house is poorly constructed, or in the case of log houses when the mud chinking falls out, flies enter through the cracks. Some houses, immaculately clean and well screened, were infested with flies. In the homes which were not screened the flies during the hot summer were a great and constant nuisance. The infrequency of sinks aggravates the fly problem, for many of the women throw the waste water out of their doors. Unscreened privies were doubtless pro-lific breeding places for flies. The unscreened homes have other intruders to contend with besides the flies. In warm weather, when windows and doors must be kept open, the chickens and pigs avail themselves of the housewife's unwilling hospitality and in spite of much shooing and chasing make themselves quite at home, especially on the sod floors.

Privies.

Although one or two well-to-do families were planning to install flushing toilets, at the time the survey was made the area had none— not even in the little villages. Slightly more than three-fourths of the families had privies. For the most part, these were deep-pit privies, closed in back, built of wood, and occasionally covered with

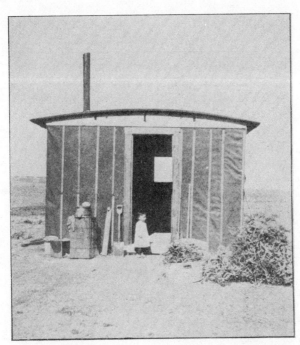

TAR-PAPER SHACK. NOTE PILE OF SAGEBRUSH.

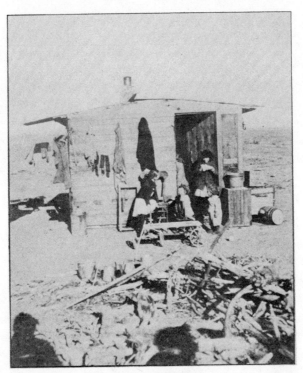

FRAME SHACK.

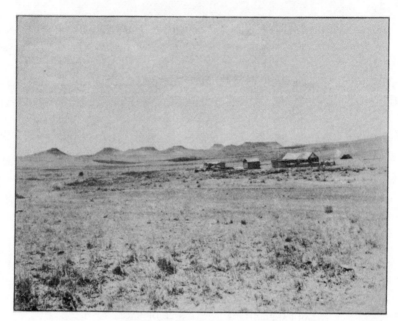

A RANCH AND A TYPICAL SKY LINE.

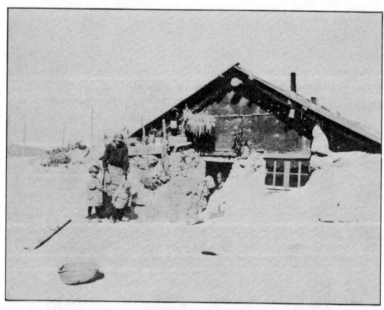

COMBINATION DUGOUT AND TAR-PAPER SHACK.

tar paper, very few being of the open-in-back type so common in southern rural areas. Often these wooden privies had no doors; in some instances a piece of burlap or sailcloth hung in the doorway provided privacy, but only a precarious protection against the weather. Some privies were found without tops, making them useless in rainy or snowy weather. Covers to the seats were often lacking—doubtless partly because of the high cost of wood.

Several privies were built of sod, and occasionally a dugout would be used as a privy. One, for instance, in the side of a hill, was part sod and part dugout. It was built mostly of sod, with a wooden roof, seat, and door. This was an insanitary arrangement, for animals could easily enter it. In most privies, however, the excreta were protected from chickens and larger farm animals, though very little effort was made to build the privies fly-tight.

One hundred and eight families, or nearly one-fourth, had no toilet of any kind. One family, for instance, had been homesteading for over three years and had not yet built one. The high cost of timber, which has frequently been commented upon in these pages, explains this lack in many cases. On the other hand, people often reported that they had had toilets, but that the high winds had blown them away.

Water supply.

Perhaps the most serious problem in sanitation is the water supply. Over the greater part of this dry country water is scarce and hard to get; and well drilling is expensive, costing $1.50 to $2 per foot, and no one knows how deep he will have to drill before he reaches water. One father drilled 200 feet for water at a cost of $300. Only 54 families had drilled or driven wells; the great majority (313) had dug wells; 62 had springs; and 32 depended on a river or creek. These figures represent the sources of water supply used during the greater part of the year.

Even dug wells are expensive and laborious to dig, and there is always much uncertainty of finding water. In one family the mother and father together dug eight wells on their homestead and yet found no water. They said that the water from a near-by creek was "bitter" and had caused the death of $900 worth of horses in two years. They haul their drinking water from a dug well 1 mile away; and the water for the stock and for household use from a similar well one-half mile away. Another family had dug two wells near the house, but both were washed in by cloud-bursts. The family has since dug a third well, 23 feet deep.

Some shallow wells which are dug in coulees depend for their supply upon day-to-day seepage; these can be used only part of the time. One family, for instance, dug such a well in a coulee a quarter of a mile from their house. For about five months of the year, in the winter and spring, they can not use it, because the coulee is then filled with snow or surface water. During this period they use creek water.

Many families use several water supplies for different purposes. Nearly all the water in the area contains much alkali or soda and some of the wells and creeks are so alkaline that they can not be used for drinking, cooking, or for the stock. One family used four separate sources—one for drinking water, one for water for washing, and two for the cattle only. Another family used a dug well for water for the stock, and because the well water had been "getting low" on account of the drought the family drinking water was carried from a relative's homestead, a quarter of a mile away. In another instance the drinking water was hauled 5 miles, and the other water 3 or 4 miles. The father said that half his time was spent hauling water and driving his horses to and from water.

In winter melted snow or ice was commonly used. Some families who lived near a river harvested as much ice as they could and melted and used it as long as it lasted in the spring. The mother in one family where this plan was followed assured the agent of the purity of the water, stating that "freezing destroyed all germs." In this same family, when the ice gave out, barrels were hauled to the top of the cliff overlooking the river, and water was dipped from the river in pails, which were carried up and emptied into the barrels. The barrels were then hauled home, a distance of $1\frac{1}{2}$ miles. This laborious method is the one usually followed by the families using river water.

The use of melted snow is common. One mother complained that in the preceding winter the snow was so deep over the spring that the family had to use snow water until the father could tunnel in to the spring. He was planning to pipe the water 300 feet nearer their house. It is now 500 feet away.

This report can make no definite statement about the pollution or purity of the water, because no samples were analyzed in connection with the survey. Although the State board of health maintains a laboratory to which people may send samples of water for analysis, there is no complete inspection of the water supply. The facts that there have been a few recent cases of typhoid fever in the area studied, that very few of the wells are protected from possible pollution, that many shallow wells are used—all lead one to think that some of the water is polluted. A few of the springs and dug wells were carefully cased, provided with pumps, and protected against dirt and surface drainage, but these were the exceptions. For the most part the wells and springs were open, sometimes accessible to the stock, and usually ready to receive the dust and dirt which the frequent high winds helped to distribute. The spring rains and the melting snows wash much surface soil into these unprotected wells. The use of buckets, whether lowered into the well by ropes or dipped in by hand, is a possible source of pollution.

To protect a dug well from pollution would seem to many families too expensive to be undertaken, partly because, since a well is in danger of drying up in summer, it does not seem worth while. There was much talk in the area of the taste of the water, but very little as to its purity.

Because the country is new and sparsely populated, few serious results have followed the lack of caution in regard to the water. Doubtless, when the area becomes more thickly settled, diseases which are attributed to impure water will become a menace to the health of the community, unless measures are taken to protect the water supply.

INFANT CARE AND THE WELFARE OF YOUNG CHILDREN.

INFANT MORTALITY.

In any discussion of the welfare of young children, the first question usually relates to infant mortality. Of the babies born in a given area how many live and how many die, and what have been the causes of the deaths? Unfortunately this question can be answered only in part, because in some cases where babies died no physician was in attendance, and the information about the causes of death is not specific. Moreover, the number of children covered by the inquiry is small and it is difficult to draw conclusions.

No attempt has been made to calculate an infant mortality rate for the period covered by the survey. This period—five years in duration—was so long that deaths which occurred four or five years prior to the time of the survey might easily have been missed.

Of the 198 live-born babies whose mothers were visited within a year after childbirth 14 died before the visit of the agent. Since none of these infants had had a chance to live a year it is probable that a few more failed to complete this period. The 14 deaths which had already occurred among the 198 infants give, therefore, a minimum infant mortality rate of 71 per 1,000.

This rate of 71, while lower than the rate for any city studied by the bureau, is much higher than the rate of 54 per 1,000 found for the rural areas studied in Wisconsin, and nearly twice as high as the rate of 40 per 1,000 found for the Kansas area.

Of the 14 babies who died all but 4 were less than 1 month old at death. There were no deaths of infants over 5 months old.[1]

Preventive medicine has shown that a large proportion of stillbirths and deaths in early infancy can be prevented by providing for the infant and its mother adequate care before, during, and after childbirth. The lack of such care has already been discussed. Some of the infant deaths in the area could probably have been prevented if the safeguards approved by modern science had been available.

---

[1] The average age of the group at the time of the survey was approximately 6 months. Probably all the deaths under 1 month in the group are included in the 14 that occurred before the agent's visit. For the months after the first, about as many deaths would have occurred after the visit of the agent and before the first birthday as already had occurred—that is, perhaps 4 deaths would have to be added to the 14 recorded to make up the complete toll of deaths in the first year of life, giving a rate of 91 per 1,000.

INFANT FEEDING.

The majority of the mothers showed great intelligence in feeding their infants. Practically all the babies received some breast feeding, all but 5 per cent being breast fed for the greater part of their first month. In the third month the proportion was still high— about 80 per cent exclusively breast fed—and in the sixth, 60 per cent. After the sixth month many mothers began to supplement breast feeding with artificial food of some kind. However, in the ninth month 22 per cent of the infants were exclusively breast fed, and only 21 per cent had been weaned before the middle of that month.

These findings are much the same as those of the Kansas survey. They are in marked contrast to some of the findings of the infant mortality investigations which the bureau has made in cities where infants were weaned at much earlier ages.

Pediatricians have long emphasized the importance of breast feeding. This survey, like the other rural surveys of maternity and infant care which the Children's Bureau has made, bears out their advice. In all these surveys the custom of breast feeding is more prevalent, and the period over which children are breast fed is longer than in the city surveys; and in spite of the many untoward conditions of prenatal, confinement, and postnatal care found in several of the rural areas studied, and notably in Montana, the infant mortality rates are in all of them lower than the rates for any of the cities studied. To be sure, many factors besides feeding affect the health of babies, but this almost invariable coincidence of a low death rate with a high percentage of breast feeding is significant.

As the Montana mothers were wise in nursing their babies, so also were they for the most part wise about withholding solid food during the children's early months. The definition of solid food as used in this connection includes such things as gravy, milk thickened with flour, cereals, or crackers, in addition to the foods which one usually considers solid. Only one baby in five had been given any such food by the end of the sixth month; at the end of the ninth month 38 per cent of the infants had not yet received any solid food.

Although the proportion of mothers who fed their babies wisely and carefully was high, there were many cases in which a child was improperly fed and in which the mother needed guidance. Thirty-two babies had been breast fed as late as their eighteenth month and nine as late as their twenty-fourth, the mothers not having realized that such late nursing was disadvantageous to the babies and to themselves. One infant, since his third week of life, when he was weaned, had been given "whatever he wanted" or whatever the family had. The mother, hearing that cereals were good for babies, had gathered some oats from her field and boiled them and fed them to him. The baby, at 10 months of age, was decidedly retarded in development and in poor physical condition. He had no teeth, was small and thin, with an unnaturally white skin, and eyes encircled with wrinkles. The mother of this child was very eager for suggestions about infant care.

Another mother, in addition to breast milk, began giving the baby tastes of food before she got up after confinement. She said she liked highly seasoned foods, and gave the baby a little of everything she ate, including wine, meat, and vegetables. Another mother, whose baby (weaned at 2 months) suffered from indigestion, did not consult a physician, but read some books which advertised prepared foods and tried to feed the baby according to these books; but the patent foods did not agree with the child. Finally the druggist suggested cows' milk and lime water, a food which at last the baby could digest. The mother commented that " one trouble with feeding a child patent food is that if the drug store runs out of it, you have to change the baby's diet, because in winter it is impossible to get supplies from the nearest city, 90 miles away."

Many mothers were eager for advice and had made great efforts, occasionally misdirected, to get information about child care. Several mothers, when visited by the Children's Bureau agents, were much worried about problems of infant feeding. One, for example, was pregnant and did not know whether or not to wean her baby. Another mother said she was afraid she " would never be able to raise her baby " because she had not had enough breast milk, and had had to wean him at 2 months. Since that time she has had much trouble finding food which the child could digest and had changed his food several times, according to the advice of the neighbors. She first used cream and water; then for a short while cows' milk; then some patent foods; and after the sixth month cows' milk again. The child was delicate until the seventh month, but a physician was never consulted.

Occasionally mothers received with surprise the advice to consult a physician about such a thing as feeding a baby. To some this seemed an extravagance, until it was made clear that good advice about the feeding and care of a child would probably keep it from getting sick and in the end be a saving of money as well as of suffering. Unquestionably public-health nurses, whom the mothers could consult about the care of their children as well as about many other health matters, would find a fertile field for their activities in the area studied and would be gratefully received by the mothers.

INSTRUCTION IN INFANT CARE.

Just as a considerable amount of reading about prenatal care was reported, so, too, many mothers (162) reported literature as a source of information about child care. Here, also, the types of reading matter ran the whole gamut from such standard works as those of Holt, and the publications of various Government and State bureaus, to quite worthless patent medicine advertising matter, and to works purporting to be of medical value to laymen but whose whole reason for existence seems to be to give employment to book agents.

One mother reported that she had followed exactly a bulletin from the Department of Agriculture on the feeding of babies. Another said that in order to rear her baby according to the advice given by a physician in a woman's magazine she had had to fight the prejudices of grandparents and neighbors, who urged the family diet for the child. Thirty-four mothers had received instruction about the care of their babies from physicians and 20 from trained or practical nurses. The majority of the mothers had had no instruction about infant care, though many of them realized their need of such information.

DIFFICULTIES OF GETTING MEDICAL CARE FOR CHILDREN.

The same limitations which make difficult the securing of medical care for mothers in confinement—weather, bad roads, lack of physicians and nurses, and expense—complicate the care of children in need of medical attention.

"Winter weather," said one mother, who lived 45 miles from a physician, "makes us prisoners. I can't tell you how I'm worrying about the winter, for if my baby should get sick I'd be helpless."

Many accounts of the difficulty of getting necessary care for sick children and of the lack of such care were given. One mother had to take a child who had appendicitis over 125 miles to the nearest hospital for an operation. The appendix ruptured on the way and the child nearly died, but fortunately recovered.

Nine of the 21 children who died were unattended at death by a physician. One 5-day-old baby became ill at a time when the Big Dry Creek had overflowed its banks and there was no way to cross it; therefore, no physician could be sent for. The baby was taken sick in the afternoon and died in the evening. In another instance the nearest physician, who lived 8 miles from the family, was away when its 18-day-old baby fell ill, and the next doctor, who lived 25 miles away, was sent for. He did not arrive until after the baby's death.

In another family, in which none of the children is robust, one child at the age of 1 year had a long series of convulsions for many days. No physician was secured for him. The nearest physician lived 25 miles away and across the river. This child recovered but is still not strong. In still another family, which lived about 40 miles from a physician, the mother and three children had scarlet fever and were for several days without medical attention of any kind. Fortunately they recovered.

The lack of medical facilities is especially serious in cases of accidents. There was one very distressing instance of this. A small child got a peanut shell in his windpipe. His parents at once took him to the nearest village, but the physician there could do nothing, and they hurried on to the county seat. There they were told that a specialist at another city, about two hours' ride away, could operate. When they reached that city they found that the physician did not have with him the necessary instruments, and the mother and baby started for an eastern city. The child became so much worse on the train that the conductor put the mother off at a small city. Physicians there operated and removed the peanut shell from the windpipe. The child died, nevertheless, a few hours later.

In another instance, a pin lodged in a child's throat, and the child had to be taken over 125 miles to have it removed; 18 hours elapsed before the family reached the physician who extracted it.

Another child fell from his sled and cut his nose badly. The nearest physician—45 miles away—was sent for. He did not arrive that day, and late the following afternoon the mother, on her way to summon him again, met him 15 miles from home. He came and attended to the wound. His charge was $45.

Sometimes, in cases of illness as well as of accident, a mother, to save time and expense, will take a sick child to a physician instead of sending for the physician and waiting anxiously for his arrival. One mother, for example, drove 7 miles one winter day with a very sick baby. The long, cold drive in the snow aggravated the child's illness, and he died after reaching the village where the physician lived.

Frequently, and especially in cases where there is no acute illness but a chronic condition, cost leads the family to neglect or postpone treatment. One mother, whose baby's feet were deformed, making it difficult for him to learn to walk, realized that something should be done, and said that if next year's crop was good, she would take the child to the nearest city for treatment. The distance—about 150 miles—was so great that the expense in addition to the doctor's bill would be very considerable. Another mother, whose child seemed to have a defective palate, said she realized that medical attention was needed, but that she could not afford it. In another family a

3-weeks-old baby had convulsions, but no doctor was sent for, partly because the family could not afford one and partly because when previous children suffered from the same symptoms physicians had said that nothing could be done.

Often families are most eager for medical attention for their children and can afford to pay a moderate price but do not know where to get any specialized care. There are no specialists within the area. One mother whose children had symptoms of adenoids did not know where she should take her children for treatment. Several families had taken their children to hospitals in near-by cities, and some to specialists in the East. A mother whose baby had stayed in a hospital for five weeks suffering from what the local physicians had diagnosed as " summer complaint " felt sure that the child would have died had she not been able to take him to a hospital.

Because medical care is so inaccessible and so expensive, and because there are no public-health nurses in the area to whom people can turn for advice, mothers are often driven to the use of home remedies or to the counsel of neighbors. These neighbors are often as uninformed about child care, first aid, and home nursing as the mothers themselves.

Occasionally the mothers take other means of securing advice. One father, while in a city, saw a physician, to whom he told his sick baby's symptoms and from whom he obtained some medicine. In another family an elaborate home treatment was applied to a child bitten by a rattlesnake. In addition to giving the antidote of whisky, the family applied the entrails of chickens and sheep to the wound. The child finally was laid inside the slaughtered sheep, that his entire limb might be in contact with it. Fortunately the child recovered.

BIRTH AND DEATH REGISTRATION.

At the end of the Children's Bureau inquiry the bureau sent to the child-welfare division of the State board of health the names of the live-born children covered by the inquiry, excluding those whose mothers went out of the area for confinement. By checking these names with the registered births the State board of health made a birth-registration test in order to learn how nearly the area studied approached the standard set for admission into the United States birth-registration area; namely, the registration of at least 90 per cent of its births.

Although Montana has practically the model birth-registration law, only 31 per cent, or less than one-third, of the live births checked for the five-year period covered by the inquiry were found to be registered. Moreover, nearly one-fifth of these births were registered after the mothers had been visited by the agents of the Children's Bureau, who pointed out to parents the need for registration and the disadvantages which a child might suffer for want of a birth certificate. Of the infants born in the year preceding the agents' visit 39 per cent were registered. The fact that a large percentage of births were not attended by a physician explains, to a certain extent, the lack of registration; not entirely, however, for of the physicians' cases 47 per cent, or nearly half, were not registered. These figures are presented not as an index to birth registration for the State as a whole—for doubtless many counties in the State have good registration—but as the findings of the test for the area studied.

A test of death registration, including maternal and infant deaths, showed that death registration was incomplete. Of 21 infant deaths, 12 were unregistered. Some of the maternal deaths also escaped registration. Several parents said that their children's deaths had not been registered and usually added the excuse that they had had no physician in attendance. In one instance, in a remote neighborhood in the breaks, a Children's Bureau agent, after having been told that there had been no death certificate for a child who had died, asked what was done when permission for burial was needed. The reply was: " Why, we can't wait for permission to bury our people when any of them die. It takes far too long. We had no certificate for my child and when Mrs. ———'s three children died a neighbor came and built coffins for them and we just took them up over the hill and buried them."

In connection with the incomplete birth and death registration it is significant that the State board of health, though it is provided by law with a bureau of vital statistics, has no special appropriation for the work of that bureau. One clerk does practically all the work of filing the birth and death certificates.

The importance of birth registration has never really gripped the attention of the United States, though it has been recognized in every other civilized country. Many parents have never heard of birth registration, and many others who do not know whether their own births are registered, and who may never have suffered as a result, are careless about providing birth certificates for their children. To some it seems the physician's business—possibly something which the law requires to prevent malpractice, perhaps merely " red tape." But many of the Montana parents who are now struggling hard to win their homesteads and to dig a livelihood from their thirsty half sections would be chagrined by the thought that a child of theirs might lose the opportunity of inheriting their hard-won acres because some one—physician, midwife, or the parent himself—had neglected to provide a birth certificate.

It is only recently, and only in certain parts of the country, that propaganda to interest every mother and father in registration of the birth of every infant has been spread. The value to the individual child is not the only stimulus which moves Federal, State, municipal, and private organizations to urge every physician to register births, and every parent to see that his child's birth is promptly registered. It is not only because a child will probably need a birth certificate to prove his legal right to inherit property, to vote, to go to work, or to be protected against premature employment, or for many other uses which could be itemized; there is a bigger and even more cogent reason for birth registration and for death registration. A count of the number of people in a country or community—of the number who are born and the number who die—is the only general measure now procurable by which we can gauge public health. Only by knowing how many babies are born and how many die in various communities and under varying social influences can we learn what conditions are favorable to infant life and what conditions are fatal to it.

Until every birth and every death is registered we have no means of measuring the infant health of a community and, therefore, are not able to improve it to the possible limit of improvement. For this reason every parent should regard it as a patriotic duty to see that the birth of his child is promptly registered.

CHILDREN'S HEALTH CONFERENCES.

The survey included a series of children's health conferences held in cooperation with the child-welfare division of the State board of health and with local committees in four different parts of the area studied. The purpose of these conferences was to demonstrate the value of a thorough physical examination of well children, and to offer to every mother an opportunity to consult with a Government physician about the individual needs of her child and about the many puzzling problems which arise in the bringing up of children.

The conferences were held for five days, and 129 children were examined, nearly all of them under 6 years of age. About one-third of these children had no defects, and of the defects found in the others many were slight, and such as could be obviated by a change in diet, or in some cases by a single visit to a dentist. On the whole, the conferences bore out the impression which all the agents making the survey had had—that these Montana babies were for the most part very sturdy and well.

The conferences were in no sense clinics, and neither treatment nor medicine was given by the physician in charge. When defects which needed the attention of a physician were discovered, parents were advised to take their children to the family doctor; or, when the defects discovered required the services of a specialist, counsel was given accordingly. The thorough and careful examinations by the physician frequently revealed a slight defect or inferiority in development which at the time was causing no distress to the child, but which might later prove a serious handicap and which by immediate treatment might be easily cured.

Several mothers who had been worried about their children, but who had not consulted a physician, were much relieved to learn that the condition of the children was not serious and could be easily and quickly remedied. One mother whose husband had died of tuberculosis was very anxious about a child who had been "ailing" and who she feared had inherited the father's disease. Her relief may be imagined when the examination revealed that the child had no symptoms of tuberculosis but had been unwisely fed and merely needed a better balanced diet. Another mother, who had thought that her child had kidney trouble, was greatly relieved to know that the trouble was much less serious.

After consultation, each mother received a written summary of the advice given her in regard to the child examined. The following few examples will illustrate the nature of these summaries:

This child is undersized and his distended abdomen indicates that he has poor digestion and that there is too much starch in his diet. His general nutrition is poor but can be improved by careful feeding. Give him only three meals a day with a cup of milk in the middle of the morning and the middle of the afternoon; let him have only stale toasted bread with his milk. Fruit juices and green vegetables would correct his constipation. Weigh him each month and keep a record of his weight to see that he gains.

This baby is very well, and normally developed. It is important to regulate his feeding so that he may remain well. Follow the advice given in Infant Care, pages 42 to 49. We shall send you another circular about feeding a baby of this age.

The foreskin should be pushed back gradually. It does not seem necessary to have the baby circumcised.

This child is in splendid condition except that his leg is paralyzed. The most important thing for this boy is to have his leg treated at once by a specialist. While the baby is young is the only time that anything can be done to improve the condition.

His tonsils are somewhat large and he seems to breathe a little through his mouth. When you have the leg attended to, it would be wise to have a physician examine his tonsils.

This child is above the average height and weight for his age and is in excellent condition. His tonsils are somewhat large but will not need attention unless he has sore throat frequently or begins to sleep with his mouth open.

Mary is a nervous child. She should have many hours of sleep every day and should live in the fresh air as much as possible. She is of normal height for her age, but is somewhat underweight. An effort should be made to have her gain in weight. Farmers' Bulletin No. 717 of the Department of Agriculture gives some useful information about food for children of this age.

Her eyes show a slight tendency to cross. If this continues, you should have an oculist prescribe treatment. Her teeth are slightly discolored and should be brushed daily. Good care of first teeth is very important.

The local committee, to whose activity the success of the conferences was largely due, helped with the arrangements, advertised the conferences, secured much local cooperation, and carried on much useful propaganda on behalf of the employment by the county of a public-health nurse. The committee for the first conference prepared a petition, copies of which were taken to the later conferences, and which were signed by nearly everyone who attended the conference, and by many other persons. It read as follows:

We, the undersigned, earnestly petition the board of county commissioners that they appoint a county nurse whose services shall be given to the western half of —— county, with —— as headquarters. The legislature of 1917, by the enactment of the child-welfare law, empowered you to make this appointment. Because of the war, physicians are being called to the service of their country and large sections of the county are left without medical attention, which will render the services of a nurse more necessary than before in giving health supervision to school children, in preventing sickness among mothers and children, and protecting the health of the community from infectious diseases.

An important part of each conference was an exhibit, in which were shown and explained many devices to lighten the mother's work in caring for her children. These included simple equipment which mothers should have to bathe the baby and to prepare his food; the proper outfits and clothing for infants, the right kind of bed, and an easily made basket bed for the small baby; effective and inexpensive methods of screening the baby; iceless refrigerators in which the baby's milk could be kept; and many other devices. Instructive posters on the care of children decorated the walls. Paper and scissors were provided for mothers who wished to cut out patterns of the model baby clothes while waiting their turn for the examination. These patterns and the life-size models of the clothes were among the most popular features of the conferences. In the afternoon demonstrations of the proper way to bathe and dress a baby were given to the school children by a nurse who used a doll. At the two conferences which were held in the largest village in the area there were afternoon and evening meetings, with illustrated lectures on the care of children, on the value of the public-health nurse, and on the Children's Bureau, and also discussion.

The fact that some families drove 25 miles each way in open wagons, and that many came over 15 miles, to have their children examined showed their general interest and enthusiasm, and gave promise that the physicians' advice would be heeded. One mother, who was seen about six weeks after the conference, said that since she had followed the doctor's advice and taken the baby off condensed milk and put her on cows' milk the child had gained a pound and one-half, whereas up to the time of the conference the baby had been losing weight. This mother said that she had written to all her relations whose babies were given condensed milk, telling them what the change to cows' milk had done for her child.

Another woman reported: " Our post office is like a different place now on mail days. The mothers who come in, and even the fathers, ask one another what they are feeding their babies and whether they took the doctor's advice."

That conversation on infant feeding should begin to compete with talk about the dry weather is excellent testimony to the value of such conferences. "Conferences like these should be held often," said one mother.

If such conferences could be held often, if a public-health nurse could follow up the cases in which medical care by a physician was needed, and help the mothers arrange for such care, if she could be available for advice at regular intervals, many of the health problems of bringing up children in this new country would be solved.

STATE AND COUNTY ACTIVITIES ON BEHALF OF MOTHERS AND YOUNG CHILDREN IN RURAL AREAS.

In any discussion of State activities it must be remembered that Montana is a young and largely rural State which was practically uninhabited until 1860 and was admitted to the Union only in 1889. These facts increase the credit for her many progressive legislative accomplishments, a few of which affect directly the well-being of mothers and babies in rural districts as well as in cities. Her active State board of health; the fact that Montana was among the first States to create a child-welfare division in the State board of health and to encourage rural public-health nursing by a law which permits counties and rural districts to employ public-health nurses; her model birth-registration law, even though it is not yet everywhere enforced—these are among the things to be mentioned.

Unfortunately, the legislature which realizes the importance of these measures fails to appropriate enough money to make them as effective and extensive as they should be to serve the best interests of the people in all parts of the State. Thus, though Montana has excellent birth and death registration laws and a law providing a bureau of vital statistics, it has appropriated no funds to be used especially for the study of the returns of birth and death registration, for the enforcement of the registration laws, or for propaganda for improved registration. The child-welfare division has carried on some propaganda on behalf of birth registration, but its duties are so many and its staff so small that its activities in this direction have necessarily been limited.

The law which created the child-welfare division and made it possible for counties and school boards to use public money to employ public-health nurses is such an important step toward the welfare of Montana children that it deserves to be quoted in full:[1]

An Act to Create a Child Welfare Division to be Under the Direct Supervision of the State Board of Health, Prescribing Its Duties and Powers and Providing for Its Maintenance.

Be It Enacted by the Legislative Assembly of the State of Montana:

SECTION 1. That a Child Welfare Division be, and the same is hereby created, which shall be under the direct supervision of the State Board of Health.

---

[1] Acts of 1917, ch. 121.

SECTION 2. The duties of this Division shall be to make and enforce regulations; to carry on a campaign of public health education and to take all possible steps for the better protection of the health of the children of the State.

SECTION 3. School Boards may employ in their discretion regularly qualified nurses, duly registered in the State of Montana, to act as school nurses. In sparsely settled communities, two or more School Boards may unite and employ a school nurse, the salary of such nurse being paid pro rata according to the assessed valuation in the school districts.

SECTION 4. County Commissioners are hereby authorized, at such time as they deem necessary, to employ regularly qualified nurses, to be known as County nurses, for duties under the Child Welfare Division.

SECTION 5. The Superintendent of Public Instruction and the Secretary of the State Board of Health, as soon as possible after the passage of this Act, shall meet and formulate rules and regulations governing the work of school, county and public health nurses, which rules and regulations, when regularly passed by the State Board of Health, shall invest the said State Board of Health with full power of supervision and regulation of said school and county and public health nurses.[1]

SECTION 6. The State Board of Health, through its Child Welfare Division, shall prepare and distribute to the school, county and public health nurses all necessary report blanks.

SECTION 7. The Secretary of the State Board of Health, subject to the approval of said Board, shall employ such officers as may be necessary to carry out the provisions of this Act.

SECTION. 8. Nothing in this Act shall be construed or operate so as to interfere in any way with the exercise of the child's or parent's religious belief, as to the examinations for, or in the treatment of, diseases; provided, that quarantine regulations relating to contagious or infectious diseases are not infringed upon.

SECTION 9. All acts and part of Acts in conflict herewith are hereby repealed.

Approved March 3, 1917.

This law makes one stride ahead of similar laws in other States which provide for public-health nurses. It centers in the State board of health " full power of supervision and regulation of said school and county public-health nurses," an excellent provision, making it possible to standardize the work of rural public-health nursing throughout the State. Even the nurses employed by philanthropic and industrial organizations are required by the rules to notify the State board of health of their appointments.

The law was passed in March, 1917. At the end of the survey two counties had already taken advantage of it and were employing nurses. In Silver Bow County, which contains the city of Butte, the work was practically " city work "; but in Teton County—a

_____
[1] See Appendix B for the rules and regulations. p. 97.

rural county with many of the same problems as the one surveyed—the nurse was doing rural work. More recently a nurse was employed in Musselshell County; and in Yellowstone County, the city of Billings and the rest of the county united to employ two public-health nurses and a full-time public-health officer.

The work in Teton County had been very recently begun, but at the time the Children's Bureau survey ended an excellent start had been made. The children of many of the rural schools had already been examined, and the nurse was hoping to visit all the schools inaccessible by railroad and examine the pupils before the winter weather set in. The county has an area of 6,566 square miles,[1] only a comparatively small part of which is within easy reach of the railroad and much of which is rough, mountainous country. The nurse used a small car for her work. She was planning, after completing her examination of school children, to broaden the scope of her usefulness to include instruction in home nursing, prenatal care, and many of the other usual activities of the public-health nurse.

Very recently the State (through the department of home economics at its agricultural college, at Bozeman), in cooperation with the States Relations Service of the United States Department of Agriculture, has employed eight home demonstration agents in various counties, and in one city, to bring to women the most recent findings of domestic science and home organization. Although the immediate purpose of this work is food conservation, it includes much instruction which should lighten the work of housekeeping. The agents have had to concentrate most of their work on the communities easily reached by railroads, and where women's clubs and other organizations already exist. Unfortunately a county such as the one surveyed by the Children's Bureau would be among the last to be served by these agents, since nearly all its area is inaccessible by railroad.

What is the county studied doing for the mothers and young children living in the area? Aside from the work on the roads,[2] which will make it easier than hitherto for some families to secure physicians, the answer is, nothing or nearly nothing.

Here, again, the factor of distance enters as a partial explanation. No part of the area studied was nearer than 65 miles from the county seat, and some parts were over 150 miles away. The people in the area go to the railroad points in other counties for their supplies, and do not even participate in their own county's fairs.

In this huge county, where means of communication are so lacking, the area studied—a region larger than the State of Connecticut—is

---

[1] County Clerk's Annual Report to the Board of County Commissioners, 1916, Teton County, Mont., p. 3.

[2] See discussion of Roads and Means of Communication, p. 17.

so isolated from its seat of government that the county health officer must delegate such duties as would fall to him in the area to local doctors, and the county agriculturist finds it impracticable to go into the area more than once or twice a year. Recently the size of the county has been given official recognition by the appointment of a deputy superintendent of schools, with headquarters in the western part of the county.

But size alone does not explain the official isolation of the western half of the county. In answer to questions about the various problems of the area—the road situation, the school situation, etc.—officials frequently mentioned that the western half, being so much more recently settled than the eastern half of the county, paid such a small proportion of the county taxes that the expenditure of these taxes in improvements was made accordingly. Of about $17,000,000 worth of taxable property, a little under $2,000,000 was located in the western half of the county. This statement surprises the casual observer, because, though the eastern half of the county is a little more thickly settled, and more plowed land and more improved farm dwellings are seen, nevertheless the country does not present any evidence of such vast difference in wealth or enterprise.

It is true that most of the homesteaders in the eastern half of the county have "proved up" and are therefore paying taxes on their land. The real explanation of the difference in assessed valuation, however, lies in the fact that one-half the land in the eastern half of the county is, or has been, railroad property, for some years ago every other section of land was granted by the United States Government to the railroad for an area extending 60 miles on each side of the track. Taxes are paid on all this land. The railroad runs through the southeastern corner of the county and the taxes paid by the railroad and on the land which still belongs or has ever belonged to the railroad are credited to the eastern half of the county. Therefore, the mere accident of the location of the railroad brings the homesteaders in the eastern half of the county greater advantages than are enjoyed by those in the western half. These advantages have expressed themselves so far chiefly in better educational opportunities, better roads, a greater proportion of the services of the county agriculturist, and practically all the services of the county health officer.

Even the eastern half of the county, however, has done very little for its mothers and babies. The county seat, a thriving city of about 4,000, is readily accessible to many, though not to the greater part of its families. In the county seat a small private hospital, with a capacity of 12 or 14, is available to those who can pay. Here, too, are several women who make a business of taking mothers in for confinement, either renting them rooms for "light housekeeping" while they await confinement or providing both board and room. In these cases the confinements are attended by local physicians. One physician stated that he had attended about 100 cases at one of these homes, but that many of the women were realizing that the cost was almost as great as at a hospital, where they could have more comforts.

The county hospital, which is on the outskirts of the county seat, does not take maternity cases except as a matter of poor relief. Only one case was attended there between January and November, 1917.

The county health officer is employed on a part-time basis. His duties of inspecting dairies, meat markets, restaurants, etc., at the county seat consume so much of his time that he can seldom go out to the other parts of the county, nor has he time to devote to public-health propaganda. He feels very strongly that a corps of county public-health nurses are needed.

SCHOOLS.

In the course of the inquiry into conditions surrounding mothers and young children there was, to be sure, frequent discussion of the family as a whole; and the question of schools was constantly brought up by the homesteaders, who urged the Children's Bureau agents not to ignore this important aspect of child welfare.

Although it was not the province of the Children's Bureau to make a study of the school facilities of the community, nevertheless the reiteration of the question, "Can't you help us to get schools for our children?" was so insistent that any discussion of this homesteading country would be wanting without at least a brief reference to the school situation. One learns from the report of the superintendent of public instruction that among the schools in a progressive State like Montana, "during the year ending August 31, 1916, there were eight schools in session one month and 175 schools in session for less than four months,"[1] and that there are thousands of children who are not provided with any kind of school.

Many neighborhoods in the area studied are confronted with serious school problems. Often parents reported that 18 or 20 children in their neighborhood had no school. In other cases the school term was very short. Even where the children had four or six months of school a year it was usually divided into two terms—one in the spring, and the other in the autumn, distances and bad weather making winter attendance impossible to many children. Nowhere was this the result of indifference or inertia.

The father of 11 children, 7 of whom ranged from 6 to 17 years of age and had no school within 6 miles, was working very hard to get one for his neighborhood. He and his neighbors were willing to give $200 toward it and to build and equip it themselves. In many instances (the county superintendent of schools states that she knows of 20 or 30 in the area) the people in a community had contributed the land, out of their private funds bought the lumber, and with their own labor built the schoolhouse. Even then they were frequently unable to secure equipment or to get a teacher for more than one or two months.

In one case where a group of neighbors supplied a school building for their 19 children, the school district furnished only four benches and desks. "After much complaint," said one mother, "we succeeded in getting a few more benches, but some of the children still have to sit on boxes or logs. For a while there was no black-

---

[1] Fourteenth Biennial Report of the Superintendent of Public Instruction, State of Montana, 1916, p. 15.

board, but the school supervisor finally took one from a school 6
miles south that had two blackboards."

A foreign-born woman, one of the oldest settlers, told of her efforts
to secure schooling for her children. In spite of much agitation, she
was unable to get any kind of school until the oldest girl was 12
years old. When it was finally established it was held in a deserted
cabin. Because she sent several children she was asked to attend to
the heating of the building in the winter. During the coldest weather
she decided to live in the schoolhouse from Mondays to Fridays, in
order to keep the children warm. This was so difficult (she had some
children under school age) that she finally offered, to be used as the
school, one room of her two-room shack, and she and her family
lived in the kitchen. At one time she and a neighbor drove 75 miles
in an open wagon to a school election, on their return bringing seats,
books, and other equipment for the school. Only recently has a satisfactory school been built at a reasonable distance—1½ miles from
her home.

In one neighborhood the agents of the Children's Bureau found
near the schoolhouse a half dozen shacks and dugouts to which families had come to live for the school term. There was also a sheep
wagon in which, the agents were told, five or six children had lived
the previous winter, the older children caring for the younger.

Some families who could afford it, or who had relatives living near a
school, had sent their older children away for the school term.
Naturally, however, many parents did not wish to let their children
go away from home, especially since it was often difficult to find a
satisfactory home for a child. Of course, the younger children were
seldom sent away.

Several families had moved away and others were planning to
leave the county because their children had no opportunity to get
an education. One family that had "proved up" had succeeded
with its farming venture; had raised prize corn; whose children belonged, by correspondence, to corn clubs; and which was altogether
an unusually intelligent and progressive family, moved away because the only school accessible to the children had a session of only
two months a year. The mother of another family said: "The hardest thing about living out here is that the children have no schooling.
My three—they're 7, 11, and 12—are the only ones of school age in
this school district, so there is no hope of getting a school very soon.
But they must have an education, even if we have to give up the
place." When the lack of educational opportunity drives such people
away the country suffers a serious loss.

These typical efforts and struggles to provide schools are convincing proof that the parents in the community appreciate their children's urgent need of an education. Why, then, are not schools pro-

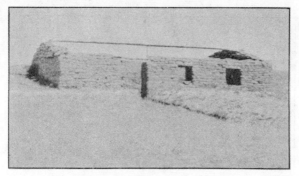

METHOD OF CONSTRUCTING A SOD BUILDING.

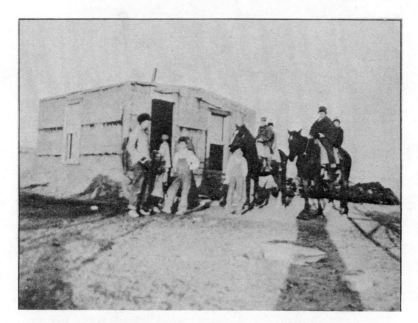

A SCHOOLHOUSE, AND CHILDREN ARRIVING.

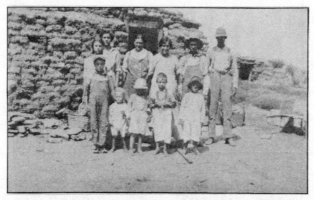

A GOOD ARGUMENT FOR A SCHOOL. THERE IS NONE
WITHIN REACH OF THIS FAMILY.

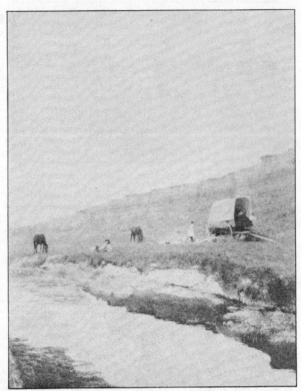

CAMPING FOR THE NIGHT ON THE BIG DRY. AN INCIDENT IN A 10-DAYS' TRIP, WITH A 4-WEEKS-OLD BABY.

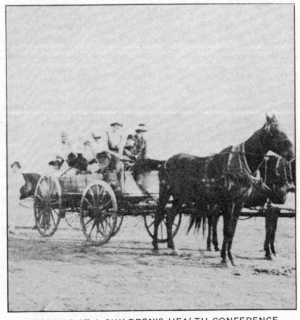

ARRIVING AT A CHILDREN'S HEALTH CONFERENCE.

vided by public money? One would anticipate the answer, insufficient public funds; and yet the answer is not altogether lack of public funds, for the superintendent of public instruction states that the county studied had at the end of the 1916 school year—August 31, 1916—a balance of $52,975.75, and that all this money could have been spent in providing schools, equipment, and teachers for children, and lengthening the school term. The answer, therefore, is to be found not in the lack of money for schools but in the distribution of the money. In a letter to the Children's Bureau, the Montana superintendent of public instruction remarks:

Rural-school problems in Montana are greatly complicated by the very unequal distribution of school funds. The general county levy of 4 mills and the State funds are distributed equally among all of the children of the county between the ages of 6 and 21. But the special levies which the school trustees themselves make, and which are the main source of revenue in many districts, are the cause of great inequalities in funds.

Many school districts have unsurveyed and unpatented lands, which, of course, are not subject to taxation. Many also possess only poor land assessed at a very low valuation. Others have most valuable lands, well improved, and possibly are fortunate enough to include within their boundaries 20 miles or more of railroad, a power plant, sawmills, a smelter and a mine or two.

It quite often happens that the district with the largest number of children possesses the lowest assessed valuation and that the school district valued at half a million dollars or more has within its boundaries not more than 6 or 8 children of school age. These conditions prevent Montana from ever giving equal opportunities in education to her children till her laws are amended.

In the county you studied all of the railroad in the county is to be found in the extreme eastern end. Schools there are well equipped and quite good salaries are paid. Educational opportunities of children are good. In the remainder of the county there is a constant struggle in many districts to provide even a short term of school and many communities are without school at all. Only a few extremely large districts in this section of the county have sufficient funds with which to maintain schools.

A larger unit of taxation with equal distribution to all children is badly needed. In a State where the wealth of counties varies so greatly, it seems the State would be the best unit of taxation for schools. However, the county would prove a far better unit than the small school district with very great inequalities of wealth and would greatly improve the educational opportunities of children in the State.

One is stirred with admiration for the intelligence and resourcefulness of the homesteader and at the same time confronted with the certainty that unless adequate provision for education is soon made the generation of children now growing up will be sadly inferior in education to their parents, and the country, now so full of promise, will suffer serious deterioration.

CONCLUSIONS.

The findings of the survey emphasize the need of a program for better protection of maternity and infancy in rural districts. Adequate care for the mother before, at, and after childbirth is most essential. In the Montana area the two most signal agencies for providing such care would be accessible hospital facilities and a public-health nursing service.

HOSPITAL PROVISIONS.

The large number of mothers who left the area for confinement; their difficulties in getting to a town in time, and the general expense of living away from home while waiting for confinement; the high cost of confinement to the mothers who were attended by physicians in the area; and the fact that most of the mothers appreciated the need of good confinement care lead one to believe that a series of small cottage hospitals—equipped especially for maternity cases, but with some provision for the treatment of accidents and other noncontagious cases—would be well patronized by the population. In addition to their use as hospitals, these cottages might serve as the health centers for a rural nursing service.

If such hospitals were provided with waiting quarters where expectant mothers could live inexpensively while waiting for confinement, they would be enabled to leave home in good season before confinement, and thus avoid the danger of being isolated by bad weather from medical care. Moreover, the last weeks of pregnancy would have the advantage of supervision as well as relief from heavy household cares.

There are in Montana, as in other States, many counties which could afford to inaugurate a system of cottage maternity hospitals and public-health nursing. On the other hand, there are counties like the one studied which, while they might have funds for one hospital, could not support a system of hospitals. In some counties it might be necessary for the State and the county to cooperate in maintaining such a service. A precedent for such cooperation of State and county is to be found in the employment of county agricultural agents, in which the United States also cooperates.

RURAL NURSING SERVICE.

This report has frequently touched upon the need of public-health nurses. Their value in safeguarding the health of mothers and young children, as well as the health of other members of the community, would be inestimably great. This has been demonstrated in New Zealand, and, since the war, England's increasing employment of public-health visitors is recognized as the great factor in her lowered infant-mortality rate.

The area studied in Montana is so large that, to cover it adequately, several nurses would be needed. The work of the nurses might include visiting mothers in their homes; bedside care in emergencies; holding, at the village or country schoolhouses, consultations in infant care and prenatal care; giving lectures on home care of the sick; and examining school children and following up the examination in the homes to see that children needing care receive it.

To quote from a previous bureau report:[1]

During the last few years it has been proved that trained nursing service is invaluable in supplementing medical supervision during pregnancy. If this is true in the city, where it is comparatively easy to consult a physician, it is still more true in the country where the distance from the physician makes it more difficult to see him regularly. A nurse who has had special training and experience in prenatal work, and who is especially equipped to discern the danger signs of pregnancy, can be of great help to the prospective mother in the country and to her physician. She will advise the mother about daily details of her care of herself so that she can avoid much discomfort and disability; she will urge her to see her physician early for a thorough preliminary examination and later when necessary; she will urge her to send samples of urine regularly to be examined, or, if asked to do so, she will make examinations of the urine and report the result to the physician. Such prenatal work may be one of the most important phases of the duty of a county public-health nurse.

In the area studied in Montana each nurse would need an automobile in order to cover her district. It is very important for the county commissioners, when appropriating money for a nurse to appropriate enough for a car and for running expenses. The commissioners in Teton County, where a nurse is employed, estimated that the car, its upkeep, and the nurse's expenses would approximate $100 a month. The employment of each nurse—including the expenses mentioned above and a salary of $1,200 or $1,500—would mean an expenditure by the county of approximately $2,500 a year. This seems a large sum of money, but the return on the expenditure in life and health and in the saving to the community of losses on account

---

[1] Moore, Elizabeth: Maternity and Infant Care in a Rural County in Kansas, p. 48. U. S. Children's Bureau Publication No. 26, Rural Child-Welfare Series No. 1. Washington, 1917.

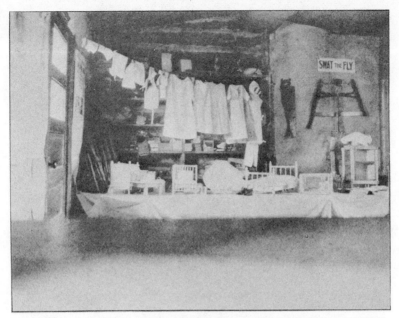

CHILDREN'S HEALTH CONFERENCE EXHIBIT HELD IN A TINY COUNTRY
POST OFFICE AND STORE.

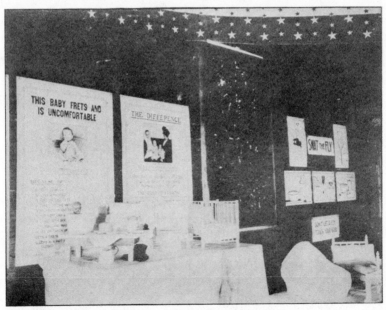

EXHIBIT IN ANOTHER VILLAGE.

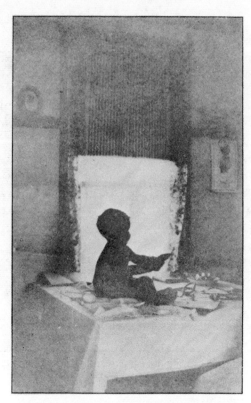

READY TO BE WEIGHED AND MEASURED.

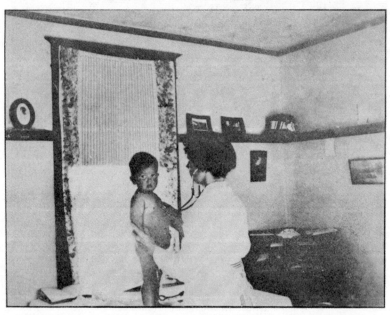

CHILDREN'S BUREAU PHYSICIAN EXAMINING BABY AT CHILDREN'S
HEALTH CONFERENCE.

of sickness would more than compensate for the original outlay. The child-welfare law already quoted [1] permits the use of public funds for the employment either by the county or by school districts of public-health nurses.

Public-health nurses would be cordially welcomed by the women in the area. The petition prepared by the local committee for one of the children's health conferences, the many signatures which it received, as well as the general comment throughout the area, reveal the eagerness of the population for such nursing service.

One mother, commenting on the needs of the area, said: " You'll find an intelligent class of women out in this county. We have to live in poor surroundings and we have few pleasures, but we're responsive to suggestions, and always eager to watch any opportunity that makes for better conditions in our families. A public-health nurse in this community would never complain of lack of cooperation."

This comment sums up very succinctly the attitude of the community toward the need of better facilities for maternity and infant care.

---

[1] See p. 82.

APPENDIX A.

TABLES USED AS BASE FOR DISCUSSION IN SECTION ON MATERNAL MORTALITY.

TABLE I.—*Death rates from diseases caused by pregnancy and confinement per 1,000 live births, in specified foreign countries for 1910.*[a]

Country.	Death rates from diseases caused by pregnancy and confinement per 1,000 live births.	Country.	Death rates from diseases caused by pregnancy and confinement per 1,000 live births.
Italy	2.4	France	4.6
Sweden	2.5	Switzerland	4.8
Norway	2.7	Australia	5.1
Prussia	3.2	Ireland	5.3
Hungary	3.4	Spain	5.3
Japan	3.6	Belgium	5.5
England and Wales	3.6	Scotland	5.7
New Zealand	4.5		

[a] Excerpt from Table XV, Maternal Mortality, U. S. Children's Bureau Publication No. 19.

TABLE II.[a]—*Average death rates per 100,000 population in certain countries from diseases caused by pregnancy and confinement, 1900 to 1910.*

Country.	Death rates per 100,000 population from diseases caused by pregnancy and confinement.	Country.	Death rates per 100,000 population from diseases caused by pregnancy and confinement.
Sweden [b]	6.0	Hungary	13.3
Norway	8.1	Japan [b]	13.3
Italy	8.9	Australia [f]	14.1
France [c]	10.3	Belgium [d]	14.8
Prussia [d]	10.4	Scotland [b]	14.8
England and Wales	11.1	United States [g]	14.9
New Zealand	12.4	Switzerland	15.2
Ireland [e]	12.9	Spain [b]	19.6

[a] Meigs, Dr. Grace L.: Maternal Mortality from All Conditions Connected with Childbirth in the United States and Certain Other Countries, Extract from Table XII, p. 56.   U. S. Children's Bureau Publication No. 19, Miscellaneous Series No. 6.   Washington, 1917.
[b] Rates based on figures for 1901 to 1910.
[c] Rates based on figures for 1906 to 1910.
[d] Rates based on figures for 1903 to 1910.
[e] Rates based on figures for 1902 to 1910.
[f] Rates based on figures for 1907 to 1910.
[g] Rates based on figures for death-registration area which increased from year to year; in 1900 it comprised 40.5 per cent of the total population of the United States and in 1910, 58.3 per cent.

TABLE III.—*Death rates per 100,000 estimated female population a aged 15 to 44 years from diseases of pregnancy and confinement, for the State of Montana and for certain foreign countries, 1910 to 1915.b*

	Years.	Rates.		Years.	Rates.
Montana............................	1910	78.9	Ireland...........................	1910	55.60
	1911	95.9		1911	52.46
	1912	89.1		1912	56.05
	1913	92.0		1913	53.81
	1914	111.4		1914	50.67
	1915	98.4			
Belgium......................	1910	56.03	Norway......................	1910	31.96
	1911	59.05			
	1912	63.79	Prussia......................	1910	43.17
England and Wales..............	1910	35.74	Scotland........................	1910	62.24
	a 1911	35.74		1911	60.99
	a 1912	36.54		1912	58.92
	a 1913	35.74		1913	62.24
	a 1914	37.75		1914	65.14
France...........................	1910	39.64	Sweden......................	1910	29.30
Hungary......................	1910	55.25		1911	29.76
	1911	53.43	Switzerland......................	1910	51.50
Italy..............................	1910	36.82		1911	57.08
	1911	34.09		1912	54.07
	1912	35.45			
	1913	35.91			

a Female population aged 15 to 44 calculated from the estimated total population for each year on the assumption that the percentage of the total population that is included in this sex and age group is equal in each year specified to the per cent included in this group at the date of the census around 1910. For Montana see note, Table IV.

b Or for the years during this time for which figures were available.

TABLE IV.a—*Death rates per 100,000 estimated female population aged 15 to 44 years from diseases of pregnancy and confinement for the death-registration States, 1910 to 1915.*

Registration States.	1910	1911	1912	1913	1914	1915
California..	51.7	57.1	57.5	61.9	56.4	54.4
Colorado...	80.5	74.4	56.9	67.1	52.7	61.1
Connecticut..	53.5	45.8	61.4	49.0	59.2	60.5
District of Columbia......................................	72.7	58.3	48.3	62.4	55.6	47.1
Indiana..	70.8	75.3	70.2	64.5	70.1	62.1
Kansas...					52.5	55.3
Kentucky...		76.4	67.2	69.2	65.2	60.4
Maine..	66.3	50.9	45.2	50.9	51.1	64.2
Maryland...	59.9	56.7	67.0	72.6	58.0	59.0
Massachusetts..	47.1	57.4	50.4	55.5	61.2	56.2
Michigan...	73.0	76.3	63.6	85.4	77.0	77.4
Minnesota..	52.4	62.6	55.3	64.6	56.4	56.2
Missouri...		70.7	67.7	71.8	67.0	59.5
Montana..	78.9	95.9	89.1	92.0	111.4	98.4
New Hampshire...	52.5	59.4	66.1	58.9	68.5	60.3
New Jersey...	61.9	64.5	60.7	64.6	58.8	57.8
New York...	58.8	58.4	52.5	54.3	56.5	54.5
Ohio...	63.2	61.7	60.8	58.1	66.0	57.8
Pennsylvania...	78.8	69.7	66.1	73.9	73.8	70.4
Rhode Island...	58.9	62.6	55.1	49.3	53.0	59.7
Utah...	84.3	71.5	72.0	71.4	55.3	81.1
Vermont..	78.2	62.6	62.4	69.8	89.8	60.5
Virginia...				83.3	98.4	93.9
Washington...	76.1	65.9	63.3	60.0	48.9	48.1
Wisconsin..	50.4	56.9	46.3	50.6	52.3	56.2

a The deaths are found in the volumes on Mortality Statistics of the U. S. Bureau of the Census. Estimates of total population, based upon an assumed constant annual increase, equal to that from 1900 to 1910, are given in Bulletin 133 of the Census Bureau. The female population aged 15 to 44 years has been computed on the assumption that the per cent of the total population in this sex and age class is the same in each year shown as in 1910 on the date of the census.

These rates are subject to error both in the estimate of population and in the assumed per cent in the special age and sex group. The latter may partly or wholly offset, or may be in addition to, the former. The later the date of the estimate after 1910 the more subject it is to error.

APPENDIX B.

RULES AND REGULATIONS GOVERNING COUNTY, PUBLIC-HEALTH, AND SCHOOL NURSES IN MONTANA.[1]

RULES GOVERNING COUNTY AND PUBLIC-HEALTH NURSES.

1. Public-Health nurses employed by city or county, philanthropic or industrial organizations shall be registered nurses of Montana; and on receiving appointment to such positions shall notify the State Board of Health of said appointment giving full name and address.

2. Those employed by towns or cities shall make home to home visits, giving actual bedside care, when necessary, and giving instruction in simple nursing service, hygiene and sanitation.

(Calls must not exceed an hour in duration, unless absolutely necessary. However, in the observance of this rule the nurse is allowed discretionary power.)

3. The nurse responds to every call but is not allowed to continue on a case unless a doctor is in attendance; except in cases of chronic patients, when the nurse follows original instructions of doctor.

4. In their work for doctors, nurses are required to adhere to the etiquette of their profession and are not allowed to prescribe in any case.

(However, when out of communication with doctors, emergencies must be met.)

5. The nurse must feel her responsibility in the sanitary conditions of the city, and report violations to the proper authorities. She must teach everywhere the relation between disease and insanitation.

6. The nurse should learn the agencies of her community and cooperate with proper authorities to improve the living conditions of her people. In cases of poverty, unemployment, overwork, bad housing, underfeeding, and such conditions, she can assist by cooperating with church, charity, and fraternal organizations.

7. Neglected and ill-treated children should be reported to the nearest deputy of Child and Animal Protection Bureau.

8. In outbreaks of contagious disease, (a) the nurse makes house to house investigations, to find early and missed cases.

(b) The nurse inspects and reports observance of quarantine. She instructs as to what constitute quarantine, proper disinfection of bed linen and clothing, of human excreta, and in good, general nursing care.

(c) The nurse must wear cap and gown and would suggest that she also wear rubber gloves to handle patient. She should use proper disinfection of nasal passages and mouth after calls.

---

[1] Montana State Board of Health, Special Bulletin No. 7 (Apr. 10, 1917), pp. 9–11.

(d) The nurse is deputy of local health officer and makes her daily reports to local Board of Health and monthly reports to State Board of Health on blanks furnished by the Child Welfare Division.

9. County nurses may at the discretion of the County Commissioners be required to perform the duties of the school nurse in one or more of the school districts of the county.

10. In order to secure uniformity of reports, the standard visiting nurse record cards should be used by all city or county nurses.

REGULATIONS GOVERNING THE WORK OF SCHOOL NURSES.

Reg. 1. As soon as a school nurse is appointed by any district, she must notify in writing the Director of the Child Welfare Division of the State Board of Health of her name and address.

Reg. 2. The school nurse shall be under the direct supervision of the Superintendent of school or schools where she is employed, and shall furnish the Superintendent with such reports as he or she may direct.

Reg. 3. It shall be the duty of the school nurse to make an examination of the children in the school or schools where she is employed and to notify the parents or guardians of the children of the physical defects and diseases from which the children appear to be suffering, and she shall call upon such parents or guardians and explain to them the nature of the defects or diseases from which the children appear to be suffering and in a tactful way advise that their family physician be consulted. The nurse must be careful not to advise the services of any one physician to the exclusion of the other physicians.

Reg. 4. Quarantine Regulations. For infectious or contagious diseases, see General Quarantine Regulations No. 39.

Reg. 5. On notification by the Superintendent or teachers of the absence from school of any child without a known cause, the school nurse, shall, as soon as possible, visit the home of such child, and if the child is found sick and gives symptons of having a contagious disease, the nurse shall immediately notify the local health officer.

Reg. 6. The school nurse shall notify the local Board of Health of any grossly insanitary condition in the community which she may find, and failing to have such condition remedied by the local authorities, she shall notify the State Board of Health.

Reg. 7. The school nurse shall make a monthly report to the Child Welfare Division of the State Board of Health on blanks furnished by that division.

O

U. S. DEPARTMENT OF LABOR

JAMES J. DAVIS, Secretary

CHILDREN'S BUREAU

GRACE ABBOTT, Chief

MATERNITY AND CHILD CARE IN SELECTED RURAL AREAS OF MISSISSIPPI

℞

By HELEN M. DART

℞

RURAL CHILD WELFARE SERIES No. 5

Bureau Publication No. 88

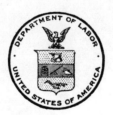

CONTENTS.

ILLUSTRATIONS.

LETTER OF TRANSMITTAL.

United States Department of Labor,
Children's Bureau,
Washington, June 14, 1921.

Sir: I transmit herewith a report entitled "Maternity and Child Care in Selected Rural Areas of Mississippi." This is one of a series of studies of child welfare in rural areas undertaken by the Children's Bureau.

The study was made under the general direction of the Hygiene Division of the Children's Bureau. The report was written by Miss Helen M. Dart, who was in charge of the field work. Dr. Frances Sage Bradley was in charge of the children's health conferences held in connection with the inquiry.

The Children's Bureau wishes to express its appreciation of the generous cooperation given by Dr. W. S. Leathers, secretary, Mississippi State Board of Health; Dr. R. W. Hall, director of the State Bureau of Vital Statistics; local physicians; school authorities; and members of the Woman's Division of the Council of National Defense.

Respectfully submitted.

Julia C. Lathrop, *Chief.*

Hon. James J. Davis,
Secretary of Labor.

MATERNITY AND CHILD CARE IN SELECTED RURAL AREAS OF MISSISSIPPI.

INTRODUCTION.

The present report upon Maternity and Child Care in Selected Rural Areas of Mississippi is one of a series of studies of the conditions affecting maternity and child welfare in rural sections of the United States begun by the Children's Bureau in 1916. That there is urgent need for the study of such problems and for the adoption of measures that will eventually lead to an amelioration of the conditions that give rise to them has already been shown in previous reports of the bureau [1] and need not be restated here in detail. A survey was undertaken under the direction of the Hygiene Division of the Children's Bureau in the spring of 1918 at the request of the Mississippi Board of Health, and the secretary of the board, in advocating the establishment of a bureau of child welfare, stated:

> This phase of health activity in Mississippi has been neglected in the past. No special provision has been made for conserving the health of the children of the State. There is no greater need in Mississippi to-day than the study of infant mortality with the hope of reducing deaths among children less than 2 years of age. * * * When it is known that thousands of children die in Mississippi from preventable causes before reaching 2 years of age, it is imperative that steps be taken to check and control this slaughter of the innocents. [2]

SCOPE AND METHOD OF THE SURVEY.

Selection of counties.—A county in the southern part of the State, where some public health work had already been done by the Mississippi State Board of Health, in cooperation with the International Health Board (formerly the Rockefeller Sanitary Commission), was chosen as the field for a series of children's health conferences, which included the examination by a Government physician of children under 6, simple talks to parents, stereopticon views, and ex-

---

[1] Children's Bureau Publication No. 26, Maternity and Infant Care in a Rural County in Kansas; Children's Bureau Publication No. 34, Maternity Care and the Welfare of Young Children in a Homesteading County in Montana; Children's Bureau Publication No. 46, Maternity and Infant Care in Two Rural Counties in Wisconsin; Children's Bureau Publication No. 33, Rural Children in Selected Counties of North Carolina.

[2] Report of the State Board of Health of Mississippi, June 1, 1915, to June 30, 1917, p. 17, Jackson, Miss., 1918.

hibits relating to child care. For the intensive survey of maternity and infant welfare a county in the northern part of the State was selected which was typical of the " hill country " of that part of the State in respect to the conditions of child care, general economic and farming conditions, and racial and industrial distribution of population. Comparatively little public health work had been done in the county, and while it was not progressive in this respect, neither was it the most backward in the State. The study was confined to rural communities in the northern county; the two county seats, towns of about 500 and 4,500 inhabitants where strictly rural conditions did not prevail, were not included in the area studied.

Sources of information.—General information was secured from the county health officer, the county superintendent of schools, the county agricultural agent, the home demonstration agent, from physicians, and from many other responsible persons in the county. But in this, as in all similar surveys made by the Children's Bureau, the information most pertinent to child and maternity care was secured through personal interviews with individual mothers by the woman agents of the bureau. Effort was made to secure interviews with the mother of every baby born in the area studied between April 1, 1916, and April 1, 1918. Information was obtained in regard to 685 babies (299 white and 386 colored) born to 675 mothers (295 white and 380 colored). In a few cases in which it was impossible to see either the mother or the father, information was secured from relatives and others in a position to know the facts sought. The local registrars for births and deaths helped in finding all the babies within the scope of the survey, and death certificates for all babies whose deaths had been registered were secured at the beginning of the work. Since birth registration was incomplete, a house-to-house canvass was made of the county.

MAIN FEATURES IN SOCIAL AND ECONOMIC BACK-GROUND OF FAMILIES VISITED.

The county in which the intensive survey was made is located in the northern part of the State and is typical of the "hill country" of Mississippi with rolling hills, open fields, broad fertile river bottoms, and a good deal of cut-over woodland.

POPULATION.

The census of 1910 showed that the percentage of Negroes in Mississippi, 56 per cent, was greater than for any other State in the Union,[1] and in the county studied more than half the total population of 22,959 was Negro.[2] Of the mothers interviewed 56 per cent were Negro, and only 1 mother was foreign born.

Urban and rural population.—About 20 per cent of the population was urban, owing to the fact that there was one city of 4,649 inhabitants.[3] In spite of its size it exerted very little more influence for progress than did the other county seat, a village of about 500 inhabitants. The population of the county exclusive of these two towns was about 17,800 in 1918. Scattered over the county there were eight small towns in which living conditions were essentially rural. They varied in size from 10 to 475 inhabitants and contained from 1 to 12 stores. None of these towns had more than one physician in regular practice, and three had no physician at all. All but one had post offices and all but two were on the railroad. Of these two, one was about 7, the other about 9 miles from a railroad station. In none of them was there a town water supply or sewerage system.

Density of population.—In 1910 the density of the rural population of the State was 34.3 persons per square mile, of the county 35.2 persons per square mile.[4] In the open country it was seldom more than a quarter of a mile from one house to the next, and even in the rougher parts of the county it was unusual to visit a family who had no neighbors in sight. This was quite different from the county

---

[1] Thirteenth Census, 1910, Population, vol. 1, p. 135.
[2] Estimated for Apr. 15, 1918, on basis of Thirteenth Census, 1910, Population, vol. 2, p. 1058.
[3] Estimated for Apr. 15, 1918, on basis of figures given, Thirteenth Census, 1910, Population, vol. 2, pp. 1035 and 1058.
[4] Thirteenth Census, 1910, Population, vol. 2, pp. 1044–1058.

9

studied in Montana, where it was unusual to find families living less than one-half mile apart. Most of the Negroes lived on the river bottoms as tenants on the large plantations, while the whites lived in the hills where the plantations had been broken up into small farms.

MEANS OF COMMUNICATION.

Railroads.—Two divisions of the Illinois Central Railroad crossed the county from north to south. Stations were only from 4 to 7 miles apart. None of the families visited lived more than 10 miles from a railroad station. The large markets were St. Louis and Memphis. Shipments of cotton, hay, cattle, hogs, and other produce were arranged for in carload lots by the county agricultural agent. Only a very small part of the stock and grain raised in the county was used by the local market.

Roads and mail service.—On account of the many hills and gullies even the public roads were winding and had many steep grades. The soil was so sandy that the roads dried quickly, and so loose that they washed out easily and needed constant care to keep them in condition. However, the main roads were usually very good and well graded, and practically every part of the county was accessible by automobile. Even in bad weather the roads were seldom impassable for more than a few days at a time, and only a few instances were reported where a father had difficulty because of bad roads in getting a doctor or midwife to attend a confinement. According to the southern custom, most of the houses were not on the main road but back on the plantations. The roads leading to them were private and not so well worn or well kept as the public roads. Some of the houses were 1½ or 2 miles from the main road; a few were almost inaccessible by automobile even when the weather was good, because the roads leading to them were rough and steep or the bridges insecure.

Good roads made possible daily mail delivery for every part of the county. No place in the county was more than 3 miles from a rural mail delivery route and most places were not so far away as this.

Telephones.—Telephone lines followed most of the main roads. Of the 675 families visited, 84 white families and 2 colored had telephones in the homes. Nearly one-half were less than a mile from some neighbor who had a telephone, 182 were 1 to 3 miles distant, and only 20 of the families (19 of them colored) were reported as living over 5 miles from a telephone. Only 4 mothers reported trouble in getting a physician for confinement because the telephone service was cut off.

FARMING CONDITIONS.

Over four-fifths of the land of the county was in farms,[5] but it was estimated by the county agricultural agent that about one-half of this land was still unimproved, although more was being brought under cultivation each year. Much of the land under cultivation had not yet been cleared of stumps, and in many fields the trees had been girdled instead of cut in order that the land might be immediately planted in cotton or corn. Nearly one-half the farm acreage of the county was in woodland.[6]

Soils.—The soil of the bottom lands, though liable to overflow, afforded some of the best farming land of the State, while the upland soil was probably more suitable for grazing than for any other purpose. To quote from the State geological survey:

Most of this region has been long in cultivation. The high, well-drained condition of the surface, the healthfulness of the climate and the fertility of the soil at an early period in the State's development invited settlement. In the antebellum days, under slavery régime, these lands were owned and worked in large plantations. As elsewhere in the State, cotton was the staple crop with just enough corn to supply the needs of the plantation. The methods of cultivation were very exhausting to the soil. Crops were, year after year, taken off the land and nothing returned to it.[7]

The report states further that the exclusive cultivation of cotton exhausted the humus and other elements of fertility. Since the Civil War the exhaustion of these lands had been more rapid than ever before, and careless terracing or circling of the hill slopes had caused many of them to wash out badly. It was only within the past few years that agricultural methods had begun to show improvement.

Climate.—Hot weather usually continues unbroken from the latter part of May to early October, and farmers count on a frost-free growing season of about seven months. The temperature does not rise any higher than it does in some northern States, but the long-continued unbroken heat and the humidity makes the climate more enervating. Only occasionally in a severe winter does the thermometer drop below zero.

The rainfall is well distributed throughout the year but the heaviest occurs in the late winter and early spring. The total precipitation for the year 1917 was 53.98 inches.[8] The snowfall is slight, even in the northern part of the State. The prevailing winds are from the south. Tropical storms and thunder showers which cause great damage to crops are not infrequent.

---

[5] Thirteenth Census, 1910, Agriculture, Vol. VI, pp. 870–871.

[6] Thirteenth Census, 1910, Agriculture, Vol. VI, pp. 870–871.

[7] Mississippi State Geological Survey, Bulletin No. 12, p. 213, Jackson, Miss., 1915.

[8] Climatological data, Mississippi Section Annual Summary, 1917, p. 101.

Crops and live stock.—Until 1911, when the boll weevil appeared in the county, cotton was by far the most important crop and a large part of the foodstuffs consumed was imported. With the dwindling of the cotton crop to about one-third its former size, other crops had assumed a greater relative importance and more attention had been given to stock raising. Diversified farming had reacted beneficially on the people as well as on the soil. They no longer staked a whole year's effort on one crop nor depended on the market value of that crop to buy their foodstuffs. One of the illiterate colored farmers said that he and his fellow tenants on the plantation had been much more prosperous and independent since each household had begun to raise its own grain and meat and garden produce. For the first time in years they had been able to get out of debt at harvest time.

There were as yet few stock or dairy farms, but practically every farmer in the county was raising a few hogs and cattle for market, and a few farmers were shipping milk to a creamery outside the county. About three-fourths of the families visited owned some cattle and about the same number were reported as keeping hogs. Some mules and horses and a few sheep and goats were raised for the market. The number of sheep had decreased considerably since the law requiring the fencing of pastures made their upkeep more expensive. Of the 674 families reporting, 280 of the white and 279 of the colored families had milch cows. In 46 cases the family did not own the cow, but had the use of her as part of the rental contract or in return for some service. Fifteen white and 100 colored families neither owned, hired, nor had the use of a cow. It must be taken into consideration, however, that not all the families reporting cows had fresh milk all the year round, and the importance of milk in the children's diet needed emphasis here as in many other farming districts.

Plantation system of land tenure.—The conditions of tenant farming in the area studied were peculiar to the plantations of the South, the form of tenure having been developed there in the reconstruction period to supplant slavery conditions. To quote from the special study of plantation areas in the South made by the census in 1910:

A large proportion of the tenants in the South actually occupied a very different economic position from that usually occupied by tenants in other parts of the country. The plantation as a unit for general purposes of administration has not disappeared, and in many cases the tenants on plantations are subjected to quite as complete supervision by the owner, general lessee, or hired manager as that to which the wage laborers are subjected on large farms in the North and West, and indeed in the South. Where this is the case a tenant is very similar in his economic position to the hired farm laborer, practically the only difference being that he confines his work to a particular parcel of land which he works by himself and that he is paid by a share of the crop instead of by wages.[9]

Along with the plantation system of land tenure was the credit system peculiar to it. From the time, early in the year, when the tenant signed the contract until the crop was marketed the landlord " carried " him. Unless the planter wished to supply the tenant from his own commissary, he arranged credit for him through either a bank or a store for a weekly or monthly allowance for food and clothing, though in many cases the arrangements were less systematic. This advance, with interest, was deducted from the tenant's share of the crop at harvest. Since the colored tenant was usually ignorant and often illiterate, the bookkeeping was completely in the hands of the landlord; and there was, without question, some exploitation. One tenant working in partnership with another reported that after deductions had been made for the debts incurred for her living expenses she received $5 and $3\frac{1}{2}$ loads of corn as earnings for the year's work.

Tenure and acreage.—The plantation system necessitated a large proportion of tenant farmers. Fifty-six per cent of the white families on farms were tenants and 89 per cent of the colored. Of the families who were reported as having farms, 75 per cent were tenants, 22 per cent owners, while for the remaining number the form of tenure was too irregular to be classified because the farmers were working farms belonging to their relatives, who in the majority of cases lived with the family but took only a minor part, if any, in the management and operation of the farm. Altogether only 45 farmers were renting on a cash basis or were paying a standard rent of a fixed amount of produce (usually a bale of cotton), while by far the greater proportion (over 80 per cent) of the tenants were renting on shares. Thirty per cent of the white and 68 per cent of the Negro tenant farmers were renting on half shares. Economically these were the lowest in the scale. The farm implements and work animals they used were owned by the landlord. More than four-fifths of the tenants of this class owned neither a horse nor a mule; about two-fifths owned no cattle; and nearly one-third owned no pigs. A quarter share rental was reported by 67 tenant farmers and 54 were paying one-fourth of the cotton and one-third of the corn. Cash and standard-rent tenants received but little supervision, but the share tenants were supervised with regard to the planting, cultivation, and harvesting of the crops.

Most of the small farms were in the rougher parts of the county, while the rich bottom lands were held by large plantation owners.

---

[9] U. S. Bureau of the Census, Plantation Farming in the United States, p. 7. Washington, 1916.

The number of small farms was large, but most of the land in the county was in large holdings. For the 121 farm owners for whom acreage was reported, 21 had farms of less than 50 acres, 28 had farms of 50 to 100 acres, and 35 had farms of 100 to 175 acres. There were 11 farms of 500 acres or more, and 2 of 1,000 or more. Farms belonging to colored farmers averaged smaller than those belonging to white farmers. The average size of farms among tenants was much smaller than among owners, because it was not customary for a man to rent more land than he and his family could work by their own labor, and furthermore rented farms included little unimproved land, while practically one-half of the land of the owned farm was not under cultivation. Of the tenants reporting acreage, 42 had farms of from 10 to 20 acres; 116 (nearly one-half) had farms of from 20 to 30 acres; and 57, farms of from 30 to 50 acres. There were only 20 tenant farms of more than 50 acres and none of more than 260 acres.

Removals from farm to farm.—As may be expected in a section where the proportion of tenant farmers is large, there was considerable moving from one farm to another. Nearly one-third of the families visited reported that they had lived in their present dwelling less than a year. Seventy-five families (1 in 9) had lived on the average less than a year in a place during married life, and nearly one-half of the families visited had lived on an average less than three years in a place. One mother said she had moved so many times she could not keep count of the number, while in another family the older daughter said they had moved every two years since she could remember. Families who move every year or two do not stay in one neighborhood long enough to get the full benefit of the schools, churches, and other community enterprises, and they have little interest in community projects, such as the building of a county hospital or the employment of a county nurse.

Removals were naturally more frequent among tenants than among farm owners. As the share tenant was supplied not only with a house but with most of his furniture, farm implements, and stock, moving was a relatively simple operation, in many cases consisting of loading all his household goods and family into a one-horse wagon and moving over to another farm without losing any time from work. The most shifting element of the population was the white tenant farmer. Only about 1 in 8 had stayed for an average of three years or more in one place. On the whole removals among the colored families were but little more frequent than among white families. The tendency to remain for a long time on one farm seemed to be stronger among the Negro than among the white families, considering the fact that the proportion of tenant families was much greater among the Negroes. Many spent their whole lives on one plantation.

Occupation of chief breadwinner.—In 93 per cent of the families visited the chief breadwinner was a farmer, farm manager, or farm laborer. Only 39 per cent of the white and 9 per cent of the colored farmers were farm owners. Of the remaining 7 per cent nearly one-half were railroad employees and the rest were professional men, merchants, salesmen, postal employees, or skilled mechanics. In 2 white and 16 colored families the mother was the chief breadwinner; 13 of these mothers were farmers, and 1 was a farm laborer.

ILLITERACY AND EDUCATION.

Illiteracy.—Illiteracy and low standards of education were serious enough in this part of the State to present a real obstacle to better health work. Many a mother refused to take the Children's Bureau pamphlets on Infant Care and Prenatal Care because she could not read and had no one who could read them to her. The percentage of illiteracy was much greater among the Negro than among the white parents, and the percentage of illiteracy among fathers was higher than among mothers. Of the white families visited, 9 fathers and 8 mothers were reported as illiterate, while of the colored families 110 fathers and 100 mothers were thus reported. In 5 white and 48 colored families neither parent could read or write. The figures for illiteracy indicate to only a small extent the ignorance which existed among most of the white tenant farmers and Negroes. These people had very few books and subscribed for practically no magazines or papers, and were unable to use readily the means which the more intelligent and progressive farmers employed to counteract the isolation of rural life.

Schools.—The schools of the county were handicapped by the lack of a compulsory education law.[10] When school attendance is voluntary it is likely to be irregular. The school session came in the months when it was least likely to interrupt farm work, and this made the term fall within the period of bad weather which caused much irregularity of attendance. The term, too, was so short that many children forgot between terms what they had learned, and many left school with only a slight knowledge of reading and writing. The term for rural schools for white children was five months in the southwestern part of the county and five and a half months

---

[10] A compulsory education law requiring 60 days' attendance, with exemptions, went into effect Sept. 1, 1918. This law was applicable only to those counties which elected to come under its provisions. (Mississippi Acts of 1918, ch. 258.) A new law requiring 80 days' attendance, with exemptions, went into effect Aug. 1, 1920. This law applied to the entire State, but permitted any county to release itself from the provisions of the act by a majority vote of the qualified electors at an election held for that purpose. (Mississippi Acts of 1920, ch. 156.)

in the northeastern, the difference being due to the additional income in the northeastern part of the county from the Chickasaw fund. Terms in the colored schools averaged about four months. Three or four districts levied a special tax for a longer term. Teachers of the first or highest grade ("grade" being based on educational requirements and type of examinations passed) were required to have only a common-school education. Practically all of the white teachers were of the first grade, with salaries averaging $50 a month. Most of the colored teachers were of the third grade, with salaries ranging from $16 to $25 a month.[11] The rural schoolhouse served to some extent as a social center for the community. Some of the schoolhouses were well-constructed buildings, while some were rough, unceiled frame houses with uncomfortable homemade benches. Several of them had no toilet facilities whatever. At the time of the survey the county had no consolidated schools, but in one or two localities there were good prospects that such schools would soon be established.

Home demonstration and agricultural agents.—The home demonstration agent of the county, employed under the joint supervision of the State and the United States Department of Agriculture, worked with the women and girls to promote better methods of household economy. She organized in close cooperation with the schools canning clubs, poultry clubs, and home economics clubs. An important part of her work was the promotion of better care and more intelligent feeding of babies and children. The first public-health nurse in the county will find her work made easier by the organizations already formed and methods already put in practice by the home demonstration agents. The agricultural agent worked with the men much as the home demonstration agent worked with the women. He made a scientific study of the soils of the county, advised the farmers in methods of cultivation and stock raising and promoted cooperative seed buying and the cooperative sale of farm products.

PUBLIC HEALTH WORK IN THE COUNTY.

The county was at the time of this survey the unit of administration in public-health work in Mississippi. One of the physicians resident in a county was appointed as health officer. His duties were to make monthly statements of mortality statistics compiled from the reports of the registrars of the various voting precincts of the county, to enforce quarantine regulations, and to act as assistant sanitary inspector in enforcing the rules of the State board of health in regard to the sanitation of public buildings, markets, milk depots,

---

[11] Statement of county superintendent of schools.

etc.[12] He was charged also with the enforcement of the law passed in January, 1916, for the prevention of blindness in the new born, which involved the recording of all cases of ophthalmia neonatorum, and the registration of the midwives of the county and their instruction in the use of the prophylactic measures prescribed by the law.[13] Most of the county health officers of the State worked only on part time and had to depend upon private practice for their living. Salaries of these part-time officers varied from $150 to $1,800 a year. The officer of the county studied received about $300 a year. In reviewing the results of this type of organization the secretary of the State board of health wrote as follows:

In many of the counties the part-time man achieves results for which he is by no means compensated. In the main, the part-time county health officers of Mississippi have been, so far as the system will permit, reasonably effective public-health workers. But * * * this business of conserving the public health requires the undivided and aggressive effort of those who serve in this capacity.[14]

Special emphasis had been laid upon campaigns against the diseases peculiar to the region—pellagra, malaria, hookworm, and soil-pollution diseases. Special effort to reach rural districts had been made through the Division of Rural Sanitation.[15] In 1914 a study of the dietary causes of pellagra was made in cooperation with the United States Public Health Service in two orphanages in Jackson.[16] Intensive work had also been done on malaria. In 1910 the State board of health, in cooperation with the counties and the International Health Board, formerly the Rockefeller Sanitary Commission, began a State-wide survey of hookworm and soil pollution. None of the intensive health work had been done in the county studied because it is not situated in the part of the State where these diseases were most prevalent. The preliminary survey had shown that the infection from hookworm based on the examination of 570 children in the county was only 2.3 per cent.[17] Nevertheless, the propaganda attendant upon this work in other parts of the State had undoubtedly had some influence. The local physicians had done some educational work in connection with their practices. One physician said that when he began to practice, most of his time was taken up with treatment of malaria. His insistent warnings against

---

[12] Report of the Board of Health of Mississippi, 1915–1917, pp. 166–201. Jackson, Miss., 1918.

[13] Report of the Board of Health of Mississippi, 1915–1917, pp. 301–302. Jackson, Miss., 1918.

[14] Report of the Board of Health of Mississippi, 1915–1917, pp. 21–22. Jackson, Miss., 1918.

[15] Report of the Board of Health of Mississippi, 1915–1917, pp. 29–30. Jackson, Miss., 1918.

[16] Report of the Board of Health of Mississippi, 1915–1917, pp. 309–310.

[17] Report of the Board of Health of Mississippi, 1913–1915, p. 26.

mosquitoes had resulted in the screening of many of the homes in his community and a decrease in the prevalence of malaria. Another, in connection with his typhoid cases, had raised the standards of sanitation and cleanliness in some of the country homes.

HOUSING AND SANITATION.

Houses.—The three-room one-story house with a wide, open passage from front to back and chimneys for fireplaces at each end of the building was the type of farmhouse most often seen. Sometimes a porch extended across the whole front of the house, sometimes a kitchen was built on at the back. Many of the larger houses were built on much the same plan, while the smaller houses had a chimney at only one end. Many of the cabins were of rough boards or logs with generous cracks between. Only about 4 per cent of the houses were plastered on the inside, and about 30 per cent were finished with ceiling. A few of the board houses were finished with a second layer of boards on the inside; some were not even clapboarded. Many were papered with newspapers to keep out the cold. Some of the poorer cabins had no glass windows, but merely holes in the walls fitted with wooden shutters; when these shutters were closed the house was dark except for the light that came in through the cracks. Comparatively few houses were painted; some were whitewashed inside and out.

The houses among the Negroes were on the whole much poorer than those of white families, many of them being old ramshackle cabins in wretched condition. Less than 1 per cent were plastered and only 21 per cent were ceiled. For the greater part of the year such houses were comfortable, but in the few winter months there was real suffering from the cold. Over 96 per cent of the houses were set up on piles so that the circulation of air underneath might make them cooler and drier; unless this space under the house was inclosed, chickens, pigs, cats, and dogs used it as a shelter. The houses of the prosperous white planters were comfortably furnished, but many of the tenant cabins had only the most necessary things—a bed, a few chairs, and a table. In some houses rough homemade benches took the place of chairs; homemade cradles, beds, and tables were often seen.

Overcrowding.—It is surprising to find that there are as serious instances of overcrowding in the country as in large cities, but the fact that there is no crowding of one house against another does not insure plenty of room inside the house. When a family of 8 members or more lives in a house of two rooms or less (17 of the families were thus reported), there is bound to be crowding, lack of privacy, and inconvenience for the housekeeper, no matter how much space there may be outside the house.

The size of the families varied from 2 persons to 16; about 85 per cent of the white families had from 3 to 8 members; most of the Negro families had from 3 to 11 members. Fifteen colored families had 12 or more members, 4 had 14 or more. The house most commonly found had three rooms, but many of the families visited were living in smaller quarters; 15 families had only one room, and 117, or 17 per cent, had two-room houses. Less than one-half of the families visited were living in houses of four rooms or more.

Forty per cent of the families visited reported 2 or more persons per room; 10 white and 70 colored families were living with 3 or more persons to a room. About one-third of the white families reported 2 to 3 persons per sleeping room; about one-fourth 3 to 4 persons per sleeping room; 28, or nearly one-tenth, reported 4 to 5 persons per sleeping room. There were 27 instances of 5 or more persons per sleeping room. Only 23 per cent reported less than 2 persons per sleeping room. Overcrowding of sleeping rooms in Negro families was still more evident. More than two-thirds reported 3 persons or more per sleeping room, and only 6 per cent less than 2 persons. In 43 families (over 11 per cent) there were 6 or more persons per sleeping room; 6 cases were found of 8 in one sleeping room, 3 instances of 9, and 3 cases of 10 persons sleeping in one room.

Screening.—Even in northern Mississippi the climate is such that screening against mosquitoes is desirable as a precaution against malaria. Flies should be kept out of the house to guard against contamination of food, and in the summer screens are very desirable to keep chickens and live stock out of the house. In one of the homes visited, a goat was wandering around inside the house, and in other cases chickens had come in and made themselves at home on the beds. Only 23 per cent of the white families and 3 per cent of the colored families were living in houses screened at all doors and windows. One of the fathers said that he had done his best to screen the house, but there were so many cracks in the walls and floor that flies and mosquitoes came in anyhow.

Water supply.—The geologic formation was such that good water was easily obtainable.[18] Flowing wells varying in depth from 160 to 200 feet were found at both county seats and along the river bottoms. Among the families visited, 41 reported a drilled well, in many cases an artesian well, as the source of water supply; 156 families reported springs; 9 secured their water from a river or creek; 16 used cisterns; 109 had bored wells; and 344 (51 per cent) had dug wells. The artesian wells furnished much the cleanest water, since they were drilled to a considerable depth and the piping kept

---

[18] Crider, A. F., and Johnson, L. C.: Summary of the Underground Water Resources of Mississippi, p. 39. Water Supply and Irrigation Paper No. 159, U. S. Geological Survey, Washington, 1906.

out surface water; river or creek water was liable to pollution from animals and fowls, and was usually muddy; springs, unless carefully protected, were likely to be dirty; and many of the dug wells were insufficiently protected from surface pollution. The bored wells were subject to much the same dangers from surface water as dug wells, but the opening was so much smaller that animals or insects were less likely to get in. Many of the dug wells were equipped with a windlass or pulley, which made them easier to use, but did not insure any more cleanliness. Eight families had water in the house, and in 21 cases the source of water supply was on the porch. For more than one-third of the families the source of water supply was less than 25 feet from the house; for more than one-half, less than 100 feet. On the other hand, about one-third of the families had to go 100 yards or more, and 53 had to go a quarter of a mile or more. Negro mothers reported on the whole longer distances from water supply. A few did not have wells on the premises, but had to go to a neighbor's for water; in some cases one well served a group of tenant houses.

Privies.—The disposal of human excreta is a particularly important problem in the South, where special precautions are needed against soil pollution diseases. The survey showed that this problem had hardly been touched in the area studied. Among white families, 61 per cent had no toilets whatever; among Negro families, 85 per cent had no toilets. Of the 166 families who had privies, 143 reported the open-back type, in which the refuse is unprotected not only from flies but also from chickens, pigs, and other domestic animals. Only two families had water-closets. The State board of health was doing effective work in rural sanitation, but thus far little of it had touched the county studied. The report of the State board of health for 1913 to 1915 [19] showed the results of an investigation of sanitary conditions in over 500 rural homes of the county; 303 had open-back privies and 270 had no privies. This gave the county a sanitary index based on the type of privies found of 5.2 on the scale of 100. The fact that this index was about the average for the whole State indicated that the problem was State wide.

---

[19] Report of State Board of Health of Mississippi, 1913–1915, p. 27.

MATERNITY CARE.

THE NEED FOR EDUCATION.

In Mississippi as well as in other parts of the country ignorance of the value of good maternity care was largely responsible for the lack of it, and several physicians in the county stated that the most important factor in getting adequate care of this kind was to educate the mothers to recognize the need of it. One physician said that when he heard incidentally that mothers were having swollen feet and other dangerous symptoms during pregnancy, he could not convince them of the necessity of reliable medical advice, and they considered visits to him unnecessary. The board of health attributed the high maternal mortality rate in the State to the fact that " a very large majority of the confinement cases among the Negroes are attended by Negro midwives, in which case little protection is afforded the patient, consequently the death rate from this cause is unusually high. It is also true that a large percentage of the confinement cases in this State as a whole are not attended by licensed physicians." [1]

MATERNITY CARE AVAILABLE.

Hospitals.—At the time of the study the hospital nearest the county was located at Memphis, Tenn., nearly 100 miles away, and the nearest one that received patients free of charge was at Jackson, over 100 miles away. Distance and expense made hospital care impossible for the great majority of mothers and children of the county. Only one of the 675 mothers scheduled had been confined in a hospital.

Physicians.—At the time of the survey there were 14 physicians in regular practice in the county, and, in addition, there were 3 or 4 who had retired from active practice, 4 or 5 who had enlisted for war work, and 1 or 2 who held no licenses but occasionally helped their neighbors in case of illness.

Midwives.—There were probably over 100 midwives practicing in the county during the period covered by the survey, and 87 of these (8 white and 79 colored) were interviewed by the agents of the Children's Bureau with the object of finding out the status of midwifery in the county. In respect to education, the white midwives

---

[1] Report of the Board of Health of Mississippi, 1915–1917, p. 111.

were superior to the colored, as all could read and write, while two-thirds of the colored midwives were illiterate; but on the whole the white midwives did not differ either in training or practice from the Negro midwives. The information gleaned from the interviews disclosed the fact that none of the midwives had had adequate training, and most of them lacked even the elementary education that would make such training possible.

Various accounts were given as to the training received to fit them for midwifery and the reasons for adopting this practice. Some of them had been taken to confinement cases and taught by physicians; some were midwives because their mothers and grandmothers had been; others had become experienced in handling emergencies or in bearing their own children; while still others said that they had been "called by the Lord." Many of them believed in various superstitions such as "Girls come at the full moon and boys on the new moon," and "Babies born on a wasting moon haven't all their senses." One midwife always cut the cord long because she had heard the saying, "Long cord, long life." Many of the midwives were very old; and decrepit, before-the-war "aunties" had more prestige among their neighbors than any of the younger midwives. One of those interviewed said: "I'm not going out on night cases any more, because I'm getting old and can't keep awake."

Some of their methods were amazingly primitive. Over nine-tenths used no antiseptics whatever in making preparations for delivery; one said: "No washing is necessary if grease is used plentifully." Various questionable expedients were used to bring the afterbirth; some of the midwives used a method of warming the patient suddenly by putting her over a bucket of hot ashes or burning feathers, while two advocated putting an umbrella or a black hat over her face. Some of the more intelligent ones knew that childbed fever was caused by uncleanliness and tried to guard against it, but among many the old custom still held of not changing the bed coverings for at least three days.

Many of them said that they always called a doctor when any complication occurred, but several told of attending cases of adherent afterbirth, severe hemorrhage, breech presentation, prolonged labor, and stillbirth without the aid of a physician, and it is probably true that many of them failed to recognize minor complications and mild cases of childbed fever. The midwife's most dangerous fault was her failure to recognize her own limitations; ignorance prevented her from recognizing cases where the attention of a physician was imperative, and in many cases it fostered a fatalistic attitude which was manifested in such expressions as "Women are born to suffer and it's wrong to interfere," and "If the baby is born to die, nothing can be done."

Several of the more intelligent midwives said that they would be glad to have a county nurse to advise them and to teach them better methods of practice. At the time of the survey there were no rural county nurses in the State, and practically nothing had been done in the area studied in regard to the supervision of midwives beyond urging them to register births. In 1916 the State legislature passed a bill for the prevention of blindness from inflammation of the eyes of the newborn, and the State board of health (1917), in the enforcement of the law, required that all midwives register with the county health officer at least once a year; that all midwives as well as physicians use a 1 per cent solution of silver nitrate in the eyes of every newborn baby, and report cases of inflammation of the eyes within six hours after they had been observed. At the time of the survey the law was not being enforced in the county, as was shown by the fact that only 3 of the 87 midwives interviewed reported having used any drops in the eyes at birth.

MATERNITY HISTORIES OF MOTHERS VISITED.

The maternity histories obtained from the mothers showed frequent pregnancies and large families. It was customary for girls to marry early and to begin bearing children when quite young. Almost one-tenth of the mothers whose ages at marriage were reported had been married before they were 16 years of age; one-third of them before 18; and slightly over three-fifths before 20. Very early marriages were more common among the colored mothers than among the white; about 1 in 8 had married before the age of 16 (two at less than 14), and nearly two-fifths when less than 18. Of the white mothers 13 said they had been less than 17 years old at the time of their first confinement, and 102 under 20. Of the colored mothers, 79 reported the first confinement at less than 17 years, and 227 under 20 years. About 1 in 7 of the mothers visited had been under 20 when the baby scheduled was born, and 28 of these had had two or three previous confinements. Nearly one-half (318) were in the age group 20 to 30 years; less than one-third were in the group 30 to 40 years. More than one-half of all mothers had had four or more pregnancies, and nearly one-fourth had had seven or more. Eighteen per cent of the white mothers and 28 per cent of the Negro mothers had had more than 6 pregnancies. One white mother and 9 Negro mothers had had more than 12 pregnancies.

Sixty-four of the 380 Negro mothers were unmarried at the time the baby scheduled was born; 52 had never been married; 6 had been married at some time previous; 6 were married after the baby was born. Half these mothers were under 20 years of age, 7 were under 17 years of age. Fifty per cent had had one or more pregnancies previous to the birth of the baby scheduled.

PRENATAL CARE.

Mothers receiving prenatal care.—The figures relating to prenatal care point plainly to the conclusion that lack of prenatal care was due in large measure to ignorance of the need for it. Only 116 mothers, about 1 in 6, had any prenatal care whatever, and of these only 9 had care because they thought that pregnancy was in itself a reason for seeking medical advice. In only 9 cases of the 116 could the care received be classed as fair, and in only 1 case was the prenatal care adequate.[2] Of these 10 mothers who had adequate or fair care, all had either had difficulties in previous confinements or such illness during pregnancy that attention from a physician seemed imperative.

The standards of maternity care were much lower among the Negroes than among the whites, the proportion of Negro mothers receiving some prenatal care being just about half that for the white mothers. Only 45 of the Negro mothers, 12 per cent, had any care at all, and only 1 of these had fair care; 10 had a physical examination and 3 a urinalysis.

While illness seemed to have been responsible for prenatal care in the majority of cases, it can not be assumed that all mothers who felt the need of care sought a physician. One white mother said that she did not feel well all through her pregnancy, though not sick enough to call a doctor. One of her older daughters was strong enough to do the housework so the family could get along. Another mother said she suffered a great deal from varicose veins but did not see a physician. Still another had no prenatal care, even though hardly able to be about during the last three months of pregnancy.

Although ignorance of the need of good prenatal care was in a large measure accountable for its lack, yet there were other factors that entered in, such as family income, distance from doctor, and traveling facilities. It is significant that the proportion of mothers receiving prenatal care was highest among families in which the chief breadwinner was not a farmer, and that they lived in or near towns, not far from a doctor. The heads of these families were for the most part ministers, doctors, merchants, salesmen, skilled mechanics, and railroad employees in the towns; over three-fourths of them were white.

---

[2] Prenatal care was classed as: *Adequate,* if there had been a monthly urinalysis, fifth to ninth months; if the mother had been under the supervision of a physician, fifth to ninth months; if an abdominal examination had been made, and, in the case of a first child, if pelvic measurements had been taken. *Fair,* if urinalysis had been made but less than five times at monthly intervals, if the mother had had some supervision by a physician, and if an abdominal examination had been made, and, in case of a first child, if pelvic measurements had been taken. *Inadequate,* if there had been visits to a physician, but no urinalysis, no abdominal examination, or, in the case of a first child, no pelvic measurements. Urinalysis with no visits to physician was also counted as inadequate care.

Analysis of care given.—In the majority of cases of women receiving some kind of prenatal care the matter ended when the mother had seen a physician. There was no realization of the importance of urinalysis, still less of abdominal and pelvic examination. Study of the number of visits, urinalysis, and kind of physical examinations made brought out the fact that 9 of the 116 mothers receiving care had urinalysis only, and did not see a physician personally. Of the 107 mothers reporting visits to or from a physician, 53 reported a single visit. Less than one-third of the 116 mothers had one or more urinalyses made during pregnancy, and 92 per cent of these mothers were white. It is interesting to consider some of the few cases in which the need of such care was realized. One mother had learned through reading and through consultation with a trained nurse that monthly urinalysis should be made, and accordingly sent specimens to her physician during the last five months of pregnancy, although she did not see him personally. In another instance the grandmother who came to stay with the mother insisted upon urinalysis because she had heard that serious complications might result from kidney trouble. One mother during pregnancy had convulsions which her physician said were caused by kidney trouble and necessitated regular urinalysis, but she insisted that they were caused by a sunstroke she had had as a girl, and refused to send specimens after the second time. Her attitude is typical of a large proportion of mothers visited. In one case a mother who had had alarming symptoms during pregnancy had been told by her physician to send specimens of urine for examination, but her husband, more through ignorance than ill nature, refused to act as messenger.

Only four of the midwives reported it as their custom to see the mother during pregnancy; six said they might make some examination if they happened to see the mother before confinement. There were often chance meetings, of course, during which the mother casually sought advice; some mothers consulted the midwife when they came to engage her, and some called her in when they were not feeling as well as they thought they should; but for the great majority of confinement cases the midwife was summoned only after labor had begun.

Use of home remedies during pregnancy.—Aside from the advice which can properly be classed as prenatal care, some mothers learned something about prenatal care through reading or took medicine not prescribed by a doctor. Two were instructed by a trained nurse. A few consulted midwives, but in the majority of cases the advice given could not be considered any better than that which might have been given by any experienced neighbor. Advice was also picked up from various other sources. One mother used liniment purchased from an agent who was canvassing the county; while another said she had written to a firm in a northern city for medicine. More than one-half (most of them Negroes) of those who used home remedies said that they took some kind of patent medicine. One mother said she had taken six bottles of a patent medicine during her last pregnancy, and another said that she had taken " more patent medicines than she could mention " during the 10 years she had been " complaining." Simple home remedies, such as castor oil, magnesia, calomel, kerosene, and camphor, were also used, and several Negro mothers said they took teas of various kinds, such as " tansy tea " or " pepper tea."

Information through reading.—Thirty-two white mothers and 14 colored had read something about the care needed by a pregnant woman. It can not be supposed, however, that the literature read was really instructive in every case, for almost none of the books mentioned were standard. Several were general " doctor books," which dealt with many subjects besides childbirth; others were pamphlets or almanacs published as advertisements; while many others were advertisements designed primarily to promote the sale of patent medicines. More than one-half of the Negro mothers who said they had received some instruction through reading had only read advertisements of this kind. Probably only the 19 mothers who read the current women's magazines and farm papers received on the whole up-to-date and authoritative instruction.

ATTENDANT AT CONFINEMENT.

Kind of attendant.—Only two-fifths of all the mothers studied were attended by a physician at confinement, while nearly three-fifths were attended by midwives. The remainder, only 4 per cent, were attended either by their husbands or by other women who were not midwives. One mother had no attendant at all. In a few instances some attempt was made to secure a physician, but the call did not reach him on account of interrupted telephone service or bad roads. In several of these latter cases the mother was attended by a wholly inexperienced person or by a Negro midwife. One mother told of being alone with her sister and husband when the baby was born. Her husband, realizing that the baby would be born before the doctor could possibly arrive, called in his wife's sister. She knew nothing about confinement cases, but " risked cutting the cord." Others told of very similar experiences.

Number and per cent distribution of scheduled mothers of specified race according to attendant at confinement.

Attendant at confinement.	Total mothers.		Race of mother.			
			White.		Negro.	
	Number.	Per cent distribution.	Number.	Per cent distribution.	Number.	Per cent distribution.
Total confinements......................	675	100.0	295	100.0	380	100.0
Physician............................	266	39.4	234	79.3	32	8.4
Midwife.............................	382	56.6	48	16.3	334	87.9
Other woman........................	24	3.6	12	4.1	12	3.2
Father..............................	2	.3	1	.3	1	.3
None................................	1	.1	0	....	1	.3

The choice between physician and widwife seemed to depend in some degree upon custom. Seventy-nine per cent of the white women were attended by physicians, while nearly 88 per cent of the colored mothers were attended by midwives. One instance was found of a Negro family who lived in town only a few blocks from a physician, but sent 3 miles into the country for a colored midwife. The proportion of native white mothers attended by a physician at confinement was the highest that had been found in any rural district studied by the Children's Bureau except the one surveyed in Kansas. However, it was lower than any of the cities studied by the bureau. A physician had been in attendance at every confinement for about two-thirds of the white mothers, but for only 3 per cent of the Negro mothers. Moreover, 11 of the 13 Negro mothers had had but one confinement. The custom among the Negroes seemed to be to call a physician only when some complication arose which the midwife could not handle. There were, however, 23 white mothers who had never had a doctor at confinement, and 14 of these had had three or more pregnancies. Of the total confinements to all mothers (3,017), 64 per cent were attended by midwifes or other women and 35 per cent by physicians. Of the remaining 1 per cent of the confinements reported, 16 were attended by the father and for 11 there was no attendant.

The difference in the choice of attendant might have been due partly to the difference in economic well-being between the white and colored families. On the whole, the Negro families were much poorer than the white, and since the midwife's fee was so much lower than a physician's the choice of attendant was in many cases conditioned by the family's ability to pay. The percentage of mothers, both white and colored, who were attended by a physician at confinement was much higher among those families living on farms of their own than among farm tenants, and was lowest among the half-share tenants.

Distance from attendant.—Another factor that entered into the choice of attendant at confinement was the distance the physician had to travel to reach the patient. Sixty-six white families were living 7 miles or more from a doctor, and on the other hand 155 white families, more than half, were less than 5 miles from a doctor. For white families the proportion of mothers attended by physicians was lower for those living 7 miles or more from a doctor than for those living nearer, and the proportion of cases attended by midwives was higher. In this connection, however, transportation facilities and the condition of the roads must be taken into account. All mothers, both white and colored, who lived in the more remote parts of the county ran greater risks at confinement than those in or near towns, because of the time and difficulty usually involved in getting a physician in an emergency, but under favorable conditions it was usually possible even for families living far from town to get a physician in time. There were, however, instances of unfortunate combinations of circumstances which prevented the mother from securing a physician for confinement. One mother told of difficulty at confinement because the first physician they called was ill and the next one was away on another case, so that she was alone with her husband and a neighbor when the baby was born. Another mother told of failure to get a physician because a man had taken down some of the telephone wire to repair his wagon. Still another had a baby born in January when a severe storm was raging. The telephone was out of order and her husband had to go through the storm to use a neighbor's telephone. He succeeded in reaching the doctor, but the latter was delayed by having to heat water in order to start his car, and when he finally reached his patient the baby had been born two hours. By that time the grandmother had cut the cord and rendered the other necessary services.

There were many midwives scattered through the different sections of the county and probably no family lived more than 2 or 3 miles from one.

CARE OF THE MOTHER AFTER DELIVERY.

Medical care.—Only one-third of the 266 mothers who were attended by a physician at confinement reported any after care by a physician; 46 received but one visit, 25 received three or more, and only five reported more than six visits. Of the 25 confinements for which the physician made three or more visits, 14 were cases in which either the mother or the baby was in a serious condition after delivery.

In 6 of the 11 remaining cases the family was living less than a mile from the attending physician, and in 3 other cases the mothers were the wives of prosperous farmers.

Nursing care.—One of the most serious obstacles to good maternity care was the scarcity of nursing care. There was no trained nurse working regularly in the area, and most of the practical nurses were midwives whose practice was largely among Negro mothers. Very few of them were really competent. Only 7 mothers of the 675 secured trained nurses, and less than one-fourth reported care by a practical nurse or midwife. It was also very hard to find anyone who could be hired to do the housework during the mother's lying-in period, and in the majority of cases the person who nursed the mother had most of the responsibility for the housework, too. This scarcity of help many times resulted in poor care for the mother and made her feel that she ought to get up at the first possible moment. One mother who had stayed in bed only a week explained that it was her custom to stay longer but that this time she could get no nurse; she was worried because the baby was not doing as well as he should, and she felt that she must get up to attend to him. Another said she had been unable to get either a trained or a practical nurse, even though all her children had whooping cough when she was confined. She finally secured a colored woman to care for her and do the housework. In another family the father nursed the mother while the older daughters, girls of 12 and 16, did all the housework and washing. One woman told of a miscarriage brought on by overwork in nursing her husband and her father at a time when no woman could be found to help with either the nursing or the housework.

Less than one-fourth of the midwives interviewed reported that they stayed in the mother's home a day or more after delivery; most of them stayed only a few hours. The majority of midwives went to see the mother afterwards from one to five times, but most of the care given during the lying-in period was for the baby rather than for the mother.

In about 1 case in 7 most of the nursing was done by the father. In about 1 case in 5 the nurse did not stay with the mother constantly, but came in for a few hours during the day. This practice was most common among the midwives, but there were other cases in which the mother depended upon daily visits from some neighbor for nursing care. In most cases such care was gratuitous—a neighborly service to be repaid only in kind. One mother said that her mother came in several times a day, but that it was a busy time on the farm and she was left alone much of the day with only the children to wait on her. Another said she secured a colored woman to come and stay with her, and one of the neighbors to come in for an hour or so every day to bathe her and the baby.

In 72 cases the nurse left before the mother was able to be up, and in only 17 cases did the nurse stay until after the mother was able to be up for most of the day. In nearly two-fifths of all cases no extra person was called in, but the mother was cared for by some member of the household. Only about 21 per cent of the mothers had paid nursing care, and only 13 per cent paid for all nursing care received.

The quality of nursing care was on the whole much poorer for Negro mothers than for white. None had a trained nurse. Less than one-third had nursing care by a midwife or practical nurse, and one-third of these mothers had practical nurses who made only a few visits and did not stay in the mother's home. The percentage of mothers nursed only by their husbands was larger among Negro than among white families. Four had only such care as could be given by a child under 14 years of age—in one instance a little girl 5 years old. Two Negro mothers had no nursing care at all. Needless to say, these mothers got up as soon as possible after confinement.

Days in bed.—As a result of the scarcity of nurses, the pressure of work, and the inadequate supervision by physicians and midwives, many mothers did not have the rest in bed after delivery that is considered essential. Of the white mothers visited, there were 20, or 7 per cent, who stayed in bed less than a week, and nearly 60 per cent who stayed in bed 10 days or more. Of the Negro mothers, 150, or 39 per cent, stayed in bed less than a week, and 30 per cent 10 days or more. One Negro mother explained rather apologetically that she had stayed in bed for a week after the last baby was born, because the weather was so cold. Ordinarily she stayed only three days. In spite of the custom among many of the Negro mothers of staying in bed only a few days, some still held to the tradition that the mother should "stay in her month." One said that she had been told by the midwife who attended her first confinement to stay in bed for a month, and she had followed this advice at each of her four subsequent confinements.

The season of the year in which the confinement occurred determined to some extent the length of time which the mother spent in bed. One Negro mother explained that she stayed in bed for only four days with a "summer-time baby," but with one born at any other time of the year she stayed in bed longer. During the busy spring and fall seasons the mother was likely to feel that she ought to help if she possibly could, and even if she did not go into the fields for work herself she might try to release for field work those who were helping with the nursing and housework.

COSTS OF CONFINEMENT.

The costs of confinement tabulated for this study include the attendant's fee, the cost of prenatal care, the cost of hospital care, and the combined cost of nursing care and help with the housework; expenses for medicine and for extra supplies or transportation are not included.

Total costs and free service.—Of the white mothers who reported the cost of confinement, 62 per cent gave totals ranging from $10 to $25, and 16 per cent reported an expense of $25 or over. Of the colored mothers who gave information on this point, 65 per cent reported a total cost of less than $5 and 25 per cent a cost of less than $2.50. These costs average lower than those found in any other rural district surveyed. In Kansas 54 per cent reported an expense of $25 or over for confinement, while in Montana physicians' fees alone were usually over $25 for confinement, prenatal care, and postnatal care. Forty-six mothers, 16 white and 30 colored, reported no money whatever paid out for the services specified. Analysis of cost by different items of expense shows that most mothers received free service of some kind. Forty received free care from the attendant midwife, and 4 paid nothing to the attendant physician. In 488 cases (three-fourths of the total reporting) there was nothing paid out for either nursing or housework. In such cases by far the largest item of expense was that for the attendant at confinement. Other costs rarely equaled or exceeded the attendant's fee, and in a great many instances it was the only expense incurred.

Costs itemized.—It was customary for the physician to charge a fee for confinement and, in addition, regular fees for each prenatal or postnatal visit, rather than a lump sum to cover all care during pregnancy and confinement. The physician's usual fee for a normal delivery was $10 or $15. Of those who reported the physician's charge for confinement alone, 193 (87 per cent) paid from $10 to $25, and only 16 paid over $25. The expense averaged higher if prenatal care had been given. Five of the nine mothers who received fair prenatal care (see p. 24) paid a physician $25 or more. About 1 in 7 of the mothers reporting inadequate care paid over $25. For the confinement fee alone only about 1 mother in 14 of those who reported paid $25 or over. None of the mothers who paid the attendant physician less than $10 received any postnatal care; approximately 28 per cent of those who paid $10 to $25 received postnatal care; and 10 of the 16 mothers who paid over $25 received postnatal care. The distance which the physician had to travel seemed to be a factor of no importance in the expense. Distances were small compared to those found in Montana,[3] where the physician's fee for mileage was sometimes greater than his fee for service. No instance was discovered in this study of a physician's making a charge for transportation or mileage.

Approximately two-thirds of those reporting payment to a midwife paid her less than $5 and in only 3 instances was the charge over $10. It is natural, therefore, that the poorer and the more ignorant families should employ the midwife rather than the physician whose fees were higher. One Negro mother stated frankly that she had tried both and preferred the midwife because she did more and charged less. The midwife's fees varied somewhat according to the difficulty of the case, the distance from the patient, and the ability of the family to pay. One midwife said she charged more for boys than for girls because "boys are harder to handle and mothers want them more."

In many cases there were informal arrangements such as exchange of services, and payments in chickens, pigs, grain, and other produce instead of money payments. One mother said she gave the midwife a bottle of snuff (valued at 25 cents) for confinement care, including nursing and help with the housework. About one-half of the white mothers and almost 95 per cent of the colored who reported on costs of confinement said that they went to no expense for nursing and housework; some of these may be included in the 71 who paid the midwife a lump sum for confinement and nursing, or in the 34 who paid her a lump sum for confinement, nursing, and housework. Many families settled the debt on a neighborly give-and-take basis which involved no money payment. One father worked his sister's crops a few days to pay her for helping his wife at confinement; another gave his wife's sister a bottle of snuff in return for her services. Negro help was often paid in left-overs from the table, milk, or second-hand clothing. Rates per week for nursing and housework varied from 50 cents to $5 or (in a few cases) more. The usual prices were $1.50, $2, or $2.50 a week. Nearly one-half the 136 white mothers who stated a definite charge for nursing and housework reported less than $5, 26 reported costs of $10 to $25, and six reported costs of over $25 for these services. Of the 20 colored mothers who paid for nursing and housework, 9 paid less than $2.50 and only 5 paid $5 or more.

Cost of confinement and economic status of family.—The percentage of white families who reported a total confinement cost of $25 or more was higher among farm owners than among farm tenants, and higher among owners of the 100 to 500 acre plantations than among the farm owners as a whole. More than one-third of the white half-

---

[3] U. S. Children's Bureau Publication No. 34, Maternity Care and the Welfare of Young Children in a Homesteading County in Montana, pp. 49, 50.

share tenants reported charges of less than $10, while about one-fifth of all white families reported charges of less than $10. The percentage of those receiving free care was much higher among half-share tenants than among any other economic group. In general the mothers of the well-to-do white families got better care than the mothers in the poorer families because they were better able to pay for it. The doctor's bill was a big item to the poorer tenant, and in many cases ignorance and poverty combined to make him feel that a physician's services during pregnancy and at confinement were an unjustifiable expense to be incurred only in cases of unusual emergency.

One Negro mother had been miserable throughout her pregnancy; she could scarcely walk, her feet were swollen, and she had to kneel in order to hoe. She seemed pitifully eager for relief, but said she could not afford to have a physician. "If I had a doctor, then when winter came there would be nothing for clothes. Poor families can't have such things as doctors." This mother had been hurt by a falling tree two months before the interview, but was still doing her house and field work, although unable to walk without the help of two homemade crutches.

Share tenants usually depended upon the landlord to advance credit for the doctor's bill and to deduct it, with interest, from the crops sold at harvest time.

MATERNAL MORTALITY.

Maternal deaths in the county.—Three mothers of the 675 for whom information was secured for this study lost their lives in childbirth, two from puerperal septicemia and one from hemorrhage following confinement. The care received by the three mothers who died was, on the whole, no better and no worse than that received by most of the mothers visited whose confinements did not terminate fatally. None of the three mothers had received any prenatal care. All did their washing, housework, and other chores up to the time of confinement and none had trained or even partly trained nursing care. Only one was attended by a physician at confinement, and in this case the mother died of hemorrhage which began after the attending physician, the only doctor within a radius of 8 or 9 miles, had hurried away on another call. One of the other mothers was attended by a neighbor because the physician who was sent for had to come 5 miles over rough roads and was an hour late; she died of puerperal septicemia about four weeks later. The other case was that of a Negro mother whose baby was born while the father was on his way for the midwife. She did not arrive until two hours later, when she found the mother and baby shivering on the floor. The mother died a few days later.

By the death of these three mothers 13 children were left motherless. Eleven were white and 2 were colored, and 10 of them were under 7 years of age.

Deaths from causes other than childbirth.—Eleven mothers who had been confined during the period covered by the survey died from causes other than childbirth before the date of the inquiry, 10 of them within eight months after confinement. In nine of these cases pregnancy and childbirth may be considered a contributing factor in hastening death. Five died from tuberculosis, all of them colored women. One mother, also colored, died of pellagra, the mortality from which is relatively high among women of child-bearing age.[4] The death of one white mother four days after the delivery of a stillborn child was ascribed to pernicious malaria. Two mothers, one white and one colored, died from nephritis, one about two months after the baby was born, the other about four months after. Two of these mothers had prenatal care of " inadequate " grade (see p. 24) ; the others had none at all. Four were attended at confinement by physicians, 5 by midwives. The deaths of these women left 40 children motherless.

Of the last babies of these mothers, 1 was stillborn, and 4 of the 8 live-born babies died under 4 months of age. One died of an intestinal disturbance two weeks after the mother's death. Another died while his mother was on a journey to see a doctor 30 miles away. One baby whose mother was too ill to nurse him " just got peakeder and peakeder and finally was nothing but skin and bone." The fourth death was that of a tuberculous mother who had been unable to nurse the baby.

---

[4] Report of the Board of Health of Mississippi, 1915–1917, p. 344, Jackson, Miss., 1918.

MOTHERS' WORK IN RELATION TO CHILDBEARING.

USUAL FARM AND HOUSEHOLD WORK.

Farm work.—Most of the mothers had been reared in the country and were used to doing farm chores and field work as well as housework. Women reported doing almost every kind of field work which was to be done—plowing, harrowing, hoeing, chopping, and cotton picking. About 85 per cent of the white mothers reported that their principal occupation before marriage had been farm work of some kind, and about 70 per cent had done field work; 8 per cent had been teachers, and a few had been employed in stores, cotton mills, or offices. Nearly all the colored mothers had done field work before marriage; a few had worked as domestic servants. About five-eighths of the mothers did field work during the period covered by the survey, and practically all of these had done farm work of some kind before marriage. Somewhat more than one-fourth of the mothers who, as girls, had worked in the fields were relieved of field work during the period studied, this being due in some instances to poor health, in others to pressure of household work, or to higher income which made it unnecessary for the mother to work in the fields. One father said he had taken work as a farm laborer rather than as a tenant so that his wife would not have to work in the fields.

The importance of the different kinds of chores as indicated by the number of mothers reporting them was as follows: (1) Care of chickens, (2) care of garden, (3) carrying water, (4) churning, (5) milking, (6) care of stock, and (7) running the cream separator. Only one-tenth of those who reported doing chores were doing less than three of those listed above, and more than one-half were doing five or more. On the whole, the Negro mothers had fewer chores to do than the white mothers, probably because a smaller proportion of the Negro families kept cows, pigs, or chickens. It was customary in most families for the women to take care of the chickens, and for the men to attend to feeding the cattle and work animals. Most of the mothers who reported care of stock took care of the pigs only.

About 79 per cent of the white mothers carried water for household use; for nearly one-half of these women the source of water supply was less than 25 feet from the house, but for more than one-fourth it was 300 feet or more from the house. About 54 per cent had a pulley or windlass to draw up the water bucket; about 40 per

cent had to dip water from the spring or pull it up from the well
by hand; only 6 of the 222, the total number reporting, had a pump.
Eighty-five per cent of the Negro mothers reported carrying water
as a regular chore. The distance averaged a little higher than those
reported by the white mothers, as more than two-thirds carried water
25 feet or more, for two-fifths the source of water supply was 300
feet or more from the house, and about 1 in 8 had to carry water a
quarter of a mile. The proportion (49 per cent) of mothers reporting
no equipment for drawing water was higher among the Negroes.

Household conveniences [1] **and household help.**—Housekeeping in
most homes was rather primitive. Some of the houses were very
barely furnished, with two or three splint-bottomed chairs, a bed, a
bench, and a rough-board table. Some mothers did most of the
cooking at an open fireplace. Of the white mothers, only 15 per cent
had more than two household conveniences, and 20 per cent had none
at all; of the colored mothers, none had more than two, and 56 per
cent had none at all. The abundance of cheap colored labor had
induced many white families to hire cheap hand labor rather than to
purchase labor-saving devices.

Sewing machines were the only modern convenience in general
use, yet only 75 per cent of the white mothers and 42 per cent of
the colored mothers had them. Eight white mothers had water in
the house, and 2 of these had a bath and sink also; 14 mothers had
washing machines and 13 had refrigerators. Many said that they
kept food cool by letting it down in the well, putting it in the spring,
or in a tub of cold water. Kerosene lamps were used for lighting in
all the homes visited. Eighty-six families had telephones and 14
had automobiles. In only 77 homes were there screens at all the
doors and windows. While screening is primarily a health precaution, it also saved the mother much annoyance from chickens, pigs,
dogs, and cats, which otherwise came in at will. It was not unusual
for the agent's interview with the mother to be interrupted while the
pig was pushed out of the door or the chickens " shooed " away from
the table.

Forty-three per cent of all mothers reported that they had some
help with the housework all the year round (as distinguished from
help during pregnancy and confinement). Three-fourths of these
mothers received help from some other member of the household—a
mother, sister, or grown daughter, who was living with the family.

---

[1] Conveniences tabulated were as follows: Water in house, bath, sink, washing machine, sewing machine, refrigerator or ice box, iceless refrigerator, fireless cooker, bread
mixer, vacuum cleaner, oil stove, furnace, gas or electric lights, engine for household use,
telephone, screens for all doors and windows, and automobile. While an automobile is
not strictly a household convenience, it was so classed because it made it so much easier
for the mother to get to market, to see her neighbors, and to reach help in time of
trouble.

Such arrangements were seldom made on a money basis, and were usually independent of the economic status of the family. Of the 123 white mothers who usually had help with the housework, nearly half had hired help. While the proportion of Negro mothers who usually had some help with the housework was slightly higher than among white mothers, none of them hired such help.

For many families the only housework for which outside help was hired was laundry work. About 88 per cent of all mothers reported that they did their own washing. The washing was usually done out of doors near the well or spring; the water was heated in a large iron kettle over the outdoor fire and the clothes were boiled over this fire.

Under the system of tenant labor on the large plantations the planter's wife was not responsible for boarding or housing the field hands. The tenant farmers and most of the farm laborers lived in houses by themselves and boarded themselves. Hired men who lived with their employer's family on a basis of social equality were practically unknown, since the great bulk of hired labor was Negro. Even the domestic servants usually lived in separate houses with their own families.

WORK DURING PREGNANCY AND AFTER CONFINEMENT.

The health of the mother and baby may be impaired by excessive work during pregnancy or too soon after confinement. Ordinary housework and the lighter farm chores are a very good form of exercise if they are not carried to the point of fatigue, do not involve heavy lifting or straining, and are not resumed too soon after delivery. It is important, therefore, to know what period of rest the mother had before delivery and how soon after confinement she had to resume full responsibility of her usual work. The time which these mothers actually spent in bed has already been discussed (see p. 30).

Mothers who could not afford to hire help and were unable to make other arrangements could not secure the desirable period of rest before and after the baby's birth. Pressure of work in the busy cotton-picking season, when all hands are in the fields, often made it hard for the mother to get help.

Emergencies similar to the following were not unknown: A mother confined in January said that during the latter part of her pregnancy her husband was taken ill, and the family was obliged to move to make room for other tenants. The mother had to assume the whole burden of moving and settling in the new home. She cut enough wood to last throughout the period of her confinement, and when labor pains began she was building a hogpen.

A few of the white mothers left home for confinement, in most cases to stay with relatives, where facilities for maternity care differed little from those in their own homes, but where they could secure a more complete relief from responsibility for the housework during the period of confinement.

Kind of household help secured.—Many of the mothers reported that it was difficult to get reliable persons to help with the housework while they were incapacitated. Only 28 per cent of the white mothers and 5 per cent of the colored reported hired help for housework. Over 35 per cent of all mothers reported free help given by an outsider. Neighbors were usually ready to come in to help when they were needed. One mother said that she and her sister who lived near had agreed that when either was pregnant the other would do the washing for both families. While there were no mothers who reported no help at all with the housework, five of the white and nine of the colored mothers said that the only help they had was from a child less than 14 years old. Such help relieved the mother of the actual work, but it did not relieve her of the responsibility. In 9 per cent of the white families and 14 per cent of the Negro families, the housework was done by the husband or son; 21 per cent of the white mothers and 41 per cent of the Negro mothers reported help given by some other adult member of the household.

Relief from work before confinement.—Of the white mothers less than one-fifth reported any relief from housework before confinement and less than one-tenth reported a relief of one month or more; about 96 per cent did some farm chores during pregnancy and 80 per cent reported no cessation before delivery. If the mother's work was lightened at all during the latter part of pregnancy it was likely to be done by relief from washing or field work. About 76 per cent of the white mothers did the washing during pregnancy, and 29 per cent of these stopped one month or more before the baby was born. Eighty-four white mothers, less than 30 per cent, reported field work during pregnancy; 39 of these had a rest of three months or more before confinement; 4 had from a week's to a month's rest; and 18 worked in the field up to the day of confinement.

Cessation of work before delivery was even less common among the Negro mothers. Approximately 93 per cent reported that they did their usual housework up to the time labor began; 89 per cent had no relief from farm chores; 79 per cent had none from washing, and nearly 40 per cent did field work up to the time of confinement. One of the Negro mothers who was confined in the cotton-picking season said she worked in a field 2 miles from home during the last day of her pregnancy; she "just did make it home" that night, but was unable to get supper for the family. Of the 320 Negro mothers who did field work during pregnancy, only 70 stopped one to three months before confinement, and only 79 three months or more.

Approximately 75 per cent of the white and 94 per cent of the colored mothers did housework, washing, and chores during pregnancy, and of these 62 per cent of the white and 79 per cent of the colored reported no cessation of any of the three kinds of work before confinement. Twenty-nine per cent of the white and 81 per cent of the colored mothers did field work in addition to their housework, washing, and chores, and of these mothers 20 per cent of the white and 42 per cent of the colored reported no cessation before confinement. The one mother who had no one to attend her at delivery hoed corn the whole day before confinement. She came home a little early and the baby was born. Her husband was still in the field and she could not get word to him.

Approximately 75 per cent of the white mothers reported cessation of some kind of work (housework, washing, chores, or field work) a month or more before confinement, and nearly 50 per cent a cessation of three months or more. Among Negro mothers nearly 50 per cent reported relief from at least one kind of work a month or more before confinement, and 27 per cent a relief of three months or more.

Resumption of work after confinement.—Among white mothers, 83 per cent reported that they resumed their usual housework less than six weeks after confinement; 19 per cent resumed it less than two weeks after. Only about 1 in 7 had a relief from housework of six weeks or more after confinement. One mother said that although she always had a hard time at confinement, she had to be up and doing all her housework within a week afterwards. Another mother who had a difficult delivery had been obliged to get up to look after the other children when the baby was 1 week old. The weather was very cold, but the family had to move when the baby was 3 weeks old because someone else was taking possession. About 75 per cent of the white mothers began to do chores less than six weeks after confinement, and nearly one-half of these began at less than four weeks. Nearly 40 per cent began to do their washing within the first six weeks; about 32 per cent of the 145 white mothers confined in the first year of the period did not do their washing in the year after the baby was born. Only seven of the white mothers worked in the field during the first six weeks after confinement. Slightly over one-fifth did field work in the year after confinement.

The proportion of mothers who resumed housework and chores in the first six weeks after confinement was approximately the same for white and Negro. Sixty-two per cent of the colored mothers began to do their washing less than six weeks after confinement, and

14 per cent began less than four weeks after. Twenty-two per cent did field work in the first six weeks after confinement. Following the tradition expressed by one mother who said, "I stayed out of the field my month," all but six did no field work during the first four weeks after confinement.

The mothers who had no rest from work before confinement were also the ones who had to begin work soon after confinement. About 75 per cent of the white and 80 per cent of the Negro mothers reported not only no relief from housework before confinement, but also resumption at less than six weeks after. Thirty-six per cent of the white mothers resumed their housework, washing, and chores less than six weeks after the baby was born, and 2 per cent had also resumed field work. Fifty-seven per cent of the Negro mothers had resumed housework, washing, and chores less than six weeks after confinement; slightly over 10 per cent resumed it at less than four weeks. In addition, field work had been resumed by 18 per cent of the Negro mothers at less than six weeks after the baby's birth.

Many mothers gave accounts of the ill effects of heavy work. One said she thought her baby had been born prematurely because of the heavy work she had been doing in the field in addition to her housework, washing, and chores. She stayed in bed 10 days after the baby was born, and in three weeks began to work in the field again. She endured the strain for a week, then had to give up, and was incapacitated for a month.

Effect of farming season on mothers' work.—In agricultural communities the work in the house is intimately correlated with the work in the fields, and pressure of work in the busy farming season is likely to mean additional work for the mother. Even if she does not go into the fields to work herself, her husband and older children have less time in which to help with the chores and housework. One mother who was confined in the winter said that although she was up in six days, she stayed in the warmest room most of the time for the next two weeks, while her husband did the housework. Another said that although she was feeling well, her husband did the work for three weeks after the baby was born, because he had no work to do in the fields at the time.

The climate was such that for only about two and one-half months in the year was it impossible to work in the fields. The busiest seasons were in May and June (hoeing time for cotton and corn), and in October and November (picking time in the cotton fields). Each season was likely to spread over two weeks before and after, and it varied with the weather and the size of the crop. Accordingly, the slack season may be considered as extending from the middle of

June to the middle of September, and from the middle of December to the middle of April.

In the case of white families the extent to which the mother might be relieved of overstrain during pregnancy and the weeks following confinement usually depended on the financial ability of the family to hire help, though in some instances economic conditions made no difference one way or the other; because the mother had relatives who came to help her; or because she was wholly incapacitated and had to be relieved whether she could afford it or not; or because at the time no help could be secured. Very few Negro families could afford to pay money to relieve the mother of her usual duties during pregnancy and after confinement.

CARE OF CHILDREN.

The connection is more or less obvious between the various subjects of the study taken up thus far—maternity care, work of the mother, housing and sanitation, and economic conditions—and the question of the welfare of the child. The lack of specialists and hospital facilities was as serious for the babies as for the mothers, and poorly built, insanitary houses made living conditions dangerous for the one as well as for the other. In this section of the report infant deaths and those elements of child care not already touched upon—feeding customs, care of sick children, home remedies used for children, etc.—will be considered.

BIRTH REGISTRATION.

Complete birth registration is a prerequisite to any adequate study of infant mortality and child welfare. Since 1912, when the State passed a law establishing a bureau of vital statistics under the State board of health, and providing for the registration of births and deaths, the board of health had been working toward complete registration, but at the time of this survey no part of the State had been admitted to the birth-registration area, and only the five largest cities to the death registration area. Only 50 per cent of the births included in this study were registered. One of the greatest obstacles to good birth registration in the county was the difficulty of getting the midwives to register births. Many of the colored midwives were illiterate, and therefore had to get some one else to fill out the certificate or report by word of mouth when they happened to go to town. Often the names were written on old crumpled slips of paper and were almost illegible. While the midwives were responsible for the greater part of the unregistered births, only 76 per cent of the births attended by physicians were registered. Only 71 per cent of the infant deaths were registered.

INSTRUCTION IN INFANT CARE.

A general lack of knowledge of child care prevailed among the mothers visited, as very few of them had received any instruction in this matter beyond what they learned from their mothers or from their own experience. Only 20 had received some instruction from a physician and 2 had been advised by a trained nurse. Fifty-eight had learned something of infant care through reading, but the high percentage of illiteracy and low standards of education prevailing in the county made instruction through reading practically unattainable for a large proportion of mothers in poor white as well as in Negro families. The literature read, however, was not really instructive in all cases, for while 2 had read books by Holt, 1 a bulletin from the Department of Agriculture, and 25 current magazines and papers, the rest had read only advertising pamphlets or almanacs or "doctor books" of one kind or another. Many mothers were very glad to receive the Children's Bureau pamphlet on Infant Care.

The methods of caring for children were in accordance with the customs handed down by other generations. The midwife's advice was often sought, especially in regard to the care of the baby during the first few days of life, and the midwives were credited with being responsible for encouraging dangerous methods of feeding and the use of filthy and dangerous home remedies.

FEEDING CUSTOMS.

The almost universal custom of breast feeding among the country mothers in the county studied probably counteracted in many instances methods of feeding unwise in other respects. The tendency of the mothers was to nurse their babies not only through the first year, but also through most of the second year or even longer. Artificial feeding was haphazard and unscientific. In many cases it included the whole range of family diet—meat, corn bread, pie, etc. Some mothers did not use cow's milk because the "bitter weed" that the cows ate made the milk bitter in taste, although not, so far as could be learned, unwholesome.

Breast feeding.—The often-repeated criticism of the feeding customs of rural mothers that they feed their babies from the table at too early an age and delay weaning too long held true in the case of the mothers included in this study. Only 14 per cent of all infants, both white and colored, for whom information was secured, were weaned before the middle of the twelfth month; two-thirds were nursed through the greater part of the fifteenth month; nearly one-half through the eighteenth month; and one-fourth through the greater part of the twenty-first month. Nine infants were nursed through the greater part of the twenty-fourth month or longer.

One instance was found at one of the children's health conferences of a child six years old who was still nursing.

The Negro mothers showed a tendency to wean their babies a little earlier than the white mothers; by the middle of the eighteenth month 63 per cent of the Negro babies had been weaned as compared with only 41 per cent of the white babies. Of the babies receiving exclusive breast feeding, the percentage was higher in each month of age for white than for colored babies; for babies receiving some breast feeding, at the sixth month the percentage was slightly higher for Negro than for white; and at 9 months the percentage (92) was about the same for both races.

Solid food and family diet.—Artificial feeding may be necessary in some cases at an early age, and, while not so good for the baby as breast feeding, does not necessarily obviate the possibility of normal development. Experts generally agree that fresh, clean, modified cow's milk is the best substitute for mother's milk, and that no solid food should be given during the first six months at least. Only one-fourth of the babies studied were receiving a strictly liquid diet at 2 months. The solid food included bread or crackers soaked in milk, gravy, or cereals, and did not necessarily include the kind of food eaten by the older members of the family. However, many mothers reported that the baby at an early age was given "tastes" of everything that the mother ate. One mother said with pride that her baby had eaten "everything" since she was 11 days old and had had all the meat she wanted since 2 months old. Another said there was nothing too hot with pepper or too sour for her 14-months-old baby to eat. Eight per cent of the mothers reported that the baby had been given family diet when less than 1 month old, 15 per cent at 2 months, and over half at 7 months. Only about 6 per cent were reported as 12 months or more of age before receiving family diet.

The tendency to give the baby solid food or family diet was more pronounced among colored mothers than among white. At the fourth month 60 per cent of the colored babies were receiving solid food as compared with slightly under 35 per cent of the white babies. Under the eighth month the percentage of colored babies receiving family diet was higher than that of white babies receiving solid food. At the end of the twelfth month nearly 80 per cent of the colored babies were receiving family diet as compared with about 60 per cent of the white babies.

CHILDREN'S ILLNESSES.

Medical care.—The accounts given by the mothers of their children's illnesses indicated the difficulties in caring for sick children in these rural districts. Children's specialists and hospitals were too far away and too expensive to be thought of by any but the most prosperous parents, and many of the poorer families living in remote parts of the county hesitated to call a doctor unless the child seemed very seriously ill. As one mother said: "A farmer only gets money twice a year, and if the children get sick between seasons they have to get along."

One mother said that her baby began to have indigestion at two months; he vomited frequently and had spasms. These symptoms continued for over three months, but the doctor was called only once. Another mother said that her baby had been ill for three weeks with some trouble in the head; she bathed the baby's head with camphor and put sweet oil in her ears but did not call a physician.

Only the two county seats had more than one physician, and families out of reach of one or the other of these towns often had to send 15 or 20 miles for the nearest physician available. Although under ordinary circumstances a doctor could be secured in two or three hours at most, there were, of course, times when this was not possible, and sometimes serious complications developed so rapidly in babies and young children that even a short delay proved serious or even fatal. The baby of a family living 4 miles from the doctor in a house back in the woods, almost inaccessible from the main road, became sick when 6 days old. The father consulted the physician by telephone, and medicine was sent, but the baby died the following day.

Nursing care.—Trained nurses were no more available for sick children than they were for mothers at confinement, and, as in other rural areas, home care was the rule when children were ill. Emergencies frequently arose when there was really acute need for trained, or even practical, nurses. One mother said that when the baby was born both the father and the other children had measles. It was an unusually severe winter. No nurse could be found nor could they get domestic help. A neighbor came in once a day for a little while, but she was too busy with her own family cares to do much. The oldest child died about a week after the baby's birth. In another case, all the members of a family were ill at the time of the mother's confinement. The father, though convalescent, was not able to do much, and as a last resort his brother came in and did the housework. In another family the mother and four children were ill with malaria. The father had to do the nursing and housework himself while he hired cotton pickers to take his place in the fields, field laborers being much easier to find than nurses and housekeepers.

Situations similar to these described were likely to be brought about whenever the mother was incapacitated. Many mothers had no one who could take their place as nurse, because relatives and neighbors were entirely occupied with their own family affairs, and furthermore many of the women, although willing to do their utmost, lacked skill and experience in the proper care of children seriously ill.

Deformities.—Several children needed special attention on account of some deformity. One white baby had deformed feet. The father had given up his farm and secured work with the railroad in order that he might earn money and perhaps secure a railroad pass to take the child to a specialist and have the deformity corrected. A mother was most anxious to know what ought to be done for her year-old baby who had a deformed hand and wrist. She brought the child to one of the children's health conferences, and the Government physician said that some manipulation and massage would do a great deal of good, but unfortunately there was no one in the county who could do it. One baby had club feet and his father, a Negro farm hand earning $19.50 a month, had never taken him to a physician. Another Negro boy about 6 years old had a stiff knee and back so that he could not stand upright and could scarcely walk. His mother said that his condition was caused by paralysis from which he suffered while teething. The family owned a small farm on the river bottom, but had never considered it possible to take the boy to Memphis or Jackson. In several other cases similar to these the need for special medical attention seemed imperative if the children were to have a fair chance in life. A public health nurse could do much toward teaching parents that it is possible to have deformities corrected and toward making the necessary arrangements with specialists and hospitals.

Accidents.—Children everywhere are liable to injury from accidents of one kind or another. But in Mississippi accidents occurring while the parents are absent in the fields are far too common. The secretary of the board of health, in commenting on the large number of deaths from burning, said: "This carelessness which resulted in the death and suffering of so many children for the last two years * * * should be given thorough study and means provided, if possible, to reduce this unnecessary mortality."[2] As the open fireplace was used for cooking in many of the cabins, the danger from fire was serious at all times of the year. It was not uncommon to find a little baby left alone in its crib while its mother was off in the fields at work. One colored mother told of the death of her oldest son from burns. She had no one to leave him with while she went out in the field to plant potatoes. Presently she heard him scream, and rushed back to find his clothing all afire. In one family visited, the baby had no toes on the right foot. The mother ex-

---

[2] Report of the Board of Health of Mississippi, 1915–1917, p. 107. Jackson, Miss., 1918.

plained that she had left the baby on the floor while she went out
for a little while, and that when she came back she found that the
baby, then 6 months old, had crawled to the fireplace and one little
foot was in the coals.

The custom of leaving infants in the care of older children too
young to accompany their mothers to the field is bound to lead to
serious results. During the hoeing season the Children's Bureau
agents often found no one at home but a little 6 or 7 year old child in
charge of one or two younger children. Sometimes he could point
in the direction in which his mother had gone, sometimes he did not
seem to know where she was. One mother left the baby with the
older children while she went to work. The baby's dress caught
fire and he was badly burned. Accidents of other kinds occurred
while older brothers or sisters were tending the baby. One baby
had been sick since the older children in their play let him fall out
of bed while the mother was working in the field. Another mother
said her baby had been very sick when 12 months old. She thought
"the children might a' dropped the baby" while she was in the
field. Such accidents as these described were more common among
Negro babies because the Negro mothers did more field work than
the white mothers. Some mothers tried to solve the problem by
taking the babies with them to the field, but with no shelter from the
hot sun this arrangement did not seem very satisfactory.

Illnesses.—The accounts of children's diseases given by the mothers
did not differ very much from those given by mothers in other parts
of the country. Colds, indigestion, and colic were mentioned frequently. In the winter previous to the survey there had been mild
epidemics of measles and whooping cough with no effective quarantine regulations. The children were, of course, liable to the diseases
peculiar to the South—malaria, hookworm, and pellagra. One
physician said he had noticed a decided tendency among mothers to
attribute almost any illness which children had to "worms" and to
persist in the belief contrary to the doctor's diagnosis. Several
mothers said that their children had had worms and that they had
used various home remedies, turpentine, soot tea, castor oil, etc.

Home remedies for children.—The great extent to which the
mothers in the area "doctored" their children presented one of the
most serious phases of child care. Home remedies have a legitimate
place in every household, but stories told by many of the mothers
indicated a widespread tendency toward overdosing and unwise selection of drugs for the home medicine chest. Patent medicines were
in common use, particularly among white mothers. The colored
mothers made frequent use of teas of one kind or another. More
or less superstition was evident in the remedies recommended by
colored mothers. The midwife instead of the doctor was frequently

summoned in case of illness, and she was often responsible for the extravagant use of home remedies.

INFANT DEATHS.[3]

In any locality where the birth and death registration is as incomplete as in the rural areas surveyed by the Children's Bureau, it is impossible to discover all births during a given period even by a house-to-house canvass. The number of omissions is probably proportionately greater for stillborn infants and babies who died early in the period included in the canvass than for the others. The returns are especially likely to be incomplete in districts similar to the county studied in Mississippi where many families live on farms remote from the traveled roads, and a large part of the population is shifting and illiterate. As a consequence, infant mortality rates for the area studied, while as accurate as any that could be secured, are somewhat lower than they would be if returns for deaths had been as complete as for births. On the other hand, figures based not on a canvass but on birth and death registration alone are likely to exaggerate death rates since death registration is usually more complete than birth registration.

Of 155 white children born alive to the mothers interviewed, 12 died in the first year of life. This number includes only children born between April 1, 1916, and March 31, 1917, the first year of the period covered by the study, since most of the children born later than that were less than 1 year old at the time the information was secured. The infant mortality rate for these white children was 77.4,[4] a rate lower than was discovered in any of the cities surveyed, but high as compared with rates for other rural districts studied. The rate found in Kansas was 40 to 1,000 live births;[5] the rate among white infants in the lowland county of North Carolina was 48.1;[6] in the mountain county of North Carolina the rate was 80.4;[6] the rate in Wisconsin was 54.[7] The rate in Montana (although based upon an incomplete record of deaths) was 71 per 1,000.[8]

---

[3] Detailed information in regard to maternal and infant care was secured only for the last confinement of each mother; in considering infant deaths, however, all the births occurring in the two years covered by the survey were included. Thus while detailed information was secured for only 664 live births, 699 live births occurred to the mothers visited during the two years covered by the survey. Six deaths occurred among these 35 nonschedule births.

[4] As in previous studies made by the Children's Bureau the rate is computed on the basis of the number of deaths at less than 1 year of age among infants born in the given period.

[5] Children's Bureau Publication No. 26, Maternity and Infant Care in a Rural County in Kansas, p. 40.

[6] Children's Bureau Publication No. 33, Rural Children in Selected Counties of North Carolina, p. 36.

[7] Children's Bureau Publication No. 46, Maternity and Infant Care in Two Rural Counties in Wisconsin, p. 69.

[8] Children's Bureau Publication No. 34, Maternity Care and the Welfare of Young Children in a Homesteading County in Montana, p. 70.

The accuracy of the infant mortality rate for Negro infants is open to more question than the rate for white, because of the greater obstacles to a complete canvass among Negro families. Therefore, for purposes of comparison, infant mortality rates are more sound which are based upon the whole maternity histories of the white and Negro mothers while resident in the area. Even these rates are likely to be an understatement of infant mortality, because mothers who had had many confinements often became confused as to the number and may have forgotten at the time to tell of the babies who died in early infancy. Since this was particularly true of Negro mothers, the figures show also an understatement of the difference between rates for white and Negro infants. The rate among white infants was 61.2 per 1,000 live births, while the rate for Negro infants was 107.3—a difference of 46.1 in favor of infants born to white mothers.

Medical care.—One of the most significant aspects of infant mortality was the small proportion of deaths attended by physicians. Information was secured as to the attendant at death for 43 of the babies who died at less than 1 year of age; only 15 were attended at death by a physician. Only 5 of the 9 white babies who died under 2 weeks of age were attended at death by a physician, and only 4 of the 6 who died over 2 weeks of age were attended by a physician. Of the 28 Negro babies who died at less than 1 year of age, only 6 were attended by a physician.

The proportion of deaths not attended by physicians was too large to be explained entirely by bad roads, poor telephone service, the distance of the family home from the physician, or by the fact that in some instances the baby died so suddenly that there was no time to call a physician. Parents often failed to realize that their children were sick, and did not appreciate the necessity of securing the best medical care possible for them.

One baby was sick for two days before death; her mother said "she seemed to have griping in the stomach and the stretches." The mother cut red onions and bound them on the child's hands and feet, but did not call a physician. Another Negro mother said she thought her baby died because she "couldn't keep the hives out on him." She said the baby was born "puny" because she had hoed right up to the time of confinement in very hot weather. This mother had had no prenatal care, a midwife had attended her at confinement, and no physician had been called for the baby. A white mother whose husband had not been able to get a physician for her confinement said that her baby had not been normal from birth, and he died when 6 days old. She seemed satisfied with the midwife's explanation that "the hives went in on it." This family lived only 3 miles from a town with six physicians in it. One colored mother said that her baby had a hemorrhage from the navel shortly after birth, and that by the time they had brought the midwife back to tie the cord again, the baby had bled to death. Two colored babies died of whooping cough without the attention of a physician.

Causes of death.—Discussion of the causes of death is hampered at the outset by lack of complete registration. For 14 of the 49 infant deaths occurring in the period no death certificate was filed, and in 20 instances, although a death certificate was filed, no cause of death was entered on it. For only 15 cases could a physician's certificate showing cause of death be secured. Eight of these deaths were due to natal or prenatal causes (four of the eight to prematurity), and five to gastro-intestinal diseases.

Among white infants who died under 2 weeks of age the death rate per 1,000 live births was 40. The stillbirth rate, based on all births in the area studied, to mothers interviewed was 2 per cent for white infants and 4 per cent for Negro. About one-tenth of all pregnancies of both white and colored mothers resulted in miscarriage, a stillbirth, or a live-born infant that survived less than 2 weeks.

Obstetricians agree that most of the deaths under 2 weeks of age are due to prenatal and natal causes and can be prevented in large measure by good prenatal care and skilled care at confinement. In rural communities, where few mothers receive any prenatal care at all and where skilled help is not available, it is to be expected that the number of deaths in early infancy will be comparatively large. Reports on prenatal care were secured from 40 mothers whose babies were stillborn or died under 2 weeks of age. Only eight had any care, and only one had care that could be classified as fair; five of those who had care sought medical advice because they were ill during pregnancy. Information was secured also in regard to the kind of attendant present at 21 of the confinements resulting in a live-born infant who survived less than 2 weeks. Six of the 9 confinements of white mothers were attended by a physician and 3 by a widwife or other woman; 2 of the 12 confinements of Negro mothers were attended by a physician and 10 by a midwife or other woman. All 10 stillbirths to white mothers and only 1 of the 11 stillbirths to Negro mothers were attended by a physician.

Improper feeding also contributed to infant mortality in the county. One of the registered deaths occurred when the baby was about 2½ months old, about 2 weeks after the mother's death. Cow's milk had been used to supplement breast milk and the baby had been given solid food some time before his death. Another baby at 2 months of age had tastes of everything the family ate. The mother said that the baby had been bitten by mosquitoes a few days before its death and she attributed death to malaria rather than to improper feeding. Another baby weaned at 3 months of age died about four weeks later. The mother said she had tried cow's milk and then malted milk. She thought that the baby had measles, but the cause given on the death certificate was ileocolitis. Another mother said: " The baby was fine and healthy, but he had one of the spells I had at confinement (convulsions) and died of that and whooping cough."

CHILDREN'S HEALTH CONFERENCES.

In order to promote interest in child welfare, a series of children's health conferences were held in two counties in the State—in the county in which the intensive survey was made and in another located in the south central part of Mississippi which contains a city of more than 10,000 inhabitants known as one of the wealthiest cities in the South. This city was very progressive; it had well-paved streets, substantial public buildings, luxurious homes, good schools, and a good city hospital of 40 beds. Outside this city, however, the county was no more progressive than neighboring counties.

PREVIOUS PUBLIC HEALTH WORK.

An intensive sanitary survey of the southern county by the International Health Board (formerly the Rockefeller Sanitary Commission), in cooperation with the State board of health, had been completed in January, 1918, shortly before the children's health conferences began. As part of the work of the survey many persons were examined and treated for hookworm and many inoculated against typhoid. The survey also included a campaign for sanitary privies both in the city and in the rural districts of the county, and special attention was given to an educational campaign against pellagra.[9] The extensive public health work done through the sanitary survey made it possible to arrange for a series of children's health conferences with a minimum of effort and with some assurance of response from the parents.

During the previous year a birth registration test had been made in the city which disclosed the fact that about one-third of the births in the city were unregistered. The births of 22 per cent of the children brought to the children's health conferences were definitely reported as unregistered.

---

[9] Report of the Board of Health of Mississippi, 1915–1917, pp. 47–48 Jackson, Miss., 1918.

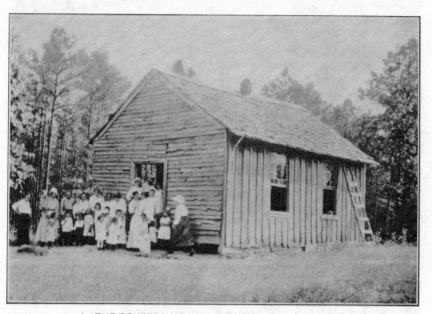

I.—THE CONFERENCE AT A COUNTRY SCHOOLHOUSE.

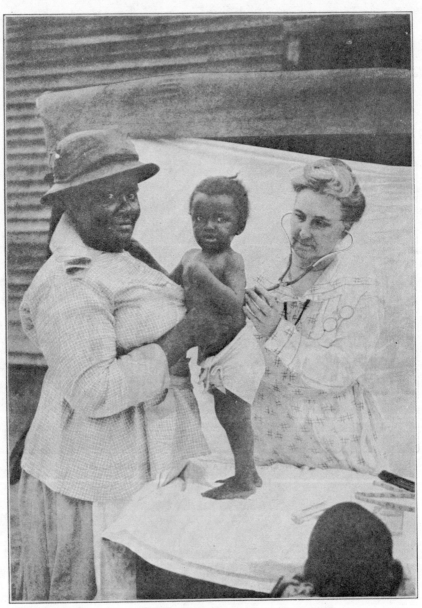

II.—AN EXAMINATION AT A NEGRO CONFERENCE.

ATTENDANCE AND PLACES OF MEETING.

The aggregate attendance at the 35 meetings held in the two counties was about 3,000. In both counties meetings were held in towns and in the country. Meetings were held in the courthouses of the county seats, in the country schoolhouses, in churches, one in an open-air pavilion in the picnicking center, and in one of the smaller towns the proprietor of a store suspended business for the afternoon and expressed pleasure in turning over his store "to the use of Uncle Sam." The babies were examined on the counter and stereopticon slides were shown in a dark corner at the back of the store. At some of the night meetings families straggled in late; having worked all day in the fields, they had then dressed the children, hitched up the horses, and driven to the conference.

EXAMINATION OF CHILDREN.

At these meetings children under 6 years of age were examined by a Government physician, and the results of the examination, together with special recommendations in regard to the care of the child, were written out and given to the person bringing the child for examination. In all, 544 children were examined by the physician, 375 white and 169 colored. If the examination revealed defects that needed special medical attention, the parents were told what was wrong and were advised to consult the family doctor. Measures were also recommended to promote better physical development. The advice given to many mothers concerned feeding alone. The physician explained to these mothers that they had been giving their children too much food, feeding them too often, or allowing them too much starchy food; and regularity of feeding and a well-balanced diet were recommended. At the end of one of the conferences one mother was heard to say emphatically that she would never have another case of "summer complaint" among her children.

EXHIBITS.

An exhibit was shown at some of the conferences of miniature models illustrating the proper clothing for a baby, baby's bed and mother's bed, and the equipment needed for bathing a baby and for preparing its food, and charts were shown illustrating various phases of child welfare. A small model of an iceless refrigerator and a homemade fireless cooker excited much interest. For conferences held at night, when neither models nor charts could be shown to advantage stereopticon slides were used. The men who attended the meetings often showed great interest in the exhibits, and said they were going to make play pens and separate beds for their babies and fireless cookers and iceless refrigerators for their wives.

RESULTS OF THE CONFERENCES.

The value of the conferences was primarily educational. The instruction received by individual parents was probably of no less importance than the impetus given to systematic public health work for mothers and children. The advisability of securing a full-time public health nurse for the county was widely discussed, and at many of the meetings the local committee circulated a petition to the county supervisors asking that such a nurse be employed. This movement was indorsed not only by parents but also by physicians and others prominent in the county. Several of the leaders among the colored people desired to secure a nurse to work among the colored people alone.

SUMMARY.

The intensive survey of maternity and child care was made in a farming section typical of northern Mississippi. Over one-half of the population was Negro, and three-fourths of the farmers visited were tenants.

Six hundred and seventy-five families were visited, and most of these were living in poorly constructed houses far too small to accommodate the whole family with any degree of comfort. Very few were plastered or ceiled on the interior, and about 40 per cent of the families were living two or more persons per room. Study of sanitary conditions disclosed the fact that only about one-fourth of the families had a privy of any kind, and of these over four-fifths had the insanitary open-back type. Only 11 per cent of the houses were adequately screened against flies and mosquitoes. Although it was possible to obtain good water by drilling deep wells, many families were using water from dug wells and from springs which were not well protected against surface pollution.

Investigation of the status of maternity care showed that the low standards were due in large measure to ignorance of the need of it, to the scarcity of physicians and nurses, and to poverty. There were 14 physicians in active practice in the area studied; there was no trained nurse working regularly in the county. The nearest hospital was 100 miles away. There were about 100 midwives practicing in the county, but a large majority of them were untrained, ignorant, and careless, and their methods were primitive and insanitary. While 79 per cent of the white women were attended at confinement by physicians, nearly 88 per cent of the colored women were attended by midwives.

Only 116 of the 675 mothers studied received any prenatal care; 9 of these received care that could be classed as fair, and only one received really adequate care. Less than one-tenth of the mothers attended by a physician received three or more calls from the doctor during the lying-in period; only 7 mothers had trained nurses; and less than one-fourth had care by a practical nurse or midwife. Most of the mothers had great difficulty in securing anyone to do the nursing or help with the housework, and the majority had to depend on relatives and neighbors. The lack of conveniences made housework a rather strenuous task, and almost all of the mothers were used to doing farm chores and field work as well as housework. As it was so very difficult to hire help, many of the mothers had neither adequate relief from work before confinement nor a sufficient period of rest afterwards.

Children as well as mothers suffered from the lack of skilled medical and nursing care. Frequently the parents failed to recognize that children were seriously ill, and they were content to use home remedies and advice from neighbors rather than to secure the best medical attention possible. Analysis of feeding customs showed that while the custom of breast feeding was almost universal the mothers tended to nurse their babies too long and give them solid food or the regular family diet too soon. Although about 85 per cent were wholly or partially breast fed during the first year, at the age of 6 months 65 per cent were receiving solid food and 47 per cent were given what the rest of the family ate. One-fifth of the children were still partially breast fed at 2 years of age.

Incomplete birth and death registration handicapped the authorities in studying the problem of infant mortality.

Standards of living were lower and the inadequacy of maternity and child care more extreme among the Negroes than among the white families. Only 8 per cent of the Negroes were farm owners, and about 57 per cent were half-share tenants—the lowest in the scale economically. Their homes were smaller and more crowded than those of the white families and sanitation was not so good. The percentage of illiteracy was high (26 per cent) among Negro mothers. Few Negro mothers had received any prenatal care or been attended by a physician at confinement. A larger proportion of Negro than of white mothers did field work, and they had less relief from work before confinement and a shorter period of rest afterwards.

Children's health conferences were held in two counties for the purpose of stimulating interest in public health activities. Children were examined by a Government physician, and exhibits were shown. The meetings had a large attendance and much interest was aroused.

In view of the conditions found to exist in the county it was evident that the most necessary steps in securing better care for the mothers and children were: The employment of a public health nurse for the county, and a county or district health officer on full time; the establishment of a county hospital, with free care available for those unable to pay; provision for the training and supervision of midwives; and the enforcement of the birth and death registration laws. In addition, it seemed imperative that steps should be taken to deal effectively with the problem of illiteracy which existed to a serious degree among the poor white and Negro families.

CONCLUSIONS.

The conditions revealed by this inquiry are by no means peculiar to the county studied; they are more or less typical of those existing in many rural communities. They call for a general constructive program for the conservation of the lives and health of mothers and babies, and of older children as well. Among the essential hygiene features of such a program are:

1. A county public health nurse (preferably one for white and one for colored), who, by doing educational work through the schools, clubs, and other organizations and by practical demonstrations of home nursing and preparation of food for babies, could accomplish much toward improving maternity and child care.

2. A well-trained public health official, devoting his entire attention to health problems in the county or the district of which it might form a part.

3. A county hospital conveniently located for all residents of the county.

4. The birth and death registration laws strictly enforced.

5. The law to prevent blindness in the new-born strictly enforced.

6. Midwifery practice controlled.

INDEX.

Family in America

AN ARNO PRESS / NEW YORK TIMES COLLECTION

Abbott, John S. C. **The Mother at Home:** Or, The Principles of Maternal Duty. 1834.

Abrams, Ray H., editor. **The American Family in World War II.** 1943.

Addams, Jane. **A New Conscience and an Ancient Evil.** 1912.

The Aged and the Depression: Two Reports, 1931–1937. 1972.

Alcott, William A. **The Young Husband.** 1839.

Alcott, William A. **The Young Wife.** 1837.

American Sociological Society. **The Family.** 1909.

Anderson, John E. **The Young Child in the Home.** 1936.

Baldwin, Bird T., Eva Abigail Fillmore and Lora Hadley. **Farm Children.** 1930.

Beebe, Gilbert Wheeler. **Contraception and Fertility in the Southern Appalachians.** 1942.

Birth Control and Morality in Nineteenth Century America: Two Discussions, 1859–1878. 1972.

Brandt, Lilian. **Five Hundred and Seventy-Four Deserters and Their Families.** 1905. Baldwin, William H. **Family Desertion and Non-Support Laws.** 1904.

Breckinridge, Sophonisba P. **The Family and the State:** Select Documents. 1934.

Calverton, V. F. **The Bankruptcy of Marriage.** 1928.

Carlier, Auguste. **Marriage in the United States.** 1867.

Child, [Lydia]. **The Mother's Book.** 1831.

Child Care in Rural America: Collected Pamphlets, 1917–1921. 1972.

Child Rearing Literature of Twentieth Century America, 1914–1963. 1972.

The Colonial American Family: Collected Essays, 1788–1803. 1972.

Commander, Lydia Kingsmill. **The American Idea.** 1907.

Davis, Katharine Bement. **Factors in the Sex Life of Twenty-Two Hundred Women.** 1929.

Dennis, Wayne. **The Hopi Child.** 1940.

Epstein, Abraham. **Facing Old Age.** 1922. New Introduction by Wilbur J. Cohen.

The Family and Social Service in the 1920s: Two Documents, 1921–1928. 1972.

Hagood, Margaret Jarman. **Mothers of the South.** 1939.

Hall, G. Stanley. **Senescence:** The Last Half of Life. 1922.

Hall, G. Stanley. **Youth:** Its Education, Regimen, and Hygiene. 1904.

Hathway, Marion. **The Migratory Worker and Family Life.** 1934.

Homan, Walter Joseph. **Children & Quakerism.** 1939.

Key, Ellen. **The Century of the Child.** 1909.

Kirchwey, Freda. **Our Changing Morality:** A Symposium. 1930.

Kopp, Marie E. **Birth Control in Practice.** 1934.

Lawton, George. **New Goals for Old Age.** 1943.

Lichtenberger, J. P. **Divorce:** A Social Interpretation. 1931.

Lindsey, Ben B. and Wainwright Evans. **The Companionate Marriage.** 1927. New Introduction by Charles Larsen.

Lou, Herbert H. **Juvenile Courts in the United States.** 1927.

Monroe, Day. **Chicago Families.** 1932.

Mowrer, Ernest R. **Family Disorganization.** 1927.

Reed, Ruth. **The Illegitimate Family in New York City.** 1934.

Robinson, Caroline Hadley. **Seventy Birth Control Clinics.** 1930.

Watson, John B. **Psychological Care of Infant and Child.** 1928.

White House Conference on Child Health and Protection. **The Home and the Child.** 1931.

White House Conference on Child Health and Protection. **The Adolescent in the Family.** 1934.

Young, Donald, editor. **The Modern American Family.** 1932.